NATIONAL HEALTHS: GENDER, SEXUALITY AND HEALTH IN A CROSS-CULTURAL CONTEXT

UCL PRESS

NATIONAL HEALTHS: GENDER, SEXUALITY AND HEALTH IN A CROSS-CULTURAL CONTEXT

Edited by
Michael Worton and Nana Wilson-Tagoe

UCL
PRESS

First published in Great Britain 2004 by UCL Press,
an imprint of Cavendish Publishing Limited, The Glass House,
Wharton Street, London WC1X 9PX, United Kingdom
Telephone: + 44 (0)20 7278 8000 Facsimile: + 44 (0)20 7278 8080
Email: info@uclpress.com
Website: www.uclpress.com

Published in the United States by Cavendish Publishing
c/o International Specialized Book Services,
5824 NE Hassalo Street, Portland,
Oregon 97213-3644, USA

Published in Australia by Cavendish Publishing (Australia) Pty Ltd
45 Beach Street, Coogee, NSW 2034, Australia
Telephone: + 61 (2)9664 0909 Facsimile: + 61 (2)9664 5420

British Library Cataloguing in Publication Data
National healths: gender, sexuality and health in a cross-cultural context
1 Medical anthropology 2 Diseases – social aspects – cross-cultural studies
3 Health – social aspects – cross-cultural studies 4 Sex – health aspects
5 Body, human 6 Body image
306.4'1

ISBN 1-84472-017-9

1 3 5 7 9 10 8 6 4 2

Typeset by Phoenix Photosetting, Chatham, Kent

ACKNOWLEDGMENTS

This volume arose out of a three-year programme on 'Gender and Literature in Cross-cultural Contexts' in the AHRB Centre for Asian and African Literatures, and especially from the three-day international workshop 'Gender, Sexuality and Health' held in London on 4–6 November 2002. We would like to thank all the participants in our programme of workshops for their contributions, insights and enthusiasm for our project.

We would also like to thank the administrative staff of the AHRB Centre, Ross Forman and Gillian Hudson, for their help in running the workshops, and Gill Rye for her very helpful comments on the Introduction.

We would like to express our especial gratitude to Andrew Pink for the background research he did for this volume and for his important contribution to the copy-editing of the chapters.

CONTRIBUTORS

James N Agar

James N Agar is Lecturer in French and Comparative Literature at UCL (University College London). He teaches BA and MA courses on modern and contemporary European fiction and film, critical theory, especially the work of Foucault, and socio-cultural discourses of AIDS. His research is focused on the work of Hervé Guibert in relation to representations of AIDS and gay sexuality. He has published articles on Foucault, constructions of masculinity with AIDS, AIDS in France, and theories of reading in relation to identity politics.

Rachel Harrison

Rachel Harrison lectures in Thai literature and film at SOAS, where she studied for her first degree in Thai and History and where she completed her PhD in 1996 on issues of authorship and identity in the fiction of the contemporary woman writer Sidaoreuang. Her book on Sidaoreuang, *A Drop of Glass* (Duang Kamol, 1994), includes translations of short stories. Inspired by feminist literary theory and gender studies, Harrison has since researched and written on the representation of prostitution in Thai fiction, the treatment of the Thai sex industry in the Western media, and issues of female sexual desire in the work of Thai women writers. As a result of her teaching of the comparative literature of South East Asia, she has also written papers on Thai literature and on the development of modern South East Asian literature from a comparative perspective. Harrison was awarded an AHRB research grant in 2002 for a four-year joint project with Dr Peter Jackson of the Australian National University in Canberra. Entitled *The Ambiguous Allure of the West*, the project traces Thailand's cultural contacts with and views of the Occident from 1850 to the present.

Margaret Healy

Margaret Healy is Senior Lecturer in English at the University of Sussex. She is the author of a study of Shakespeare's *Richard II* (Northcote House, 1998), and of *Fictions of Disease in Early Modern England: Bodies, Plagues and Politics* (Palgrave, 2001). She is currently writing a book on the body in the English Revolution.

Deborah Kirklin

Deborah Kirklin is a family physician in London with postgraduate training in medical ethics and law. She is Senior Lecturer in Medical Humanities and Director of the Centre for Medical Humanities, Royal Free & University College Medical School, UCL. In addition to overseeing the educational programme of the Centre, where she is actively involved in the development, delivery and evaluation of arts and humanities-based education for healthcare professionals, she also teaches medical ethics at undergraduate and postgraduate level. Her research interests include an examination of how the ethical issues related to the new genetics, organ donation, end of life issues and women's health can be illuminated by analysis of the use of metaphor, narrative and framing within medical and medico-ethical discourse. Her publications include two books co-edited with Ruth Richardson, *Medical Humanities; A Practical Introduction* (Royal College of

Physicians, 2001) and *The Healing Environment: Without and Within* (Royal College of Physicians, 2003), as well as chapters and papers in both clinical and humanities textbooks and journals.

Shigehisa Kuriyama
Shigehisa Kuriyama is Associate Professor at the International Research Center for Japanese Studies. He received his PhD in the History of Science from Harvard University, and has taught previously at the University of New Hampshire and Emory University. In 2001, his book, *The Expressiveness of the Body and the Divergence of Greek and Chinese Medicine* (Zone Books, 1999), was awarded the William Henry Welch Medal of the American Association of the History of Medicine. His article,'The historical origins of *katakor*', in *Japan Review*, 9 (1997), is representative of his work on the history of the body in Japan.

Philippa Levine
Philippa Levine teaches history at the University of Southern California. She has published widely on Victorian feminism in England and on sexuality and medicine in the British Empire. Her most recent publications include *Prostitution, Race and Politics: Policing Venereal Disease in the British Empire* (Routledge, 2003) and an edited volume on gender and empire for the *Oxford History of the British Empire* (OUP, 2004).

Nicola Mai
Nicola Mai is Morris Ginsberg Fellow in the Department of Sociology at the LSE. His doctoral research was in Media and Cultural Studies, and focused on the multiple ways in which the Italian media were involved in the Albanian migration to Italy. During his doctoral fieldwork he was the director of a development project aimed at the setting up and management of four youth social and cultural centres in Central and Southern Albania. From April 2001 to July 2003 he was Research Fellow at the University of Sussex, working on a project on the experience of social exclusion of Albanian migrants living in Italy funded by the Leverhulme Trust. His most recent publications include *Exploding the Migration Myths* (Oxfam/Fabian Society, 2003), a co-authored book on the Albanian migration to the UK; and several articles on different aspects of the Albanian migratory flow. He is currently working on the relation between social change, transnational media consumption and migration by comparing his research on Albania with the Cuban and Moroccan contexts.

Lynda Morgan
Lynda Morgan completed her PhD in South African settler fiction at SOAS in 2003. Her particular interests are in representations of bodies, boundaries, sex and disease. She is currently publishing papers on these topics, and is extending her work into comparative study of South African and Australian settler fiction. She will present a paper on this subject at the 2004 International Comparative Literature Association Congress in Hong Kong. She is Field Chair in English Studies and Creative Writing at Buckinghamshire Chilterns University College, an Associate Lecturer with the Open University, a teaching consultant on an Open University course team preparing a major new course in twentieth-century

literature, and resident academic on the BBC/OU web discussion site for the 2004 Reith Lectures. She is also a published poet.

Audrey Prost
Audrey Prost has recently completed a PhD in Social Anthropology on the topic of social change and health among Tibetan exiles in India. The thesis examines how the predicaments of exile have impacted on health in the community of Dharamsala, and investigates the construction of symbolic meanings around diseases such as tuberculosis. As a recipient of an AHRB Fieldwork grant, Audrey returned to Dharamsala in order to conduct research on the creation of Tibetan scientific vocabulary in the fields of Physics and Medicine, exploring the cultural construction of Tibetan scientific language. She is currently a temporary lecturer in Medical Anthropology at UCL.

Stephen Quirke
Stephen Quirke is Curator at the Petrie Museum of Egyptian Archaeology and Lecturer at the Institute of Archaeology, UCL. He studied Egyptology at the University of Cambridge (BA, MA, PhD). His research focuses on the cursive 'hieratic' script derived from hieroglyphs, and in particular on the written record of the Middle Bronze Age in Egypt (Middle Kingdom) within the context of other archaeological evidence for the social history of that time and place. He has published extensively on ancient Egyptian administration and religion.

George S Rousseau
George Rousseau has been Professor of Eighteenth-Century Studies at UCLA and Regius Professor of English at King's College Aberdeen in Scotland. He is currently a member of the Faculty of Modern History at Oxford University and was the holder of a Leverhulme Trust Award 1999–2001 for research on the cultural understanding of disease conditions of cholera, nostalgia and tuberculosis. His often-cited 1981 article, 'Literature and medicine: the state of the field' *Isis* LXXII (September, 1981): 406–24, is considered to have charted a new academic field, and his article on configurations of same-sex arrangements in the Enlightenment won the James L Clifford Prize for the best article of the year in the USA. He is the author of many articles and books dealing with medicine and the humanities, most recently (with Roy Porter) *Gout: The Patrician Malady* (Yale University Press, 1998) and *Framing and Imagining Disease in Cultural History* (Palgrave, 2003). He recently retired.

Nahid Toubia
Nahid Toubia, founder and President of RAINBO, is a medical professional and a women's rights activist. She is a fellow of the Royal College of Surgeons of England and was the first woman surgeon in Sudan; she also has a degree in Health Planning and Financing from the University of London. She lived in New York for 10 years during which time she was Associate for Women's Reproductive Health at the Population Council leading the work on unsafe abortion worldwide, and an Associate (now Adjunct) Professor at Columbia University School of Public Health. She was also an advisor to the WHO, UNICEF, Human Rights Watch, and the Global Fund for Women. In 1994, Dr Toubia established RAINBO,

and in 2000 oversaw the establishment of AMANITARE, a network of African women's NGOs on Sexual and Reproductive Health and Rights in Africa. She has written extensively on reproductive health, women's rights and gender inequality issues with a focus on Africa and the Middle East.

Caroline Warman
Caroline Warman is Tutor in French at Exeter College, Oxford. She has written a book on Sade and materialism and also works on the cultural history of medicine.

Nana Wilson-Tagoe
Nana Wilson-Tagoe is a senior lecturer at SOAS. She was born in Ghana and was educated there and in Britain and the West Indies. She has taught at universities in Africa, the West Indies, the USA and the UK. She has received Rockefeller, Fulbright, Chapman and Cadbury awards for research in the USA and Britain and has published several articles and books on Caribbean and African literature. Her most recent publication is *Historical Thought and Literary Representation in West Indian Literature* (University Press of Florida/John Currey Oxford, 1998). She is currently completing a book entitled *History and Imagination in African Literature.*

Michael Worton
Michael Worton is Vice-Provost and Fielden Professor of French Language and Literature at UCL. He has written extensively on modern literature and on issues in critical theory and gender theory. His publications include *Textuality and Sexuality: Reading Theories and Practices*, co-edited with Judith Still (Manchester University Press, 1993), *Michel Tournier* (Longman, 1995), *Typical Men* (Nottingham: Djanogly Art Gallery, 2001; catalogue of the exhibition *Typical Men: Recent Photography of the Male Body by Men*, co-curated with Judith Still), and *Women's Writing in Contemporary France*, co-edited with Gill Rye (Manchester University Press, 2002). He is the director of 'Individuality, Identity and Culture in Modern Europe', a five-year UCL/Mellon Post-Doctoral Fellows interdisciplinary programme examining key themes in the construction and representation of identity. He is currently preparing a co-authored book with Judith Still, *Real Men and Others: Essays in Masculinities.*

LIST OF ILLUSTRATIONS

CONTENTS

INTRODUCTION

Michael Worton

We are made for togetherness
Archbishop Desmond Tutu[1]

The underlying premise of this book is that socio-cultural systems and attitudes have a major impact on the ways in which disease and healthcare are conceptualised and experienced. This is not to contest the importance of scientific, evidence-based approaches to illness. Rather, this book seeks to show how an awareness of cross-cultural and trans-historical issues, with especial reference to gender and sexuality, can help us better to confront and live with illness and can contribute to the shifting of focus from a narrowly body-centred conception of health to a more holistic notion of well-being. In other words, this book is a contribution towards the establishment of what might best be called Cultural Medicine.

In today's globalised world, it is essential that we understand at least something of the otherness of different societies and of their beliefs, histories and practices of expression and representation. While many of the contributors are writing from a Western perspective, we are acutely aware that our conceptual frameworks are inevitably based on assumptions that are culture-specific rather than on universal truths or laws. For instance, the primacy of the individual is an essentially Western notion, and we need to remember that the individual is not universally considered to be the centre of human agency, responsibility and decision-making: there are many societies in which the individual is seen rather as a social being whose motives as well as actions are determined collectively by the community and through cultural tradition. This is particularly important in the context of medicine and healthcare, where the dominance of Western medicine has tended to promote and impose particular expectations of the doctor/patient relationship as well as a determinedly scientific approach to medicine.

All too often, even in enlightened societies, misunderstandings and prejudices can lie behind an apparent inter-cultural understanding, notably with regard to questions both of gender, which is differently constructed in different societies according to local conditions and traditions, and of sexuality, which is frequently implicated in the social structures of control, management and even oppression.[2] The feminist philosopher and psychoanalyst, Luce Irigaray, has convincingly argued that, in both political and ethical terms, sexual difference is perhaps the

---

1 Said by Archbishop Desmond Tutu in his sermon at the inaugural Mass of the Spring Term at King's College, London, on 14 January 2004.

2 For illuminating discussion (and examples) of many of the socio-cultural and ethical issues involved in healthcare research in a cross-culture context, see Calman *et al* (2002), especially pp 39–53.

most urgent issue to address in the modern world.[3] Masculinity and femininity are, unquestionably, culturally-specific ideologies and contextually-determined practices. Furthermore, identity is itself fluid and performative rather than stable and fixed – and in most present-day societies, which remain fundamentally patriarchal, it is usually reactive in its performativity. This said, it is equally important to remember that the biological body has a more than symbolic role in these ideologies and practices. In seeking to explore and assess gender and sexuality, we need therefore to take account of the body's physicality as well as of the ways in which it presents itself and is presented and performed. Nowhere is this more significant than in sickness and in the domain that we call 'health' (which is itself a construct). In other words, both sickness and health are cultural as well as physical states. There is a great paradox in the fact that, on the one hand, as Roy Porter has pointed out, Western medicine is unique in being the 'the only [medical] tradition which has succeeded in globalising itself',[4] yet on the other hand, as Tony Barnett and Alan Whiteside stress: 'Public health systems are underfunded: politically they attract few votes and in parts of the world they are close to collapse. For the moment, there is only a mere intimation of any system of *global* public health.'[5]

Globalisation is often thought of as an essentially economic phenomenon, whereby market forces (or, quite simply, capitalism) hold sway and local specificities and differences are blurred and frequently diminished. This is particularly significant when it concerns healthcare, a field where the interests of multinational pharmaceutical companies, for instance, can have more influence over the destiny of a particular nation's people than its own government. However, we would insist on the fact that globalisation is more than an economic phenomenon. Its principal ideological foundation is undoubtedly that the international distribution of goods and services is best achieved when left to market forces. In this, it had much in common with capitalism – and also with imperialism, but we should remember that underpinning globalisation is also an ideology of social co-ordination – which is best effected and managed through the free movement of individuals that trade facilitates. The impetus towards greater freedom of movement and the vision of a more integrated socio-cultural world are admirable goals and have much in common with the aspirations of many societies and cultures. The difficulty is that globalisation operates in a partial and asymmetric way, whereby the rich get richer and the poor get poorer. Globalisation as it currently operates is ensuring that the West's values and way of life take on hegemonic power and authority; cultural differences are being blurred, linguistic individuality is being made subservient to the ubiquitous American-English, and social beliefs, codes and customs are ineluctably being homogenised. Put simply, globalisation poses a challenge, even a threat, to many of the identities that have determined us over the past few centuries. Also, we need to remember that such other crucial parts of our identity, such as our gender,

---

3 Irigaray (1993a) p 5.

4 Porter (2002) p 1.

5 Barnett and Whiteside (2002) p 27.

sexuality and our relationships with our bodies, are also affected by globalisation. It is for this reason that we need to be aware of, and reflect on, historical and geographical differences, and take full account of the implications of losing local specificities in the interest of creating and being part of that wider 'commonwealth' of humanity that globalisation seems sometimes to promise.

In the domain of health, cultural expansion or imperialism is currently proving almost as problematic as its historic military precedents, in that conditions such as obesity, heart disease, hypertension, diabetes and emphysema, which have for several decades been rampant in the wealthy West, are now taking their toll in the Third World, as people there increasingly seek to imitate and adopt the lifestyles that they associate with wealth and modernity. The 'McDonaldisation' of the world is more than a (worrying) joke-alternative to the capitalist or military globalisation of the world: fast food (in the sense of 'junk', fatty, salty, sugary food) is becoming the norm throughout the world, accompanied by the prevalence of primary colours and tawdry give-away toys, and is bringing new diseases to developing countries, just as military and economic colonisation has done for centuries.[6]

On the other hand, over the past few decades, there has been a substantial interest in alternative medicine: in the UK today, for instance, more than 25% of citizens use complementary medicine and there are now fewer GPs (General Practitioners or physicians) than there are registered practitioners of 'alternative' or 'complementary' therapies. One reason for this may be the move of emphasis towards the specialist physician even if, in countries like the UK (unlike the USA), primary care remains firmly in the hands of generalist family doctors. Another reason advanced for the rise of alternative medicine is that acupuncturists, art and music therapists, herbalists, homeopaths, etc, are perceived as being more willing to *listen* to the narratives of their patients and thus treat the whole person, with all of his or her emotional and even spiritual anxieties and aspirations. There is also growing interest in the modern West in traditional Chinese medicine, which identifies and offers methods of treating some diseases and conditions that Western medicine does not, whereas, on the other hand, it does not itself recognise some conditions that are identified and treated by Western medicine (such as depression), since they do not accord with or fit into its framework of 'Chi' (a mystical form of bio-energy), which seeks to improve bodily harmony through the growth and flow of Chi energy.

This book is certainly not an *apologia* for alternative medicine of whatever kind; indeed, it refers to alternative therapies only occasionally and then only for the purposes of historical or cross-cultural analysis. However, in setting the gendered patient, either real or represented, at the heart of our explorations, we necessarily also highlight the cultural, rather than the clinical, dimensions of health issues and therefore need to be attentive to the complex multiplicity of approaches that have been and are still employed. We would thus propose that

---

6 We are, of course, aware that not all fast food is necessarily unhealthy (eg, much Indian, Japanese or Thai food offered as fast food), and there is a growing market in the USA, for instance, for 'healthy' fast foods.

the active recognition of cultural and gender difference and diversity in both the conceptualising and the treatment of illness should ideally be a part of the experience of doctors and patients alike.

Much important research work is currently being done on the nature and the dynamics of the doctor-patient relationship.[7] We would argue that it is not a question simply of learning how to communicate and how to listen; it is a question of addressing how the various subjectivities involved in clinical encounters can be recognised and mobilised. In 1834, the French doctor Pierre Louis distinguished clearly between symptoms and signs, arguing forcibly in his *Essay on Clinical Instruction*[8] that the clinician should treat symptoms with some scepticism, because they were only what patients felt and sensed and were therefore highly subjective and variable, whereas signs were discovered through the process of physical examination by a scientifically-trained clinician. For Louis, these signs constituted objective data and therefore were to be considered as the only basis for diagnosis and for decisions regarding treatment. In an essay on narratives in medicine, Anna Donald offers an example of this familiar to us all: 'while the patient might *feel* pain, fever and an aching throat, the clinician *sees* viral proliferation.'[9] While we would in no way challenge the importance of the scientific approach, we would nonetheless maintain that doctors need to admit of subjectivity, not only in their patients but also in their own responses to their patients and to the symptoms and narratives that they present. This is not to diminish the importance of scientific objectivity and the need for a certain emotional distance in such encounters. However, it is vital to understand that medical practice is itself informed by subjectivity and, more fundamentally, that the complex ways in which we perceive, experience and understand our own bodies and the health of our bodies are at one and the same time highly subjective and culturally shaped. Furthermore, it is critical also to recognise that each of us has several identities (nationality, gender, ethnicity, age, faith, profession, etc) and that these identities may lead to different engagements with our individual bodies and states of health at different times and in different situations.

In today's climate of aggressive litigation, the doctor/patient relationship can all too easily be damaged, with the disappearance of the trust that is at the heart of that relationship. While we would agree with Brian Hurwitz, who, in his fascinating article on medical negligence and the creative potential of narratives, suggests that the granting of more time to *listen* to patients in consultations and thereby to build empathy could reduce the numbers of patients who become litigants if a cure is not promptly found for them,[10] we would emphasise again that consultations are increasingly held in a bilingual way, with an advocate or

---

7 See, for instance, Aldrich (1993), Korsch and Harding (1998), Ley (1988), Luckmann and Tindell Nobles (2000), Minardi and Riley (1997), Northouse and Northouse (1992), and Redleaf and Baird (1998).

8 Louis (1834).

9 Donald (1988) p 23.

10 Hurwitz (1998) pp 244–45.

third person acting as interpreter for the patient. In these cases especially, it is not enough for the doctor to listen to a patient's story in order to develop empathy; s/he must also have sensitivity to, and understanding of, the cultural otherness of a patient which may mean that the story has a radically different sense and significance than in a Western context. So, added to the need to have mastery of a panoply of scientific knowledge is the need to be actively aware of cultural difference. Clearly, no single doctor can be expected to understand the full range of cultural diversity encountered in today's globalised cities, but it is essential that there be at least a sense of working with the implications of cultural difference.

The role and the place of the doctor are changing as society develops and becomes more complex and diverse and also as patients have ever higher expectations and, furthermore, are increasingly concerned with self-diagnosis through a variety of self-care books and especially through the internet. The doctor's authority is therefore no longer what it was in the previous century (although it is much better and stronger than it was in, say, the seventeenth century, when doctors were the butt of many jokes and lampooned in such plays as Molière's *The Flying Doctor* (date unknown; probably the early 1650s), *The Doctor in Spite of Himself* (1666) and, most famously, his last play, *The Hypochondriac* (1673). In today's world, patients in the West increasingly expect doctors to be both scientifically up-to-date physicians and also sympathetic and thoughtful comforters and advisers. The decline in the importance accorded to the accounts told by patients of their symptoms and suffering is often linked to the rise in hospital-based medicine, in which clinicians see great numbers of patients of whom they have no knowledge other than the notes of the referring doctors and with whom they therefore have no real bond or shared history. Their concern is thus not the individuality of the patient, but the ways in which the same disease manifests itself across people of different sexes, age groups, classes, etc. As Foucault argues when thinking about nineteenth century hospital medicine (and it holds true for much of today's patient 'care'), the sick person was redefined as 'the accident of his disease, the transitory object upon which it happens to have seized'.[11] Patients in the West now expect much more of their doctors and, in the UK, the National Health Service is now explicitly committed to providing a patient-centred service – although one cannot help but wonder who or what else could legitimately be at the centre of such a Service! This means that doctors are explicitly encouraged to be more focused on their patients and their needs, and there is an increasing willingness amongst some clinicians to recommend complementary therapies.

It is important, though, to remember that the ways in which doctors and indeed medicine itself are regarded vary enormously between continents, between countries and regions within continents, and even between different towns or villages within a single country. While it is true that modern, Western medicine has globalised itself, this is essentially the case with regard to acute conditions (because of the effectiveness of antibiotics in rapidly eliminating

---

11 Foucault (1973) p 59.

infections).[12] However, in many parts of the developing world, sufferers frequently believe that chronic conditions or recurring problems are caused by social, moral, emotional, or even religious factors, and practitioners of alternative therapies are often consulted. This sometimes means that the pathway chosen by patients is first of all to consult alternative medical practitioners and only later to consult modern, scientifically trained healthcare practitioners – in a sense, the reversal of what can happen in the West.

One of the greatest problems or paradoxes of pain is that it is experienced in a very individual way, even if it often disrupts and even shatters one's sense of selfness as one's entire being can come to centre on the pain or suffering. However, these experiences can be talked about, described, explained, even to oneself, only through the clichés and dead metaphors that are conventionally used in Anglophone societies, such as 'a dull pain', 'a shooting pain', etc. This means that, as Howard Brody suggests, the individuality and uniqueness of the pain are diminished, even eradicated, by the very fact of the experience being contained within a social framework. For this reason, it is even more urgent for patients to find ways of reconstituting their sense of selfness through their constructions of individual narratives that can forcefully communicate in the clinical encounter what they are really feeling. Brody, interestingly, if provocatively, argues that it is the meaning that an individual accords to an experience of pain that produces suffering – and so this meaning, if properly understood, harnessed and directed, could ultimately provide a means of alleviating the suffering.[13] Although Brody would not claim that any meanings ascribed are the sole causes of pain and suffering, we would endorse the emphasis on the semantically determined dimension of pain, whilst also arguing that the process of striving to understand and to give meaning to experiences of illness is necessarily a dual one, in which there is a dominant socio-cultural determinism but also a strong individual drive to assert and communicate one's subjective physical and mental suffering.

There is no need, for example, to be an anthropologist to realise that physical pain is a very relative experience: it depends on situation and context. A wasp sting, for instance, is hardly noticed if it occurs in the midst of an arduous climb through bushes of gorse on the way up a mountain, whereas it is experienced as very real pain if it happens when one is lying tranquilly in the sun reading a novel. Furthermore, pain is very dependent on culture and context: thresholds of acceptable pain and suffering are much higher in the Far East or in Africa than in the modern developed West, where individuals consult doctors for conditions that their parents or grandparents would have shrugged off as just part of ordinary life, as merely part of the human condition. Things are made even more

---

12 We would point out in passing that the term 'antibiotic', coined by Selman Waksman (1889–1973) in 1941, literally means 'destructive of life', in that one organism destroys the life of another in order to preserve its own. Waksman was awarded the Nobel Prize for Physiology or Medicine in 1952 for his discovery of streptomycin, the first specific agent effective in the treatment of tuberculosis.

13 See Brody (1987) pp 26–30.

complex by the fact that in situations of suffering the sense of meaning itself becomes unclear and uncertain; as the medical anthropologist David B Morris argues: 'Pain in effect spends its existence moving in-between the extremes of absolute meaninglessness and full meaning.'[14] In extreme situations, this 'moving in-between' is true of language almost as much as it is of pain. Indeed, language inevitably proves inadequate as a means of *saying* pain, suffering, or even discomfort, since we try vainly to communicate our own very private, personal experience, yet we are also aware that others too have suffered similarly and so we believe that we should be able to use a common, shared language – or that such a vocabulary has been (or should have been) created somewhere by someone. From this point of view, it is useful to consider, as do several of the contributors of this volume, the practice of writers who, when sick, seek to invent new terms and images or, more frequently, to revitalise stock metaphors in order to convey their sense of distress and of physical and mental degradation. Interestingly, this is often more striking in such writers' journals, diaries and letters than in their literary works intended for publication and public consumption – as if such exploratory experimentation is a personal rather than a professional, communicative necessity.[15]

A further factor that needs to be taken into account when considering the relationship between illness and language is the impact of time. The temporal sequence of communicating our experience of illness usually begins with describing it to relatives or close friends before 'explaining' to a doctor who then tends to fit it into a scientific framework in order for him or her to understand it and decide how best to treat the condition. For scientific reasons, the doctor ineluctably locates the individual's experience within a pattern. However, of late, researchers and writers have increasingly shown interest in the ways in which story-telling or narrative occurs in the encounter between doctor and patient, and in the (very different) narratives that the doctor and patient tell after that encounter.[16] We would suggest that it is now urgent explicitly to recognise that the ways in which patients speak about their illnesses change over the course of time, as their conditions improve (or not), and that they also develop different expectations as they gain more knowledge about possible treatments and certainly greater awareness of their own bodies and often even accurate and specific ways of speaking about them. In other words, there is a temporal dimension that should not be neglected in patient care, where the dimension of history is not simply the medical history of the patient but the history of his or her gradual entry into the (scientific, cultural and linguistic) worlds of illness and of medicine. Susan Sontag opens her seminal essay, *Illness as Metaphor*, with the following striking metaphor: 'Illness is the night-side of life, a more onerous citizenship. Everyone who is born holds dual citizenship, in the kingdom of the

---

14 Morris (1991) p 35.

15 A particularly interesting example is the nineteenth-century writer, Alphonse Daudet (1840–97), whose work *La Doulou*, published posthumously in 1930 (*In the Land of Pain*, 2002) describes his suffering from *locomotor ataxia*, which he knew to be the tertiary stage of syphilis.

16 See, for instance, Greenhalgh and Hurwitz (1998).

well and in the kingdom of the sick.'[17] Sontag's notion of dual citizenship is a striking one, which emphasises the fact that to be born is to be destined at some point to fall ill and ultimately to die. However, we would want to modify somewhat her image of us *belonging* to these two different worlds and would, rather, emphasise that the experience of illness is a *journey* into a foreign country. It involves entry into otherness, physically through altered bodily sensations and deteriorations and through the need to inhabit doctors' surgeries and hospitals, and emotionally through the encounter with the culture and the language of medicine, which are very different from those to which one is accustomed in everyday life. Furthermore, in our multi-cultural and multi-ethnic societies, for many people it is an uncomfortable confrontation with inappropriate, if well-meaning, presuppositions about what is helpful. For instance, many hospitals in the UK now have advocacy teams, which provide interpreters for the many patients from around the globe who attend but do not speak English fluently or even at all. It is, of course, costly and, in logistical terms, very difficult to provide interpreters for all patients who attend clinics, especially those attending Emergency Departments, so several hospitals have taken to publishing in several languages information leaflets on the most common conditions and on key healthcare issues. This initiative is admirable, but it does not take into account that there are many cultures which are essentially oral rather than text-based, and so work is now being done on providing alternative linguistic solutions, such as audio tapes, image-based 'pick-and-point' leaflets, speaking signs, etc. These developments are particularly important in our globalised world, since they serve to diminish in small but practical ways the sense of trepidation and even alienation that patients can all too easily have when entering the impersonal, if highly sophisticated centres of technology that are today's hospitals. After all, the experience of serious illness can involve a mentally painful entry into alienation from the self, since one can no longer define oneself – or even recognise oneself – through one's stable, physical state as one had previously been able to do.

Culturally, it is clear that illnesses have always been seen as having a meaning beyond the purely physical. Some have been presented as 'disgraceful' diseases: leprosy, for instance, is stigmatised in the Bible and was feared and regarded with revulsion for centuries; syphilis was seen as a form of moral leprosy or divine judgment for inappropriate sexual behaviour; more recently, AIDS continues to be stigmatised by some as a 'divinely wrought gay plague', despite the ongoing ravages of AIDS within heterosexual communities throughout the world, notably in Africa; in the nineteenth century, tuberculosis was often used as a metaphor for venereal disease. On the other hand, strange as it now may seem, some diseases have been coded as positive and almost desirable. The most striking example is tuberculosis, which, in the nineteenth century, was coded positively as well as negatively. It was imagined to be an aphrodisiac and to confer upon the sufferer extraordinary powers of seduction. Known as consumption (from the Latin *consumere*, to waste away), it was also associated with Romantic genius, as in the case of the Keats or Chopin, or with moments of intense being-in-the-world just

---

17 Sontag (1979) p 3.

before death, as in Alexander Dumas's *La Dame aux Camélias* (1852), translated by Verdi into the opera *La Traviata* (1853), or in Puccini's opera *La Bohème* (1896) – and here it should be noted that in literature, opera and painting, artists tended to portray dying heroines, thereby gendering the disease as feminine, even although many male artists actually died of it. The positive, aestheticising symbolisation of tuberculosis or consumption has often been considered a peculiarly European cultural construction. However, this phenomenon is also to be found in other cultures. For instance, in Japan from the late nineteenth century onwards, the 'pale and interesting' appearance of tubercular female patients was seen as fascinating and beautiful, as Mahito Fukuda has shown,[18] and in this volume, Audrey Prost shows how popular perceptions of tuberculosis amongst the Tibetan exile communities in India have become stamped with socio-cultural meanings that can affect the way in which sufferers are perceived and treated.

Gout is another, very different, example of the positive social coding of an illness. Gout is one of the most common forms of arthritis, usually affecting the feet and ankles, with the big toe the site most frequently affected. Although acutely painful, it was known as 'the disease of kings and the king of diseases' and was often seen as the mark of a gentleman who knew how to live well, because of its association with alcohol and rich foods. It has a certain celebrity, having famously plagued the lives of such as Immanuel Kant, Samuel Johnson, Benjamin Franklin, Thomas Jefferson and Robert Browning, and in the eighteenth century it was used mercilessly by such satirical artists as William Hogarth to lampoon members of the aristocracy. Gout is a mainly male condition; it can affect men of any age and is much less common in women, who can be affected by it only after the menopause. Again associated with Western culture (and, indeed, with an elitist patriarchal West), largely as a result of the work of writers and artists, it is nonetheless very common in other parts of the world – for instance, in New Zealand, it is particularly prevalent in Maoris and Pacific Islanders, where it has been shown to be present in up to 10% of adult males.

Throughout history, as medicine has developed, it has always been mediated not only through changing notions of the body but also through broader cultural perspectives and preoccupations. In Europe, the first major figure, one who even today presides over medicine through his celebrated Oath, was Hippocrates (c 460–377 BC), who gave medicine its own independent place in society by separating it from philosophy and who promoted 'natural' theories of health and sickness and 'natural' modes of healing.[19] Hippocrates is many ways a construction rather than being a historically locatable individual in Ancient Greece. While he is said to have written about 60 works, these texts lack internal coherence and the sense of a single voice; like the books of the Bible, they were almost certainly composed by many different people and over a considerable period of time. However, the central principle of Hippocratic medicine was to

18 See Fukuda, *A Cultural History of Tuberculosis in Modern Japan*.

19 Galen (c 129–216 AD), the most important figure in medicine after Hippocrates, argued that medicine should be informed by philosophy and that the physician should both heal and work in the disciplines of logic, ethics and physics. He too took an ethical stance, insisting on the all-importance of trust between doctor and patient.

dominate Western medicine right up until the eighteenth century. This principle (known as *humouralism*) was that health and illness can be explained through the four *humours* (or key fluids): *blood*, the source of life and vitality; *choler* (or bile), the gastric juice; *phlegm*, which lubricates and cools; and *melancholy* (or black bile), the most problematic of all the humours, which is not a pure liquid, but one that darkens other liquids, producing states of suffering. The Hippocratic system offered a convincing explanatory system, largely because it was based on a series of binary oppositions (hot vs cold; wet vs dry; liquid vs solid, etc). This determined binarism was to dominate medical thinking for centuries, but we should also recognise that this same binarism is the core of much philosophical thinking and is in many ways at the heart of the Cartesian philosophy led by René Descartes (1596–1650) that underpinned the Enlightenment and opened the way for much modern philosophy.[20]

One of the most influential tenets of Hippocratic medicine was its insistence on bringing together in its analytical frameworks domains often considered to be irrevocably separate: the physical and the emotional (which included the mental and the psychological); the natural and the man-made; the healthy and the sick. In this sense, although wholly outdated scientifically, it can be seen as having heralded and prepared the way for the holistic approach to healthcare which is so important today. One further point to be stressed about Hippocrates and his followers is that, unlike many 'magical' healers, they never claimed to make miraculous cures. At the centre of their concept of medical care was the principle of *primo, non nocere* (above all, do no harm), and they privileged the welfare of the patient above all else, whilst also insisting on the doctor's healing impulse and vocation. Their position as doctors was an essentially – and committedly – ethical one, as is manifested in the Hippocratic Oath.

Almost every day, the Western media address medical issues, whether it be abortion and women's rights, obesity, teenage sexual behaviour, the MMR jab (against measles, mumps, rubella), the use of transplant organs, cloning, or whatever. Medicine and healthcare are now major foci of public debate, and increasingly debates are driven by ethical and socio-cultural concerns. It is perhaps thus not surprising that, as Vivian Nutton has pointed out, the

---

20 The central idea of Cartesianism is that the mind is separate from the body. It proposes that the mind can be better and more fully understood than the body, that internal mental processes have more reality than physical, bodily processes, and that a human being's essential identity is his or her mind. Consequently, subjectivity or what one *thinks* is more important than objectivity or what *exists* in the phenomenal world. This emphasis on the mental and the subjective as superior to the physical led to the development in the Enlightenment of the concept of the subject, which underpins all Western culture, philosophy and politics; it also enabled the development and maintenance of capitalism. Descartes also developed the notion of the body-machine, and still today we often unconsciously think of a machine and use metaphors from the world of machines to describe our bodies when they become ill or quite simply old. The privileging of the mind over the body was also a means whereby men were privileged over women, since the Enlightenment valued the mind (promoted as rational – and associated with men) over the body (considered to be irrational – and associated with women). Contemporary feminist theory and philosophy has done much to deconstruct this opposition; see, for instance, Irigaray (1985, 1993a and 1993b).

Hippocratic Oath, the single most famous document in the history of medicine, should have been taken most seriously and even been sworn as part of the ceremonies by which one becomes a doctor from the second half of the twentieth century onwards.[21] As Nutton makes clear, the Hippocratic Oath 'has not, and never has been a fixed unalterable document', but is, rather, a document that has been interpreted, re-interpreted and even modified over the centuries by different societies as they sought to graft their own values and preoccupations onto it.[22] The late twentieth and early twenty-first centuries have seized on it because it places concern for the patient's welfare at the heart of medical practice and promotes an ethical approach to medicine. However, there are particular problems for today's society or, at least, for certain parts of contemporary Western society, in that there is an explicit commitment not to 'use the knife' (that is, do surgery) and not 'to give to a woman an abortive remedy'. Furthermore, the classical version of the Oath makes quite clear that doctors are all men, that their knowledge is to be shared only with other men, and that the practice of medicine is a profession which is intended to be self-regulating. This last dimension of the Hippocratic vision of medicine is one which can cause alarm: 'The medical oath has been seen as an invitation to a medical conspiracy to murder, and a mark of a closed-shop unionism that bans competition, imposes the physicians' writ on all other healers, and closes ranks against the outside world, especially in the face of patients' complaints.'[23]

The very variability of the Hippocratic Oath across the ages (and across countries) testifies to the interactions between societies and the medical practices that inform and support them. There is a common thread of ethical concern for the patient in all societies. However, it is important to recognise that this concern is variable and culture-specific, just as apparently immutable and foundational ethical positions are always determined and shaped by the moral and socio-political issues that are dominant in a society at any particular time.

At the heart of medicine lies the human body. This may seem a platitude, but it is important to think through the implications of this statement. The body is not a mere physical entity; it is also a cultural construct and is bound up in a complex of beliefs, assumptions, protocols, etc, of the society in which it is found. Furthermore, sickness, disease and suffering are not exclusively the domain of doctors and patients; they are also inherently – and profoundly – shared cultural phenomena. Each of us is situated in a cultural matrix, whereby the conjunction of the 'vertical' axis of history and the 'horizontal' axis of society determines much of what and how we think and behave. In situations of illness, we feel particularly vulnerable: after all, medicine tells us that illness is a dysfunctioning of the body. However, to be ill is also always a highly subjective, emotional and mental experience. This apparent truism is all too often forgotten. Illness makes us

21 Nutton (1995); see also Loudon *et al* (1994). Many but by no means all medical schools in the USA and in Europe today administer a form of the Oath, although the wording varies considerably.

22 Nutton (1995) p 519.

23 Nutton (1995) p 523.

acutely aware of our bodies, whereas in the West we have culturally been distanced from them; this is especially true of men who since the eighteenth century have been taught and programmed to distance themselves from their bodies. On the other hand, illness is an experience which often can make us acutely aware of the *community* within which we live: the experience of many ill people includes discovering who their true supportive friends are and who can be with them and offer support only when they are in the less demanding states of not being ill. To be ill therefore is to be simultaneously living an experience that is intensely personal and living one that is culturally shaped.

It is equally true but often forgotten (or not realised) that the body itself is not regarded in the same way over time and across the globe. For instance, in the Egypt of the Pharaohs, one of the key positions in the household of the Pharaoh himself was Iri, Keeper of the Royal Rectum, who was the Pharaoh's expert in enemas. One might smile at the idea of a present-day monarch or national president having, as one of their main medical carers, a keeper of the rectum, but let us not forget how important colonic irrigation was to Princess Diana and thereby to a whole generation. On a more ethical level, dissection was for centuries forbidden by Islam and Christianity alike. Whatever the religious, moral or legal framework may be at any point in any society, the question of dissection is always a fraught one. For this reason, the example of Gunther von Hagen's 'Body Worlds: The Anatomical Exhibition of Real Human Bodies' is striking. Consisting of authentic anatomical specimens donated by individuals during their lifetime and plastinated,[24] the exhibition is intended by von Hagen to have not only an educational, but also a moral and even an edifying role. Seen by an astonishing number of people worldwide (more than 13.5 million) since its first showing in Mannheim in 1997, the exhibition might seem to prove, as its creator argues, that the general public is eager to learn more about the structure and function of their bodies. However, it is also a testament to the public's fascination with the morbid and with the *monstrous*:[25] playing with a variety of taboos, it is above all a *spectacle*, one in which the human body is exposed, literally flayed and probed and offered to voracious, voyeuristic gazes. Whether educational or exploitative, the exhibition has undoubtedly raised many questions about the (literal) place of anatomy in society's daily life.

The body, living, suffering and dead, has been the subject of much religious, moral and philosophical debate across cultures and throughout the centuries. However, one particular legal problem was not resolved in the UK until an important case was heard in 1999. At the January 1997 London Contemporary Art Fair in London, an artist, Anthony-Noel Kelly, exhibited cast body fragments which were much praised for their realism and for the way in which, through his

---

24 See the 'Body Worlds' website, www.koerperwelten.com/en/pages/plastination.asp, for details of the process of plastination that enables the preservation and display of biological (and human) specimens. Plastinated specimens are dry and odourless; they are identical with their state prior to preservation, to the extent that even microscopic examinations of them are possible.

25 'Monstrous' derives etymologically from the Latin *monstrare* (to show or display).

sculptures, the artist had confronted the issues of illness, suffering and death through his sculptures. However, it soon became apparent that the sculptures were in fact cast from parts of dead bodies. Kelly had smuggled the dissected human remains of up to 40 bodies out of the Royal College of Surgeons in order to make his artworks, with the aid of a hospital worker, Neil Lindsay, who had naively agreed to help him as he wanted to ensure that the remains were finally given a proper burial. Kelly was sentenced to nine months in jail for his crime of smuggling out these body parts. However, the verdict was possible only after a landmark ruling by the judge, Geoffrey Rivlin QC, that human remains used for medical research could be classed as property and could therefore be treated as stolen in this case. This ruling ended more than 100 years of uncertainty over the legal status of human remains. For example, in the eighteenth and nineteenth centuries, those found guilty of body-snatching were not charged with theft but only with lesser offences such as outraging public decency.[26]

The importance of the 1999 Kelly case is that it raised in a very public way the question of the ownership of the body. Recent developments in bio-medical research have engendered other anxieties and provoked further debates on and around ownership of the body and its constituent parts. For instance, the cloning of Dolly the sheep has raised questions about what will happen when cloning of human cells takes place. Who will be the 'owner' of cloned cells and how will this ownership translate into intellectual property rights when pharmaceutical and other bio-medical products created as a result of genetic manipulations start to be marketed? Indeed, in terms of human rights and the experimentation on human embryos up to the age of 14 days, when does life (and thence the capacity to own) begin? Who should (or who can) decide these issues? Governments? Churches? Philosophers? Moralists? Doctors? Lawyers? There is no single answer yet to these questions, but it is certain that no one group of professionals or indeed any single culture can decide finally on these issues.

All histories of medicine (like all historical accounts) are culture-specific. It is easy to forget or ignore, for instance, that in Europe in the Dark Ages, medicine was practised and developed only by monks and priests who were the only truly educated men in the West, whereas the classical medicine of Hippocrates and Galen was in the same period being developed in what was then the much more advanced Islamic world (modern-day Egypt, Iran, Iraq and Syria). The cross-cultural exchanges in medicine between the Christian and the Islamic world over the centuries still need serious exploration, as do the exchanges between the

---

26 In the nineteenth century, dissection was illegal unless the bodies of hanged criminals were used, so British doctors took to breaking the law. The so-called 'Resurrection Men' hunted round looking for recent burials, dug up the corpses and sold them to a doctor for £3 a body (a considerable sum at the time). The activities of the Resurrection Men became so unpopular that they ran the risk of being torn to pieces if caught by a mob, and churchyards were surrounded by huge iron railings and guarded by watchmen to prevent the thefts. The most notorious Resurrection Men were William Burke and William Hare, who, when stocks ran short for a famous Edinburgh surgeon, Robert Knox (1791–1862), provided fresh bodies: instead of digging up corpses, they plied their victims with whisky to get them drunk, strangled them and then sold them for the princely sum of £7/10s, that is, more than twice what had been the 'standard price' per corpse.

Eastern and the Western medical traditions. There is much yet to learn from the different ways in which each tradition perceived and enabled the development of healers. Although we do not have space here to explore this topic in any depth, we would draw attention to the female figure of Peseshet, who was one of the Pharaoh's senior physicians in Ancient Egypt. Peseshet had managerial as well as medical skills, being the director of more than a hundred women doctors, and she was also director of the soul-priestesses appointed to tend the funerary cults of private persons. This figure is of great importance as she is the first female physician recorded in African or, indeed, world history; she is also evidence that, whereas in the West, medicine was, from Ancient Greece onwards, an essentially male-dominated profession, the Ancient Egyptians recognised formally throughout their society that women had an important medical role to play – and not simply in midwifery or nursing, which were in a sense essentially extensions of their social and gender roles as mothers, daughters, sisters and wives.

Before the nineteenth century, when women in the West did engage in medicine, they were marginalised, ostracised, stigmatised and even killed as witches. As Margaret Healy shows in her study in this volume of the meanings and myths of menstruation in fifteenth- and sixteenth-century England, women were usually silent about medical issues, even about this purely female condition. 'Wise women' did practise medicine, often, although by no means always, of a herbalist nature, and they were able and willing to enter into and negotiate 'taboo' areas feared by men (such as menstruation), although they were resented by men for the very fact of their daring to transgress in order to treat and cure. The exclusion of women from medicine continued until the nineteenth century, when barriers slowly came down, largely because women began to be admitted to universities.

In the West, the nineteenth century finally saw the admission of women into medicine as doctors. The UK was slower in moving forward than other countries, and the following pioneers born in England all had to go abroad to qualify: Elizabeth Blackwell (1821–1910) in America; Elizabeth Garrett Anderson (1836–1917) in France; and Sophia Jex-Blake (1840–1912) in Ireland. Significant pioneering work was also done by women in reforming nursing and healthcare more generally. Three figures stand out. The American Dorothea Dix (1802–87) spent more than 20 years campaigning to improve the treatment and conditions of the mentally ill, initially in North America and later in Europe, and, perhaps more importantly, working tirelessly to convince people that mental illness is not incurable. The Jamaican Mary Seacole (1805–81) became an expert in dealing with cholera, and during the Crimean War she travelled to England at her own expense to offer her services at the War Office, who rejected her offer because of her ethnicity. She then travelled, again at her own expense, to the Crimea, where she gave medical treatment to wounded soldiers of both sides on the battlefield itself. She became a national heroine in England, where she was known as the 'black Florence Nightingale'. Florence Nightingale (1820–1910), the celebrated 'Lady with the Lamp', radically improved not only the quality of nursing in military hospitals as a result of her experiences in the Crimea, but also the image and status of nursing, hitherto associated with working class women. As a result of the work of these three women, nurses came to be regarded as having equal importance with doctors in healthcare, even if there continued to be a hierarchy in which male power and authority prevailed. Indeed, it was not until the last decade of the twentieth century that, for the first time, women represented more than 50% of the intake into British medical schools, where the vast majority of tenured professors continue to be men.

Inequalities abound in healthcare, but it is important also to recognise that illness often makes the ill person both socially vulnerable and liable to be marginalised or made to feel inferior. Illness and infirmity are conceptualised as deviations from biological, psychological, or physical norms. More than this, they are seen as deviating from socio-cultural norms in the sense that the ill are, all too often, not (allowed to be) fully participating members of their society. There is also an ethical dimension to the marginalisation of the ill, in that they can be seen as not fully pulling their weight, being a burden on society, etc. It is for this reason that it has been necessary to pass legislation such as the UK Disability Discrimination Act 1995, in order to ensure not only that discrimination does not occur, but that it should slowly be helped to change. Furthermore, the language of health and healthcare is often not neutral and can stigmatise illness precisely by presenting it as a deviation from the norm.

Illness also raises the question of what the 'normal' is. Current debates about obesity, for instance, in both the UK and the USA are leading to increased awareness of the importance of diet, but they also presuppose – and *impose* – a norm that stigmatises those children and teenagers who only 20 or 30 years ago would have been seen as 'healthy eaters', children who 'enjoy their food'. We need to remember that it is actually very difficult, indeed impossible, to speak with any authority about what is the norm in regard to health and well-being. Indeed, even in clinical medicine, norms are a problematic concept even though they are widely and authoritatively use. What is normal blood pressure, or a normal cholesterol level? As soon as one takes into account cultural differences, notions of 'the normal' become problematic. For this reason, we hope that this book with its focus on cross-cultural and trans-historical issues will help to offer insights that enable such problematising to be seen as something potentially creative. It is, of course, essential to have definitions in medicine and healthcare, and there needs to be some sense of what in broad parameters can be seen as normal. Nonetheless, we would argue that it is vital that within medical structures and practices there is an equally important need to recognise that each individual sick person has a unique identity, a specific socio-cultural framework and a highly particular way of engaging with and responding to illness.

In his seminal work, *The Normal and the Pathological*, Georges Canguilhem makes the following argument: 'Health, taken absolutely, is a *normative* concept defining an ideal type an organic structure and behaviour.'[27] We therefore need to question what health itself is and to find ways of defining as something more than the simple absence of illness. Notions like normality and regularity are brought

27 Canguilhem (1991) p 137; added emphasis.

into play here. The normal is something which is 'standard', the condition which is the most frequent or habitual. Another way of defining the normal is the natural, but this poses a further problem in that the natural is in no way a simple state against which things can be tested in order to determine rules. In other words, it is impossible to determine a universal norm against which everything else is judged and from which all difference would be a deviation. We would argue very strongly that in socio-cultural terms – and consequently in terms of health – there is no such thing as a universal law. As Canguilhem suggests, 'the abnormal is not what is not normal, but what constitutes another normal'.[28]

While statistics and references with regard to a norm are useful, perhaps even essential, for doctors and other healthcare workers, we must remember that the experience of illness is simultaneously relational and culture-determined and also highly individual. However, we would add that it is also – apparently paradoxically – *not* relational, in the sense that the patient does not worry about whether he or she is either more or less sick than someone else; rather, he or she experiences the illness with regard to his or her own previous or usual state of well-being. And in coming to terms with the emotional as well as the physical reality of the illness, the sufferer often has to contend with a society that can seem unsupportive and even hostile in its playings with the construction of health and disease.

In his fascinating if sometimes chilling book, *The Biotech Century: Harnessing the Gene and Remaking the World*, Jeremy Rifkin draws attention to a worrying intervention by commercial pharmaceutical interests into the conceptions and definitions of illness, one that has particular resonance for our concerns. In the 1980s, two companies, Genentech and Eli Lilly, were given patents in the USA to market a new genetically engineered growth hormone to children suffering from dwarfism. The market for the hormone was considered to be very small, so both companies were awarded 'orphan' drug status, which gave them a monopoly on sales of the product as recompense for having invested so heavily in a drug with limited market potential. The hormone outdid all market expectations, and by 1991 it had become one of the best selling pharmaceutical drugs in the USA with the two companies sharing a market of approximately $500 million. The reason for this was that, while dwarfism is a very precise medical condition, many children were considered by their parents (or considered themselves) to be too short. In the USA, tallness is seen as desirable, and so many parents asked their doctors to prescribe the hormone for their children, and some children even began to take it illegally. Furthermore, the two companies then decided to lobby for 'normal' shortness to be defined officially as an illness. This decision was made, of course, on commercial grounds but the National Institutes of Health (NIH), an agency of the USA Department of Health and Human Services, decided to set up a twelve-year research project to examine the effects of human growth hormones on children born into families with a history of shortness. This posed a serious ethical issue in that the NIH is legally prevented from experimenting on healthy

---

28 Canguilhem (1991) p 203.

children, yet had precisely committed to do so. At the time, an NIH spokesperson offered the following astonishing argument: 'These kids are not normal. They are short in a society that looks at that unfavourably.'[29]

What is particularly disturbing about this example is that it goes further than defining as abnormal children who simply do not meet the expectations of average height: it defines their condition as an illness. In other words, the pharmaceutical industry joined forces with the medical community to promote what is no less than a form of eugenics aimed at creating human beings who match up to notions of normality (or perfection). What enabled this manipulation is the socially promoted perception that illness is somehow 'bad'. However, there are other ways of looking at this. Madness, for instance, is one of the most frightening of illnesses, and yet it has for several centuries and in several cultures been associated with divine inspiration and, in the Christian mystic tradition, physical suffering is often regarded as a path to saintliness and a true understanding of God. On the individual level, it can also be argued that illness enables (or perhaps obliges) the sufferer to think more closely about his or her body and to enter into a more creative and thoughtful relationship with the body – which can enable the sick person to re-conceptualise himself or herself both as subject and as object. In our society, we are all too often reduced to the position of objects, especially, perhaps, with regard to our bodies, and so the experiential (and existential) solitude and isolation that accompany serious illness can actually help us to re-establish a sense of selfness and, paradoxically, of autonomy.

We would certainly not argue that illness or infirmity are desirable in and of themselves, but it is important to recognise that they have the potential, if lived out and reflected upon positively, to help us to grow as individuals and to engage more thoughtfully with the society in which we find ourselves. In other words, we would argue that health is not purely a physiological and medical issue; it is also a cultural and ethical one.

---

29 See *Wall Street Journal* (1992) p A1, footnote 76. For further details, see Rifkin (1998) pp 139–44.

Bibliography

Aldrich, Clarence Knight, *The Medical Interview: Gateway to the Doctor-Patient Relationship: a Manual for First or Second Year Medical Students*, foreword by Pellegrino, Edmund D, 1993, New York, London: Parthenon Publishing Group.

Barnett, Tony and Whiteside, Alan, *AIDS in the Twenty-First Century: Disease and Globalisation*, 2002, Basingstoke and New York: Palgrave Macmillan.

'Body Worlds' (no date), www.koerperwelten.com/en/pages/plastination.asp (accessed 27 March 2004).

Brody, Howard, *Stories of Sickness*, 1987, New Haven, CT: Yale University Press.

Calman, Sir Kenneth C *et al*, *The Ethics of Research Related to Healthcare in Developing Countries*, 2002, London: Nuffield Council in Bioethics.

Canguilhem, Georges, *The Normal and the Pathological*, translated by Fawcett, Carolyn R, in collaboration with Cohen, Robert S, with an introduction by Foucault, Michel, 1991, New York: Zone Books. (Originally published as *Le Normal et le Pathologique*, 1966, Paris: Presses Universitaires de France.)

Daudet, Alphonse, 'La doulou' in *Oeuvres complètes illustrées*, vol 17 (1930) Paris: Librairie de France. (Translated by Barnes, Julian, as *In the Land of Pain*, 2002, London: Jonathan Cape.)

Donald, Anna, 'The words we live in', in Greenhalgh, Trisha and Hurwitz, Brian (eds), *Narrative Based Medicine: Dialogue and Discourse in Medical Practice*, 1988, London: BMJ Books, pp 17–26.

Fukuda, Mahito, *A Cultural History of Tuberculosis in Modern Japan*, www.lang.nagoya-u.ac.jp/~mfukuda/english.html (accessed 27 March 2004).

Foucault, Michel, *The Birth of the Clinic: An Archaeology of Medical Perception*, translated by Sheridan Smith, AM, 1973, London: Tavistock Publications. (Originally published as *Naissance de la Clinique: une Archéologie du Regard Médical*, 1963, Paris: Presses universitaires de France.)

Greenhalgh, Trisha and Hurwitz, Brian (eds), *Narrative Based Medicine: Dialogue and Discourse in Clinical Practice*, 1998, London: BMJ

Hurwitz, Brian, 'The wounded storyteller: narrative strands in medical negligence', in Greenhalgh, Trisha and Hurwitz, Brian (eds), *Narrative Based Medicine: Dialogue and Discourse in Clinical Practice*, 1998, London: BMJ, pp 234–46.

Irigaray, Luce, *This Sex Which Is Not One*, translated by Porter, Catherine, 1985, Ithaca, NY: Cornell University Press. (Originally published as *Ce sexe qui n'en est pas un*, 1977, Paris: Éditions de Minuit.)

Irigaray, Luce, *An Ethics of Sexual Difference*, translated by Burke, Carolyn and Gill, Gillian C, 1993a, Ithaca, NY: Cornell University Press. (Originally published as *Éthique de la différence sexuelle*, 1984, Paris: Editions de Minuit.)

Irigaray, Luce, *'Je, Tu, Nous': Towards a Culture of Difference*, translated by Martin, Alison, 1993b, New York: Routledge. (Originally published as *Je, Tu, Nous, pour une Culture de la Différence*, 1990, Paris: Grasset et Fasquelle.)

Korsch, Barbara, and Harding, Caroline, *The Intelligent Patient's Guide to the Doctor-Patient Relationship : Learning How to Talk So Your Doctor Will Listen*, 1998, New York, Oxford: Oxford University Press.

Ley, Philip, *Communicating with Patients: Improving Communication, Satisfaction and Compliance,* Series: Psychology and Health, vol 4, 1988, Cheltenham: Stanley Thornes.

Loudon, Irvine *et al* 'The Hippocratic Oath' (1994) 309 *British Medical Journal* 414 (6 August), and (1994) 309 *British Medical Journal* 952–53 (8 October).

Louis, Pierre Charles Alexandre, *An Essay on Clinical Instruction,* translated by Marin, Peter, 1834, Reigate: Highly and Allingham. (Original French version never published.)

Luckmann, Joan and Tindell Nobles, Sylvia, *Trans-cultural Communication in Health,* 2000, Albany, NY: Delmar.

Minardi, Henry, and Riley, Martin, *Communication in Health Care,* 1997, Oxford: Butterworth-Heinemann.

Morris, David, *The Culture of Pain,* 1991, Berkeley, CA, Los Angeles, CA, Oxford: University of California Press.

Northouse, Peter and Northouse, Linda, *Health Communication: Strategies for Health Professionals,* 1992, Norwalk, CT: Appleton and Lange.

Nutton, Vivien, 'What's in an oath?' (1995) 29 *Journal of Royal College of Physicians* 518–24.

Porter, Roy, *Blood and Guts: A Short History of Medicine,* 2002, London: Allen Lane.

Redleaf, Angelica, and Baird, Susan, *Behind Closed Doors: Gender, Sexuality and Touch in the Doctor/Patient Relationship,* 1998, Westport, CT, London: Auburn House.

Rifkin, Jeremy, *The Biotech Century: Harnessing the Gene and Remaking the World,* 1998, New York: Jeremy P Tarcher/Putnam.

Sontag, Susan, *Illness as Metaphor,* 1979, London: Allen Lane.

Sontag, Susan, *AIDS and its Metaphors,* 1989, London: Allen Lane/The Penguin Press.

Wall Street Journal, 'NIH hormone tests with children draws criticism of group' (1992) *Wall Street Journal* (Eastern Edition) p A1 (25 June).

OVERVIEW

Nana Wilson-Tagoe

The chapters of this volume are significant in the ways that they explore gender, sexuality and health from a variety of disciplinary and cultural contexts. In linking sexuality to gender, illness and health, they move it from an essentially biological conception into areas of sexual experience mediated by social, cultural and political realities. They locate bodily experiences like menstruation, childbirth, and disease firmly in the arena of sexuality and link them meaningfully to the languages, codes and myths that define them in gendered terms. All the chapters here raise fundamental questions about constructions of gender and sexuality, about the power relations involved in such constructions and about the factors that mediate them in specific cultures and historical moments.

Nicola Mai's chapter foregrounds several of these issues in its exploration of the cultural, social and epidemiological implications of sex as a strategy of survival among Albanian migrants in Italy and Greece. Focusing on a particular context of upheaval in Albania and the massive migrations of Albanian young men to Italy and Greece, Mai examines how notions of masculinity and hegemonic articulations of gender and sexuality are negotiated in the marginal worlds of Albanian migrants. Based largely on his research among Albanian sex-workers in Italy and Greece, his chapter uncovers an ambivalence towards established canons of masculinity and morality that has implications for attitudes to homosexuality, the practice of safe sex and HIV/AIDS transmission among migrant sex-workers. As he argues, the endurance of patriarchal roles and values even within the emasculating contexts of social exclusion and exploitation prevents a true assessment of HIV transmission patterns and hinders real knowledge of protective modes of sexual behaviour.

Philippa Levine's chapter presents another context in which gendered notions of sexuality and colonial power relations distort understanding of disease transmission. The many-layered perspectives of her chapter demonstrate how the intersection of law, politics and medicine in the nineteenth-century Contagious Diseases Acts in Britain and its Empire targeted female sexual activity as virtually the sole agent of disease transmission. In foregrounding the different assumptions that overlaid these legislations in the Empire and in Britain itself, Levine reveals how the control of women's sexuality in both contexts was mediated by the politics of gender and imperialism. As she suggests, colonial notions about the natural promiscuity of women prostitutes in the colonised regions could conceivably have inspired the less stigmatising and redemptive rhetoric that surrounded the Contagious Diseases Acts in Britain. Levine's inferences point not only to the convergence of politics, race and gender in the construction of women's sexuality but also to the instability and vulnerability of the notion of sexuality itself.

Nahid Toubia's chapter confirms this instability as it explores the cultural divergences and power politics that mediate perceptions of female circumcision in the West and in Africa. It is through locating female circumcision in the context of women's reproductive health and rights and within a broader campaign for social change that Toubia distinguishes the different prejudices and agendas that have mediated the discourse on female circumcision since the turn of the twentieth century. In her view, the attempts of Western commentators to direct and manage the histories and narratives of this practice do not escape the age-long biases that have always defined Africa as 'Other'. Indeed, in controlling the dissemination of views on the subject, Western scholars and writers distance the experience and knowledge of Africans and move debates on the subject away from their true contexts in the social dynamics and power in African communities. Toubia's chapter, like Levine's, exposes the determining power of language in shaping the discursive forms through which notions of sexuality are conceptualised and disseminated.

The relationship between sexuality, medicine and the social management of disease reveals the extent to which the practice of medicine is frequently mediated by social and cultural conditions and biases. Audrey Prost's chapter, based on her research among Tibetan refugees in India, demonstrates how the epidemiology of tuberculosis is transformed by the social meanings given to it by the community. In linking the disease to conditions of migration, Prost explores a connection between tuberculosis and the distress and disorientations of displacement. Her case studies are significant in revealing how Tibetan communities – even when displaced – construct their discourses in terms that are mediated by gender considerations privileging men's experience, for while the tuberculosis of adolescent boys is seen in terms of the suffering of exile, the infection of girls is seen in negative, disapproving terms as a disease of dieting and a sign of disintegrating moral values among Tibetan girl migrants.

Images, taboos and myths built around bodily functions throughout time have important implications not only for human health but for the social constructs that societies build around bodies and the anxieties that generate them. Margaret Healy's inter-disciplinary approach to researching the subject of menstruation in early modern England yields valuable insights into the ambivalent and paradoxical meanings inscribed in the myths and discourses around menstruation. Her decision to explore these myths through religious, medical, philosophical and fictional material allows her to read the myths and discourses around menstruation from multiple perspectives. On a major level, she reads the myths and taboos as deriving from a general belief in the fundamental weakness and the potentially corrupting nature of women's bodies. Such beliefs, her analysis demonstrates, underlined women's inferiority and 'justified' men's dominance over them.

What makes Healy's research valuable are the different and often contending perspectives she foregrounds in her analysis. Her recognition of other discourses that refuted the venomous aspects of menstrual blood, together with her suggestion that taboos and prohibitions actually privileged women's private spaces as well as their fertility and potency, reveals a far more complex dynamic at work in early modern England than is often acknowledged. Indeed, Healy's work reveals the extent to which the science and practice of medicine were frequently mediated by the humanistic discourses of philosophy and religion. At a methodological level, it exemplifies the inter-disciplinary thrust of this book in its suggestion that only such multiple approaches can unravel the complex processes involved in the intersections of disease, medicine and the social construction of gender and sexuality.

A similar sense of the dynamic forces at work in relationships between women's bodily functions and discourses of sexuality emerges in Shigehisa Kuriyama's chapter on 'Angry Women and the Evolution of Chinese Medicine'. His account of the history of the imagination of fire in Chinese philosophy and medicine reveals close links between the pathology of fire and the disorders of women. As he argues, the rise of the discourse of fire was influenced and inspired by a new consciousness of congestion (conservation of semen, conservation of vitality) and new anxieties about depletion of male semen and male energy.

George Rousseau's chapter connects logically and thematically with these approaches and presents other dimensions and contexts for exploring the links made between disease, culture, and sexuality in nineteenth-century Europe as he examines the ideologies and biases that mediated medical discourses around cholera. Working from the premise that disease in human history is mentalised and conceptualised before being diagnosed and treated, Rousseau traces the complex processes through which cholera came to be associated with primitiveness and homosexuality. His analysis of the medical literature on cholera between 1752 and 1842 reveals how the association of cholera with the fundament or anus was influenced by perceived threats from the 'barbarous' East and the 'degenerate' homosexual. In linking this sense of threat to colonising ideologies of the nineteenth century, to the development of sexology and the notion of a 'third sex', Rousseau's chapter, like others in the book, demonstrates significant correlations between science, politics and sexuality that underpin the multi-disciplinary thrust of our book.

The chapters in this book do not only straddle disciplinary and cultural boundaries; they also cut across temporal and historical moments. Rousseau's focus on the shifting conceptualisations of disease and health in different historical moments of European history finds a resonance in Stephen Quirke's chapter and in the challenges of reading and interpretation demanded of us by the issues he raises. Quirke's reading of gender in ancient Egyptian writing on healing identifies the challenges that such a healing script presents to modern manipulators of gender and Western definitions of medicine. His open-ended reading of the Petrie papyrus identifies a variety of possible gendered readings as well as attitudes to homosexuality that may appear uncomplicated on the surface. However, his analysis of factors and contexts that inspired the writings on healing forces our appreciation of the extent to which a healing script bears or does not bear gender already inscribed during the processes of writing. Indeed, his discussion of the papyrus on healing suggests that what appears in the writings as gendered inscriptions of a male-dominated literary elite should be read against factors that differentiate our modern contexts of reception from notions of literacy, concepts of medicine and categories of social differentiation that prevailed in ancient Egypt. The issues of translation and interpretation that Quirke raises here are crucial not just for comparative explorations of different temporalities but also for the inter-disciplinary criss-crossing that lies at the heart of this book.

The sociological factors that Quirke identifies in ancient Egyptian conceptions of history find an interesting resonance in Deborah Kirklin's chapter, which explores links between medical science, sociology and politics. Working from the premise that a shared understanding of health and well-being is central to the construction of a medical culture, she demonstrates how such a culture may be enhanced by being grounded in the day-to-day realities of medical practice as they touch particularly on attitudes to sex, gender, and sexuality. Drawing from her experience in teaching medical humanities, Kirklin explores several areas of medical practice in which sex, gender and sexuality may determine the quality and justness of healthcare provision. Her chapter demonstrates, with close reference to her classroom experience, how literary texts can illuminate complex issues of disease and health by exploring representations of individual experiences that transcend the purely scientific and clinical aspects of illness and health. Kirklin's chapter is tentative and exploratory, but in its awareness of links between imagination, representation and the practice of medicine, it looks to the future and to further possibilities of the mutual illumination of literature and medicine. It thus illustrates an important aspect of this book's approach: the combination of literary representation and social science approaches to gender and sexuality in order to validate a social imaginary beyond the actualities of empirical research.

In this volume, analyses of visual and literary representations of gender and sexuality sit alongside empirical studies, but they do represent different orders of knowledge and illumination. The traditional opposition between the social sciences (centred on empirical knowledge) and art (deriving from the interplay of experience and imagination) has been blurred by recent moves towards narrative in the social sciences and by the increasingly socio-cultural focus in literature. However, the two disciplines still have different modes of narrative and different expectations from it. Artistic representations like photography may, for instance, appear to issue directly from the physical world, yet, as Michael Worton's chapter makes clear, the physical world it represents is also an intervention, a manipulation of the world of empirical experience. It operates as a translation of reality that is, as he argues, semantically mobile. Literary representation as opposed to photography is sometimes even less dependent on empirical experience. Its value, as with all representations, lies in the kind of distance it sustains between experience and its formulation and between how we see the world and what that world may be or become. In imaginative literature it is the power of language and the play of dialogic interactions that makes a transformative and Utopian vision possible. A book on gender and sexuality that combines social analysis and consideration of artistic representation therefore has the benefit of multiple illuminations about reality as it exists and as it can be made to be.

These multiple perspectives are what Michael Worton's chapter, 'Behold the

(Sick) Man' offer readers of this book. It situates itself between the biblical context of *Ecce Homo* and the artistic genres it inspired in Western art, in order to explore the radicalising of both theme and genre in the photographic works of four contemporary male artists. Taking as his starting point the cultural force of the story of Christ, displayed and mocked as an object of monstrosity, Worton examines the problematics of representing illness by calling into question the Christian and Hellenic traditions of representing suffering. Against the tendency of such codes to foreclose areas of human pain and suffering, Worton opposes the capacity of art to open up the various conflicting and contradictory feelings that criss-cross in our expressions of suffering. Worton's chapter draws on both literary theory and theories of photography to examine the paradoxical realism of the art of photography. The distinctiveness of this medium, he argues, lies in its particular and problematic realism – its ability to communicate an effect of the real rather than represent an imitation of it.

The challenge that such a representational medium offers is the challenge of using the familiar codes of *Ecce Homo* to re-think and re-focus on the male body. The significance of Worton's chapter lies in the way it demonstrates how this re-thinking disrupts traditional certainties about masculinity and re-positions questions of gender. It is again, in Worton's view, the ability of photography to modify reality that enables all four artists not so much to conceptualise AIDS, smallpox and varicose veins as to present them in acts of witnessing that see something other than what seems to be represented. These artistic and representational dimensions of the interplay of gender, sexuality and health complement the book's empirical analyses and investigative case studies by offering other kinds of insights that move us beyond the realities we deal with.

Following a mode of exploration and interpretation similar to Michael Worton's, James Agar's chapter provides remarkable insights into the interplay of gender, sexuality and health in imaginative literature. Although his specific focus is on two works of European fiction and how they figure, appropriate and interpolate Africa into their representations of AIDS, he is also fundamentally engaged with examining how literature can contribute to our understanding of the complex interweaving of gender and power that shapes our understanding of AIDS and mediates narratives that attempt to represent it. Agar works with the premise that fiction can provide a reflective and critical space for interrogation and speculation, and that, through language and narrative construction, literature contributes to the very essence of what AIDS is, what we understand by it, and how we live (with or without it).

Reading fictions about AIDS, Agar argues, allows for a critical re-reading of some of the seemingly dominant issues inherent in AIDS discourse. His chapter should be read in relation to chapters in the book that investigate the handling and management of disease in different periods of human history, for there is a sense in which his reading of Adam Mars-Jones's 'Slim' and Hervé Guibert's *Paradise* has resonances with the historical and sociological studies of Philippa Levine, George Rousseau and Nicola Mai, whilst also providing other illuminations that only the narrative and reflexivity of art and literature may yield. The crucial point underlying Agar's analysis holds true for all the other chapters on disease in the book: the need to make a dreaded disease foreign is common to the cultural construction of a range of plagues; different cultures construct AIDS as though it is a foreign condition, a viral threat from abroad to the boundaries of the domestic space. Agar's reading of the two texts examines the contradictions inherent in narrativising a European experience of AIDS through a trope of Africa perceived as taint, disease and contagion.

Lynda Morgan's critical exploration of South African settler fictions of the nineteenth century echo several of the issues raised in James Agar's chapter and should be read in relation to it and to George Rousseau's and Philippa Levine's reading of colonialism and discourses around infectious diseases. In their different communicative and performative forms, all three chapters illuminate the different ways in which ideas that circulated in centres of European colonial power were embodied in a variety of different discourses across the empire. If the medical literature that Rousseau analyses demonstrates the certainties of colonial epistemologies, the South African fictions that internalise colonial discourses on disease reveal no such assurance. Rather, their obsessions with bodily integrity and coherence as expressed in representations of miscegenation reveal the vulnerability of white settler identity itself. Morgan reads these fictions from a variety of theoretical perspectives in order to illuminate the paradoxes, the anxieties and the unconscious fantasies about blackness that underlie representations of miscegenation. Images of disease in these fictions, she argues, intersect with those of blood, semen and dirt, to construct a hierarchical system of racialised, class-infected and gendered bodies. Yet, as she demonstrates, sexual relations across the racial divide are contested exchanges, and white fantasies about blackness expose fractures in the notion of a white South African identity that indicate a profound psychological anarchy.

The kind of psychological perspectives that Lynda Morgan deploys in her reading of South African settler fiction are to be seen also in the chapters of Caroline Warman and Rachel Harrison as they explore three sets of confessional works. Confessional writing has been instrumental in exploring relations between texts and the innermost fears, anxieties and aspirations of writers. Caroline Warman's chapter offers valuable insights on how two generations of francophone men use the form to deal with their fragile sexuality, and her case studies of Astolphe de Custine and Henri-Frédéric Amiel show how the diary form can become the arena of psychological and literary modernism.

Rachel Harrison's chapter on moral degeneracy and erotic excess in a contemporary Thai novel focuses on another kind of confessional writing that reveals contrasting relations between text and experience within a different culture and time. In the nineteenth-century European works that Warman explores, the confessional enacts a private, non-patriarchal self that would be imperilled and torn apart in the public domain. In the modern Thai context of *Jan Daraa*, the novel that Harrison explores, confessional writing works rather to transgress taboos about sexuality by placing representations of sexuality squarely in the public domain. As Harrison argues, such a transgression is consistent with the novel's foregrounding of the multi-layered tensions and contradictions that co-exist with Thai attitudes to sexuality. The novel's own preoccupations,

Harrison argues, demonstrate these contradictions by enacting a trajectory of erotic adventures and justifying them by referring back to Thai classical works and the erotic episodes of its highly poetic conventions. Thus, rather than textualising private alienations from dominant sexual discourses, they expose simplistic Western notions about Thai sexuality and reveal the multiple locations and expressions of sexuality that Thai society continually suppresses.

The nineteenth-century European texts and the twentieth-century Thai novel explored, respectively, by Caroline Warman and Rachel Harrison all address constructions and internalisations of gender and sexuality by reorganising relationships which are in tension with the normative spheres of the public domain. In all three cases, such relationships are nonetheless inspired by the social organisation of gender and sexuality and the dominant discourses they produce. Nana Wilson-Tagoe's chapter on the semantics and politics of childbearing and motherhood in contemporary African literature provides other contexts in which the cultural concepts that encode notions of sexuality are negotiated through confrontations with the language, codes and myths that shape them. Her chapter focuses particularly on women's writing because, as she argues, women's social place in African societies has been and continues to be defined by their biological functions and sexual roles. Examining contemporary women's negotiation of these dominant discourses from the combined perspectives of semantics and politics, she argues that a focus on semantics provides a key to the production of sexual meanings and at the same time reveals gaps between the language of culture and the alternative meanings created in imaginative literature. Wilson-Tagoe's reading of Buchi Emecheta's novel, *The Joys of Motherhood*, and Yvonne Vera's *Butterfly Burning* draws on the different historical contexts of Nigeria and Zimbabwe to tease out the imperatives as well as the linguistic forms that shape the negotiations of gender and sexuality in the writing of two generations of contemporary African women.

In identifying and distinguishing the social science discourses from the artistic discourses within the various cultural contexts of the chapters in this volume, this summary aims not to emphasise their separateness as disciplines but, rather, to highlight how the interplay of their different illuminations can help us better to understand how healthcare operates and is mediated through gender and sexuality.

PART I
THE POLITICS OF SICKNESS AND HEALTH

CHAPTER 1

FEMALE GENITAL MUTILATION: CONTESTING THE RIGHT TO SPEAK OF WOMEN'S BODIES IN AFRICA AND THE WEST

Nahid Toubia

In my capacity as founding director of RAINBO,[1] I have been concerned with the practice of female circumcision (FC) or female genital mutilation (FGM) for nearly 20 years.[2] As a Sudanese woman, physician, activist, researcher and scholar – an unusual combination of roles – every aspect of my life has been closely involved in some way with one or other of the social orders which promote FC/FGM. I find myself constantly faced with the difficult choice of whether to continue focusing RAINBO's limited energy and resources on the work of advancing the rights of African women to control their own bodies – including the right to freedom from genital cutting – or whether to respond to the barrage of enquiries from those in the West who are 'interested' in FGM. Most of the time, I choose the former. In this chapter, however, I will take the (rare) opportunity to pause and reflect on my experience of the latter, focusing on the way individuals and institutions – mainly in Europe and the USA – have behaved in relation to the practice of FGM. In doing so, I make no claim either to reflect an analysis of scientific data or to make a thorough review of published literature. I simply draw upon the accumulation of my personal and professional experiences as an African woman responding to Western interest in FGM.

As the head of an organisation which has gained international recognition for its leadership in campaigning against the practice of FGM, I have come across every conceivable medium of Western communication on the subject: magazine articles, radio, television, websites, academic journals, student papers, public presentations, 'educational' material, health professionals' training sessions and public debates, as well as increasingly combative and far-reaching proposals for legislation against FGM. I have worked on this issue at an international, executive level, not only in the USA and the UK, but also in Australia, Canada, Denmark, France, Germany, Italy, New Zealand, Norway, Spain, Sweden and even at the United Nations. At the same time, at a practical, national level, RAINBO provides

1 RAINBO (www.rainbo.org) is an international organisation, started in 1994 and lead by African women to advance women's rights in Africa. Its aim is to highlight issues relating to women's health and rights, and to redress the imbalance in the way these issues are reported in a world dominated by Western media and Western interests.

2 RAINBO is clear in its use of terminology: female circumcision (FC) acknowledges – and respects – the intent of those who practise female genital mutilation; the term female genital mutilation (FGM), by contrast, reflects our strong opposition to FC. We also encourage researchers and physicians to use the local terms used by the communities they are working in. Female genital cutting (FGC) is more increasingly accepted as a neutral non-judgmental term in international circles.

technical help and financial support for groups in Africa that work against FGM and for women's rights to their sexual and bodily integrity. The organisation engages with African individuals, African professional and community organisations, African governments and the African feminist movement. Thus, when I travel in Africa, I speak not only to the 'structures' but also, and much more crucially, directly to women and girls about their lives and how the fact of FC/FGM plays a role in shaping them.

As a result of my direct experiences of life in the West and in Africa, I am all too aware of the tension that exists between what I see as the Western need to understand and legislate, and Africa's need for action to implement social change. Although genuine and respectful dialogue between those 'interested' in FGM in the West and African women (and men) is possible, such dialogue does not occur very often. The principal reason for this, in my view, lies in the underlying motivation of those people in the West who are drawn to the issue. Many of these people engage with FC/FGM out of self-interest, rather than out of real concern for those who are part of the practice. Some are motivated by the desire to sell magazines, make good radio programmes, turn in good term papers, or write PhD theses on an 'exotic' theme. Others are drawn to the subject as a means of developing their careers, gaining access to funding opportunities, or – more rarely, but most alarmingly of all – of reinforcing the superiority of their own identity over that of the perceived African 'other'. These Western 'motives' are, of course, diverse, complex and multi-layered, but they share one common element: namely, the fact that they are less concerned with facilitating the removal of a violation than with promoting self-interest.

It has been a long journey from my early years with RAINBO, when I spent many sleepless nights struggling with the hurt, anger and humiliation I felt after trying to engage sensibly and fairly with people on the subject of FC/FGM. I now have a thicker skin and a personal 'toolkit' of rationalism, wit, sarcasm and provocation with which to protect my African self and to create a space that encourages others to listen, however briefly. However, despite my use of these intellectual tools, a persistent ache remains, impossible to dull, which is deepened by the lack of sensitivity in others. It is a pain that I share with my activist African sisters and with people from other cultures who have the sensibility and humility to listen, share and understand.

In late 2002, the cultural clashes and racial politics of the FGM debate were at an all-time high and the fight for access to funding was all too apparent. I returned to London to find radical proposals being made for the revision of the UK's 1985 FGM law. For the networks of activist African women, the motives for this amended legislation were unclear and highly suspect.[3] The two sides of the 'FGM

3 See [UK Parliament] (2000). The Prohibition of Female Circumcision Act was passed in 1985. It was brought forward on 11 December 2002 to strengthen the UK's position on FGM. The Female Genital Mutilation Act 2003 (which repeals and re-enacts the Prohibition of Female Circumcision Act 1985) gives extraterritorial effect to the existing provisions. This means that any of the prohibited acts done outside the UK by a UK national or permanent UK resident will be an offence under domestic law and can be tried in the courts of England, Wales and Northern Ireland (the Act does not extend to Scotland). The Act also increases the maximum penalty for FGM from five to 14 years' imprisonment. For the updated legislation that came into force on 4 March 2004, see [UK Parliament] (2003).

world' appeared as far removed from each other as ever. For me, the haunting memory of this moment is of an image seen during a night of fitful sleep and restless dreams: in one dream, I saw Africans sitting inside a behaviourist's examination room surrounded by two-way mirrors. The intention was to confront them with reflections of their disturbed, uncivilised and sick state of being. Meanwhile, on the outside, the 'others', mostly Westerners, looked in through the glass, unable to see themselves. They appeared confident and impassive as they scrutinised the Africans with the cold gaze of self-assured Western professionals. If this image is indeed the model for interaction between cultures, how will there ever be a true dialogue between them, between the 'self' and the 'other' on both sides?

I fear that the current Western interest in FGM – couched as it is in terms of 'cultural sensitivity' and 'concern for human rights' – is in fact a thinly disguised re-enactment of the old colonialist project of 'saving the souls of the barbaric African'. If this is the case, Western concern about FGM, operating on the basis of self-interest, lacks any of the necessary elements of mutual respect, dignity or honest dialogue between equals. If there is no attempt to 'look into each other's eyes' – that is, if there is no attempt by the West to see Africa with all its strengths, vulnerabilities, confusions and certainties – then there can be no genuine, human interaction. The discovery of commonalities and differences between cultures will give way to the calculated materialist ethics of the West's dominant and expanding worldview.

History of Western writing on FC/FGM

A decade ago, few in the West would have heard of FGM. Today it is clear that, of all the topics concerning African women's health and African women's rights, it is now the one most frequently written and talked about. Virtually every time I tell people that I work on women's health and rights in Africa, the first response I get is: 'OK, so you work on genital mutilation.' In other words, people forget all too easily the deaths from pregnancy and childbirth that claim the lives of at least a quarter of a million women in Africa every year. They forget about women's vulnerability to HIV/AIDS, caused by the fact that the primary means of livelihood for most women in Africa is giving sexual favours to men either within or outside marriage. They ignore the violence against women in armed conflict and civil unrest. The list goes on and on. These issues and many others that affect women are all linked to issues of sustainable (and non-dependent) economic development, on the equitable distribution of resources, on democracy and good governance, and on gender inequalities, about which the West remains ambivalent in the work that it does through and with international assistance funds. We live in a post-colonialist, post-World War II world, in which the dominant liberal discourse frowns upon views that maintain and express ideologies of superiority and inferiority. Nonetheless, many such views still prevail, albeit tacitly but in various degrees of intensity; the fact that they remain unexpressed (except by the radical right) means that they remain ultimately unexplored and unchallenged.

One does not need to scratch too deeply below the surface of individual and institutional ethos to realise that convictions regarding which is the superior or inferior culture (European vs African), race (Caucasian vs Negro) or religion (Judaeo-Christian vs Islam) continue to be alive and thriving. Indeed, the tabloid media maintain such oppositional views quite shamelessly. Issues such as FGM and women's treatment under Islam are particularly attractive to proponents of such views, since it enables them to articulate their views with apparent impunity, hence the widespread attention that FGM receives. Put crudely, FGM is presented as providing indisputable proof of Africa's barbarism, and the treatment of women by fundamentalist political Islam provides ample ammunition for the Western propaganda machine in its campaign to assert cultural dominance: there is a repeated – and wilful – association between FGM and Islam, despite the fact that evidence is repeatedly provided to the contrary. The well-oiled and highly efficient machine of cultural dominance continues to operate with the same vigour today as it did in the time of colonisation, although the environment is now one of satellites and the internet.

The earliest documented evidence of female circumcision was written at the turn of the twentieth century by colonial missionaries such as the Woolfe sisters.[4] The fact that the sisters documented the practice – it would previously have been recorded only in songs or folk-tales – established them as the first objectors. In the 1940s and 1950s the anti-slavery movement raised the issue in the British Parliament and the British Colonial administration was obligated to respond.[5] The great debate of whether the West has the right to interfere in local culture, not unlike the one conducted today, had started and resulted in the passing of the 1946 law against the severest form of the practice (infibulation) in Sudan.[6] Sudanese-nationalist leaders, mostly men fighting for independence, used the opportunity to rebel against the law as a way to mobilise resistance against the colonial administration. We now have undisputed evidence that during this time many mothers were resisting the practice within their families – some at the risk of severe social penalties.[7]

From the 1930s through to the 1990s a few Western physicians, or their well-trained male African counterparts, made a name for themselves by publishing studies on the clinical complications of female circumcision.[8] Most of these studies were of poor quality and contained questionable data and conclusions, yet

---

4 Miss Woolfe was a British midwife who, together with her sister, wrote some of the earliest documented reports on female circumcision in the 1920s (Sudan Archives Cir Sec 44/2/12); see Rahman and Toubia (2000) pp 215–18.

5 *Report on Female Circumcision in the Anglo-Egyptian Sudan*, Khartoum: Sudan Medical Service, 1 March 1945. in reports 4/1/1, Sudan Archives. For details, see Rahman and Toubia (2000) pp 215–18.

6 Penal Code 1974 (1974 Act No 64), art 284A(1); see [Sudan] (1977–81), volume 9.

7 This evidence comes from the stories of second-generation African women activists whose mothers and grandmothers stood against the practice. Unfortunately, none of this evidence is documented in writing.

8 Examples are in Aziz (1980), Daw (1970), Diejomaoh and Faal (1981), Dirie (1985), Dirie and Lindmark (1992), Iregbulem (1980), Modawi (1973), Roles (1967), Shandall (1967), Verzin (1975) and Worsley (1938).

they remained uncontested for over two decades and were used as the primary evidence for campaigning and legislating against the practice. It was not until the late 1990's that the data in these studies was questioned by Makhlouf (a Harvard anthropologist of Lebanese origin) in an extensive review of the evidence on medical complications.[9]

In the late 1970s an Austrian-American architect, Fran Hosken, working for the United States Agency for International Development (USAID), stumbled on the practice of FC/FGM while on a mission to Africa. She went back to the USA, raised money for a tour of several African countries to investigate this practice and produced *The Hosken Report: Genital and Sexual Mutilation of Females*.[10] The title of the report and its contents speak volumes about the 'motivation' of this particular European-American woman's interest in FGM. Through her writing style, the values embodied in the book and the organisation she built on it, Hosken claimed monopoly 'ownership' of FGM, which she aggressively tried to maintain through the publications of the second and third editions of her report and the monthly newsletter *WIN NEWS*.[11] In personal interactions and correspondence, she systematically attacked African women who were interested in dealing with the practice in their own country and ignited a 20 year conflict between African women's rights activists and Western FGM crusaders (I use the word 'crusaders' to label this brand of interest in FGM in the West deliberately). Until the end of the 1980s, the broader feminist movement in the West had not been engaged with the issue and only a handful of FGM careerists, such as Hosken, were posing as representatives of all Western women and claiming to be the undisputed salvation missionaries against this barbaric practice.[12] By 1993, the world was changing and African women were working closely with the global feminist movement on issues of women's rights towards the Vienna conference on Human Rights where I presented the issue of FGM as a violation of human rights at the non-governmental Tribunal together with my first publication on FGM.[13] At the end of my presentation in Vienna, tens of African women came to hug me in tears mostly saying 'thank you for claiming ownership of this painful issue for African women and for putting it in the appropriate context'. This change in the international feminist discourse forced the Western crusaders to change their language considerably as can be detected in the fourth edition of the Hosken Report.[14]

On another front, a minor media interest was aroused in the British press in the 1980s by a fabricated conflict between the so-called 'African cultural apologists' and the 'Western Women Liberators' – a misrepresentation of events at the

9 Makhlouf-Obermeyer (1999).

10 Hosken (1979).

11 Women's International News Network, 187 Grant Street, Lexington, MA, 02420–2126, USA.

12 Also see Lightfoot-Klein (1989).

13 Toubia (1993). A copy of the video of the Vienna Tribunal is available from the Center for Women's Global Leadership, Douglas College, Rutgers University, NJ, USA.

14 Hosken (1994).

Copenhagen Conference of the Mid-decade for Women (1975–85). Similar media campaigns where Western liberators were set against African defenders of FC were repeated many times over the years in Norway, Sweden and other Western countries. I myself was the victim of this when interviewed by the US issue of the *TIME* magazine in early 1994: I was presented as the cultural apologist against the 'saviour' Alice Walker as part of the promotion campaign for one of her two books on FGM.[15] On reading the finished article, I was shocked by misquotations which effectively negated my views and belittled my life's work against the practice. I decided to investigate what had happened and discovered that the junior researcher who conducted the interview had presented my words honestly, but was overruled by the editor who needed to generate controversy in order to sell the magazine. In the face of an influential Western publication, I, as an African woman, felt utterly frustrated and powerless.

Another area for Western writing started to emerge in the 1980s among (mostly female) anthropologists who found numerous ways to study FGM for their PhD theses and peer-reviewed journal articles. The relentless pressure on these academics to publish and distinguish their voices in a field already over-saturated and highly competitive drove them to search for an exotic subject, which FGM then was and continues to be. As a result, there are scores of lengthy theoretical and ethnographic studies which seek to explain the role of the practice within African culture. Given the sheer volume of anthropological literature on FGM in various languages, I cannot undertake a detailed critical analysis of their content. However, despite their tendency to focus on 'exotic' traditional culture rather than understanding the dynamics of present-day society, some of these studies have proved a useful means of furthering my understanding of the mechanisms that promote and preserve the practice.[16] Some of these anthropologists became so possessive of their cultural 'subjects', and the need to preserve them, that they in fact became a strong voice against any attempts to stop the practice. At a populist level their position was championed by the controversial and outspoken Germaine Greer who argued that African women are happy with their status as circumcised, or in a polygamous relation, and that outsiders should leave them alone.[17] The difficulty with Germaine Greer's attempt at open-minded and fair analysis is that she transformed African women into the objects, not subjects, of her observations and did not reflect on the nature of African societies which, like her own and every other, consist in a complex and dynamic system of power relations and group interests.

The 1990s saw a significant improvement in communications and ease of movement across continents. It was also the age of media dominance and 24-hour news satellite TV. In 1993 USA soldiers entered Somalia and, as part of its temporary focus on Africa, the US media 're-discovered' FGM and Islamic women. The issue of FC/FGM as presented to the American public tends to exclude the voices of African women, or to use them to enact a pre-determined

---

15 Gregory (1994). See also Walker (1992) and Walker and Parmar (1993).

16 Boddy (1989), Gruenbaum (1991), Sanderson (1981).

17 Greer (1999a). See also Greer (1999b).

scenario in which they are presented as the victims of a barbaric culture that is saved by the brave heroes of American modernisation. I have frequently found myself forced to choose between the roles of a victim or the detached medical professional as the only two possible options. I was not allowed to be my complex self and never an African activist. This occurred in interviews with New York 1, ABC and NBC Television stations in 1995, and even on the famous Oprah Winfrey show.[18] Sadly my experience of the Oprah show was as painful as that at *TIME* magazine. With two other interviewees cast as the victims I was cast as the medical doctor. When I attempted to speak of African women's activism and struggles against the practice my interventions were edited so badly that the program shows visible and unprofessional cuts to remove what I said.

The New York Times published a series of articles in a period of over a year on FGM by the columnist Abe Rosenthal, who never once mentioned attempts by Africans to stop the practice.[19] After repeated attempts, the editors of the newspaper finally accepted a piece by a group of African women activists and scholars opposed to FGM to present a more balanced point of view.[20] One notable exception to this relentless media misrepresentation in the USA was an interview I recorded on National Public Radio with Terry Gross.[21] Thanks to her humanity and professionalism, my sense of dignity and trust in communication across cultures was restored.

With the publication of her two books on FGM,[22] Alice Walker, the renowned African American feminist writer, entered the arena and raised the profile of the issue among the broader Western feminist constituency, as well as in gender and women's studies circles in American universities. My personal encounter with Alice Walker and my reading of her books has convinced me that, in the West, a sense of cultural superiority is much stronger than allegiance to skin colour. This is borne out by the fact that the feminist journal *Ms. Magazine* chose to promote only Walker's point of view – Walker being one of its cult heroes – and so offered a perspective no less biased than that of Abe Rosenthal while proving less liberal than *The New York Times* by blocking any attempts at parallel publishing of African feminist points of view.[23] International sisterhood and solidarity has not, in this case, crossed the cultural and political divide with the result that the one-sided journalistic, academic and popular deluge continues unabated.

There remains no satisfactory explanation for this level of obsession with the issue of FC/FGM, yet somehow it still manages to grab attention and stay in the

---

18 Oprah Winfrey show, aired on Thursday 7 September 1995.

19 Rosenthal (1993a; 1993b; 1993c).

20 Dawit and Salem (1993).

21 Interview with Terry Gross, aired in the programme *Fresh Air*, 27 March 1996 and rebroadcast on 4 February 1997.

22 Walker (1992) and Walker and Parmar (1993).

23 The same group of African activists who submitted to *The New York Times* also submitted a longer piece to *Ms. Magazine* in November 1993. These included Seble Dawit, a human rights lawyer and FGM activist, Mekuria Salem, an Ethiopian film-maker, Mecere Githae-Mugo, a writer and scholar from Cornell University, and Nahid Toubia. It was not published.

memory of readers of women's magazines who typically are interested only in the colour of their make-up and the size of their hips.[24] Do any of these women know, care about or even imagine the life of African girls and women? Would they be at all interested to hear their side of the story? I am left wondering what the Western obsession with FC/FGM is all about. Is it because the subject appears tantalising and exotic? Does it provide comforting reassurance that to be born in the West is to be born lucky? Is it an amnesic device to help the West forget its own shameful history of the treatment of women? Is it a way to re-ignite a sense of superiority over others in an age of lost identity and lost causes? Why is it that a story of children dying and disabled by measles, or women dying of childbirth, is just not as interesting? Is there perhaps a pornographic element that fires the imagination?

What do African women think of FGM?

This is a question that I am asked frequently and that I can never answer simply because there is no such thing as 'the African woman'. We are individuals and groups as diverse in our opinions and interests as other individuals and groups in other dynamic and changing societies. The African feminist movement, otherwise unified in its understanding of gendered power relations, holds divergent views on whether to prioritise FGM as an issue worthy of attention. The majority of women in African communities that practise FGM continue to use it as an important negotiating tool for social acceptance and survival. Some women who have gained education or wealth still believe in the importance of the practice as part of their identity. Many others, however, are pioneering change: ordinary mothers, for instance, who have decided to protect their daughters from their fate; or women teachers, nurses or doctors who have more information and the social standing to enable them to speak out. In addition, there are many African men who defend women's rights and lend their support to the anti-FGM cause. These diverse African voices need to be heard and respected in order to create the space for social dialogue that propels change. However, the existence of such diversity amongst African communities is denied by the hegemonic portrayal of the African as uniformly stagnant and bound to culture and tradition needing to be saved against themselves, as in the writings of Abe Rosenthal, or must be kept intact and preserved as in anthropological studies including seemingly liberal points of view such as those of Germaine Greer. Evidence to the contrary is systematically buried – especially when it is not presented in written form in the first place.

Historical evidence of African women's voices, for example, is found in their songs and stories where they resist social conventions such as arranged marriage, polygamy and wife-inheritance. Forms of resistance such as this were not documented by Western writing and so it was assumed that they did not exist and that all African women have been, and will continue to be, subservient to and compliant with their cultures. This is not the case. Since the 1950s, many African

24 Bardarch (1993).

women who became mothers have resisted the circumcision of their daughters against tremendous odds, risking their own lives or livelihood in the process. Three of these women (from Kenya, Sudan and Somalia) were celebrated on 4 February 2003 at the African Women's Health and Rights Day celebration, held in Johannesburg by the *AMANITARE* Network (African Partnership for Sexual and Reproductive Health and Rights of Women and Girls).[25] Another is the renowned Egyptian activist, Marie Assaad, who celebrated her 83rd birthday in 2003 and is still one of the most dynamic leaders in the African movement against the practice and for gender equity. In 1979, at the World Health Organisation's first international meeting on FC in Khartoum, a group of African women attending the meeting refused to accept a suggestion that FC may be performed in hospitals by doctors to avoid complications.[26] In taking a stand, these women won the first decisive victory over FGM in the form of an international agreement that all forms of female circumcision are wrong and must be banned.

Looking forward

The Western media has never given African women adequate space in which to voice their point of view. For those who stand for women's rights in the West, perhaps a dialogue with African women writers and scholars would prove informative and enable them to present a more balanced picture. However, to engage in such a dialogue is to admit that there are equivalent minds and fighting spirits among the women's movement and intellectuals in Africa, or to admit that such Africans even exist. In Africa today there are many women, girls and men struggling with their own experiences of FGM, with their loyalties to their families and their discontent with the status quo. Many are questioning other issues of gender and social power relations as they also struggle for peace and democracy. They are the engines of the social change that is taking place in Africa on a daily basis – and are certainly not subjects willing to pose for anthropologists in search of a traditional, static 'photo opportunity with the natives'.

Is it possible, I wonder, for such anthropologists to use their research money as a means of understanding the function of FGM in society, rather than simply framing ethnographic portraits? Few studies, if any, look at the social role of FGM within gendered power relations, or document the emerging resistance to the practice within families and communities as part of a process of social change, and yet, I would argue, activists and scholars can and should work together to promote such change. If scholars use their skills to understand and document the social dynamics and power relations which promote and preserve FGM, activists will have an excellent weapon with which to defend their corner.

The 1990s saw the rise of two international women's rights movements: the Women's Reproductive Health and Rights Movement, which evolved out of Latin America; and the Women's Human Rights Movement, within which individuals

---

25 For more information, see AMANITARE (2003).

26 [WHO] (1979).

and groups from the global South were prominent.[27] Within this context, the work of African women on FC/FGM over the past two decades has resulted in its inclusion as a principal means of bringing violations of a woman's right to bodily integrity in all cultures to the fore. As mentioned above, FC/FGM was one of the testimonials on violence against women presented to the World Conference on Human Rights in Vienna in 1993, and in 1994, at the International Conference on Population and Development in Cairo, the work of African activists drew attention to FC/FGM as a reproductive health and rights issue. At last, African women's activism acquired an international profile which encouraged many thousands of women in Africa to continue resisting the practice in their homes through their work and by speaking out against it.

There is a small body of writing by African women during this period which can be found in specialised publications and interview articles in journals and magazines. Although this material is accessible, it is not as easy to find as Western writing on the same subject and – apart from a small elite – remains far beyond the reach of most African women. Meanwhile, diasporic African scholars have produced a stream of writing reacting to Western concern with FGM, labelling it imperialistic and defending the national right of Africans to preserve their culture.[28] Writing from their new Western homeland, however, these present-day writers of the African diaspora tend to fall into reductive 'us and them' binary structures and so continue to frame an image of race and ethnicity that is, at best, unhelpful.

Conclusion: two questions

'Should I, as an outsider give myself the right to study, comment on, or act against FGM?' My simple answer is 'Yes!'. Yes, if you want to add your skills and your resources to help those working with the FC/FGM practising community. Yes, if you stand side by side with them, look into their eyes and speak with them using the same human language. Yes, if you do not view them through the glass shield as 'other'. Yes, if you do not believe in your own superiority. Yes, if you will actively seek out and facilitate the rich and diverse voices of African women. Yes, if your action will allow those you study to enhance their sense of dignity and humanity.

'What do African women want?' I cannot speak for all African women, but I can speak for those with whom I share similar beliefs and values. As an African feminist I believe that our views and choices, individually and collectively, should command the same respect as the views and choices of women in the West. We need to be able to engage with the world as equals, free of Western prejudices and patronising attitudes,[29] and as women we need the space to reflect on our own

27 For example, see Abdalla (1982); Sillah (1996); Kere and Tapsoba (1994); Seif El Dawla (1999).

28 Ahmadu (2000).

29 Akale (1999).

situation, to interact with and challenge the political and social systems that define our lives. We need the time and space to go through our own learning experiences and to share them with others from Africa and beyond. We demand respect and insist that we are allowed a voice and that that voice is heard. We believe in our right to celebrate our achievements and successes and not to be portrayed either simply as victims or as receivers of charity. We are learning to take part in intercultural dialogue and, since writing and publishing is an important means of furthering that dialogue, we will write and publish our views.[30]

Bibliography

Abdalla, Raqiya Haji Dualeh, *Sisters in Affliction: Circumcision and Infibulation of Women in Africa*, 1982, London: Zed Press.

Ahmadu, Fuambai, 'Rites and wrongs: an insider/outsider reflects on power and excision in female "circumcision"' in Shell-Duncan, Bettina and Hernlund, Ylva, *Female 'Circumcision' in Africa: Culture, Controversy, and Change*, pp 283–312, 2000, Boulder, CO: Lynne Reinner Publishers.

Akale, Catherine Mudime, *Who Has the Right to Name Female Genital Mutilation a Crime?* (1999), www.skk.uit.no/WW99/papers/Akale_Catherine_Mudime.pdf (last accessed 15 January 2004).

AMANITARE (2003) 3 *Voices* (July), www.amanitare.org/linked%20documents/newsletters/AMANITARE%20Voices,%20Issue%203,%20July%202003.pdf (last accessed 12 February 2004).

Aziz, FA, 'Gynaecologic and obstetric complications of female circumcision' (1980) 17 *International Journal of Gynaecology and Obstetrics* 560–63

Bardarch, A, 'Tearing off the veil' (1993) *Vanity Fair* 122–27 and 154–58 (August).

Boddy, J, *Wombs and Alien Spirits: Women, Men, and the Zar Cult in Northern Sudan*, 1989, Madison, WI: University of Wisconsin Press.

Daw, Edward, 'Female circumcision and infibulation complicating delivery' (1970) 204 *The Practitioner* 559–63.

Dawit, Seble and Salem, Mekuria, 'The West just don't get it'(1993) *The New York Times* (7 December).

Dirie, Mahdi Ali, *Female Circumcision in Somalia: Medical and Social Implications*, 1985, Mogadishu: Somali Academy of Sciences and Arts.

Dirie, MA and Lindmark, G, 'The risk of medical complications after female circumcision' (1992) 69 *East African Medical Journal* 479–82.

Diejomaoh, FME, and Faal, MKB, 'Adhesion of labia minora complicating circumcision in neonatal period in a Nigerian community' (1981) 33 *Tropical and Geographical Medicine* 135–38.

Greer, Germaine, *The Whole Woman*, 1999a, New York: AA Knopf.

Greer, Germaine, 'Why genital cutting goes on' (1999b) *Newsweek International* (5 July).

30 See, for example, the publication of AMANITARE Voices at www.amanitare.org (last accessed on 15 January 2004).

Gregory, Sophfronia, 'At risk of mutilation: can a woman win asylum for fear of 'circumcision' in her home country?' (1994) *TIME* magazine (21 March).

Gruenbaum, Ellen, 'The Islamic movement, development and health education: recent changes in the health of rural women in Central Sudan' (1991) 33 *Social Science and Medicine* 637–45.

Hosken, Fran, *The Hosken Report: Genital and Sexual Mutilations of Females*, 1979, Lexington, MA: Women's International Network News.

Hosken, Fran, *The Hosken Report: Genital and Sexual Mutilation of Females*, 1994, fourth edition, Lexington, MA: Women's International Network News.

Iregbulem, LM, 'Post-circumcision vulval adhesions in Nigerians' (1980) 33 *British Journal of Plastic Surgery* 83–86

Kere, LA, and Tapsoba, I, 'Charity will not liberate women', in Nataraj, Shyamala (ed), *Private Decisions, Public Debate: Women, Reproduction and Population*, 1994, London: Panos, pp 43–56.

Lightfoot-Klein, Hanny, *Prisoners of Ritual: an Odyssey into Female Genital Circumcision in Africa*, 1989, New York : Harrington Park Press.

Makhlouf-Obermeyer, Carla, 'Female genital surgeries: the known, the unknown, and the unknowable'(1999) 13 *Medical Anthropology Quarterly* 79–106.

Modawi, Suliman, 'The impact of social and economic changes in female circumcision' in *Proceedings of the Third Congress of Obstetrics and Gynaecology*, Sudan Medical Association Congress Series, No 1, 1973, Khartoum: Sudan Medical Association, pp 242–64.

Rahman, Anika and Toubia, Nahid, *Female Genital Mutilation: A Guide to Laws and Policies Worldwide*, 2000, New York: Zed Books.

Roles, RC, 'Tribal surgery in East Africa during the nineteenth century, part two: therapeutic surgery' (1967) 44 *East Africa Medical Journal* 17–30.

Rosenthal, A, 'Female genital mutilation' (1993a) *The New York Times* (4 December).

Rosenthal, A, 'Female genital torture' (1993b) *The New York Times* (12 November).

Rosenthal, A, 'The torture continues' (1993c) *The New York Times* (27 July).

Sanderson, L, *Against the Mutilation of Women: The Struggle to End Unnecessary Suffering*, 1981, London: Ithaca Press.

Seif El Dawla, Aida, 'The political and legal struggle over female genital mutilation in Egypt: five years since the ICPD' (1999) 7 *Reproductive Health Matters* 128–36.

Shandall, AA, 'Circumcision and infibulation of females: a general consideration of the problem and a clinical study of the complications in Sudanese women' (1967) 5 *Sudan Medical Journal* 178–212.

Sillah, MM, 'Bundu trap' (1996) 105 *Natural History* 42–51.

[Sudan], *Laws of the Sudan* (1977–81: fifth edition), Khartoum: Khartoum University Press.

Toubia, Nahid, *Female Genital Mutilation: A Call for Global Action*, 1993, New York: RAINBO.

[UK Parliament], *Report of the All Party Parliamentary Group on Population, Development and Reproductive Health; Hearings Held on 23–24 May 2000*, www.appg-popdevrh.org.uk/Publications/FGM/FGM_surveyreport_00_APPGPDRH.pdf (last accessed 15 January 2004).

[UK Parliament], *Female Genital Mutilation Act 2003*, 2003 www.hmso.gov.uk/acts/acts2003/20030031.htm (last accessed 15 January 2004).

Verzin, JA, 'Sequelae of female circumcision' (1975) 5 *Tropical Doctor* 163–69.

[WHO], 'Traditional practices affecting the health of women and children (female circumcision, childhood marriage, nutritional taboos, etc. Report of a seminar, Khartoum, 10–15 February)', (WHO/EMRO technical publication, no 2), 1979, Alexandria: World Health Organisation, Regional Office for the Eastern Mediterranean.

Walker, Alice, *Possessing the Secret of Joy*, 2002, London: Cape.

Walker, Alice and Parmar, Pratibha, *Warrior Marks: Female Genital Mutilation and the Sexual Binding of Women*, 1993, New York: Harcourt Brace.

Worsley, Allan, 'Infibulation and female circumcision: a study of a little-known custom' (1938) 45 *Journal of Obstetrics and Gynaecology of the British Empire* 686–91.

CHAPTER 2

ALBANIAN MASCULINITIES, SEX-WORK AND MIGRATION: HOMOSEXUALITY, AIDS AND OTHER MORAL THREATS

Nicola Mai

This chapter aims to explore the cultural, social and epidemiological implications of the way sex-work has emerged as a strategy of survival for some Albanian young men in the context of their migration to Greece and Italy.[1] The interlocking of the common association of AIDS with an understanding of homosexuality in terms of a moral disease, and the repressive and 'heteropatriarchal'[2] nature of Albanian society, can be seen as shaping the dynamics of HIV/AIDS diffusion among the Albanian population. Since the chapter focuses on the way in which the relationship between gendered identities and sexual practices is negotiated across the migratory process, it is divided into four main parts. The first focuses on the concept of identity and outlines the theoretical framework of this chapter. The second analyses the way in which the relationship between gender and sexuality is negotiated in Albania, with particular reference to same-sex practices. The third section explores the way in which the articulations of gender and sexuality which are hegemonic in Albania were negotiated in the context of emigration to Italy and Greece. The final section analyses the interconnection between mobility, sexual cultures and epidemics by focusing on the relation between the Albanian hegemonic understanding and experience of masculinity, sex-work and the risk of HIV/AIDS diffusion in the context of emigration in Albania.

It is important here to provide an overview of the main dimensions and destinations of the Albanian migratory flow, in order to contextualise the specificity of the social group under examination within its complexity. Whereas during communism emigration was forbidden, nowadays more than one in five of the current Albanian population lives abroad and migrants' remittances are a

1 This chapter is one of the outcomes of the research project, 'Albanians in Italy and Greece: a study in migration dynamics and social exclusion', financed by the Leverhulme Trust, 2001–03, and is based on 45 interviews and other fieldwork material gathered between March 2002 and February 2003 in Rome and Athens. Specifically, in Rome, the sample population was composed of 20 male sex-workers from Albania and Romania, between the ages of 16 and 24, working mainly in the streets. In Athens, most of the 20 interviewees were Albanian men between the ages of 17 and 25, working in gay venues. In both settings, doctors working for HIV/AIDS clinics and directors of NGOs working with gay people, migrants and in the field of HIV/AIDS prevention were also interviewed.

2 Wilton (1997) p 31.

key strategy of economic survival for Albanian households and society more in general. The Albanian migration of the 1990s began with the collapse of the Albanian communist regime in early 1991. By the end of 2000, about 800,000 people out of a total population of 3.8 million were living abroad – 500,000 in Greece, 200,000 in Italy, 50,000 in other European countries and 50,000 elsewhere, mainly in North America.[3]

Although Albanians' experience of emigration was characterised by a rapid emancipation from an initial condition of social exclusion and marginalisation,[4] it was also subject to a stigmatising representation by the Italian and Greek media, as Albanians rapidly became the migrant group to be most readily associated with violent crime in general and to trafficking and exploitation of women in particular.[5] It is with reference to these stigmatising discourses disseminated by the Italian and Greek media and to their role in enforcing social vulnerability that it must be stressed how only a minor fraction of Albanian male migrants actually sell sex. Moreover, those who do are further discriminated against by both their own migrant group and the host societies. Because of their ambivalent relation to the hegemonic canons of masculinity in Albania and of homosexuality abroad, and of their experience of multiple marginalisation, Albanian male sex-workers find themselves in a condition of extreme socio-cultural and epidemiological vulnerability.

Homosexualities, masculinities and safer sex practices

The main aim of this section is to explain the way that the relationship between identities and sexual practices will be understood in this chapter, with particular reference to its epidemiological implications. According to Stuart Hall, in the last two decades the concept of identity has been the focus of an anti-essentialist critique from different perspectives and disciplines. The definition of identity Hall proposes as a synthesis of these debates is 'not an essentialist, but a strategic and positional one'.[6] This implies that it is only in relation to a 'constitutive other' that a positive identity can be constructed and that therefore 'the internal homogeneity, which the term identity treats as foundational, is not a natural, but a constructed form of closure'.[7] Applying these now familiar considerations to the analysis of masculinity and considering the different dimensions (class, gender, ethnicity, sexuality, etc) implicated in the formation of men's identities must lead us to decline the term 'masculinity' in the plural, as a way of acknowledging the implicit plurality of experiences and trajectories it encompasses.[8]

---

3 Barjaba (2000) p 69.

4 See Melchionda (2003) and Hatziprokopiou (2003).

5 For an analysis of the Italian media's coverage of Albanian migrants, see Mai (2002). For an overview of the Greek media's attitude towards ethnic difference in general, see Triandafyllidou (2002).

6 Hall (1996) p 3.

7 Hall (1996) p 5.

8 Ghoussoub and Sinclair-Webb (2000) p 7.

As far as the relation between sexual practices and masculinities is concerned, this too should be seen as historical and contextual, rather than fixed. For instance, most researchers of the history of homosexuality, influenced by the work of Michel Foucault, agree that it was only in the second half of the nineteenth century that the concept of 'homosexuality' emerged in the West as an identity formation associated with a specific sexual choice. According to Foucault, this association was made possible by the encounter between two modes of production of truth (procedures of confession and scientific discursivity) and was consistent with the increase in the regimentation and surveillance of the self brought about by modernity.[9]

In his analysis of the way in which, in modern times, sexuality became a primary locus of personal identification and social control, Foucault looked back into history, and in particular to the Greco-Roman world, to trace different articulations of the relation between morality, identity and sexual practices. In particular, his analysis of Athenian homoeroticism underlines that, whereas in modern times sexual identities are defined confessionally and introspectively, on the basis of the subjects' sexual orientation, amongst the Greeks they were defined performatively, on the basis of the distinction between active and passive sexual roles.[10] According to this understanding of ancient Greek mores, it was socially acceptable for men to have sex with other men as long as they respected the dividing line between the subjects of sexual activities, adult free men, and their object-partners: women, boys and slaves.[11]

Although Foucault's understanding of Greek sexual mores provides us with a rigid picture of Athenian masculinities and femininities and was criticised from different perspectives and disciplines,[12] his analysis is still useful for the argument of this chapter as it seems to capture the two main articulations of subjectivity, sexuality and identity ambivalently co-existing in Albania, Greece and Italy today. Contemporary attitudes towards sexual practices can be related to the survival of ancient performative comprehensions, as Faubion argues in the case of contemporary Greece and as Lambevski's work suggests with reference to most Mediterranean, Middle Eastern and Balkan societies.[13] While the modern and the ancient experiences of masculine identity are harnessed to very different relations to the self and are consistent with different social and cultural worlds, they should not be seen as mutually exclusive, but as having co-existed contradictorily and ambivalently across different historical and social contexts. As I explain later, Albanian male sex-workers' experiences of (homo)sexuality and identity emerge from the encounter between contradictory regimes of subjectification and discursive resources both at home and abroad. However, while in contemporary Albania masculinity is embodied and experienced predominantly according to the performative model outlined by Foucault with

---

9 Foucault (1981) pp 64–65.
10 Foucault (1990) p 30.
11 Foucault (1990) p 47.
12 For a good overview of these debates, see Larmour *et al* (1998).
13 See Lambevski (1999) p 403.

reference to ancient Greece, the modern confessional model of 'homosexuality' is now hegemonic in Italy and Greece.

Because of its centrality in Albanian young men's understanding of their moral selves, the concept of honour and its relation to the cultural construction of Albanian masculinities need also to be clarified. The honour-shame complex has traditionally been studied as *the* mechanism of 'social evaluation' of Mediterranean societies, where members of a social formation are usually measured according to a unified 'type of personality considered as representative and exemplary'.[14] The most important implication of this literature for my purposes is that it analyses the honour-shame complex as a (hetero)patriarchal ideology based on the celebration of masculine moral and sexual potency as the 'natural basis of authority' and on 'the defence of familial honour' through men's control of female sexuality.[15] According to this masculinised ideology, the honourable behaviour of men and women differs, since men's relation to honour is based on the performance of an active and dominant role, whereas women must preserve their purity by adopting a passive and submissive position.[16]

Against this scenario of cultural fixity and historical immobility, and in line with the conceptualisation of identity outlined above, this chapter addresses 'tradition' and 'honour' as dynamic discursive repertoires and practices which are deployed strategically by both female and male actors in order to respond to new priorities and emerging needs. The masculinised honour ideology used by Albanian male sex-workers to morally justify their behaviour is consistent with social values and practices which have been historically hegemonic within Albanian culture. However, the re-deployment of these resources in the sex-work and emigration contexts responds to a mutated socio-cultural landscape and is related to the emergence of new social subjects and opportunities within the recent phase of post-communist transformation.[17]

Finally, the way in which sexual acts are related to gendered identities and ultimately to the understanding and experience of the body in any socio-cultural setting is important when analysing the diffusion of HIV/AIDS and other sexually transmitted diseases (STDs). In this respect, men's sexual habits, especially when they are consistent with a cultural construction of masculinity in sexually active, penetrative and dominating terms, deserve particular attention as the 'inability to question the performances of power and dependency in accepted gendered sexual behaviours inevitably favours [...] the passing on of the HIV virus'.[18] Thus, analysing the way in which homosexualities are culturally constructed is key to understanding the way in which masculinities and femininities are articulated, negotiated and experienced. Although 90% of infections are believed to occur through sexual transmission via unprotected

---

14 Peristiany (1965) pp 9–10.

15 Pitt-Rivers (1965) p 45.

16 Pitt-Rivers (1965) pp 45–46.

17 For an analysis of the re-deployment of 'tradition' in the phenomenon of trafficking and exploitation of Albanian young women, see Mai (2001a).

18 Lewis (2002) p 16.

penetrative sex between men and women, men's sexual practices and the way in which these are harnessed to culturally-sited notions of masculinity tend to remain unquestioned and unchallenged by HIV/AIDS prevention discourses and literature.[19] As I show later, being a man in Albania means continually to prove one's difference from stigmatised non-masculine others, and this impacts in direct ways on the practice of safer sex both at home and abroad.[20]

Albanian (homo)sexualities

This section analyses the seemingly contradictory way in which Albanian young men seem to experience and understand homosexuality at home and when they are involved in migration abroad. According to the cultural construction of masculinity hegemonic in Albania, homosexuality is still highly stigmatised and refused at home and Albanian 'gay' people are forced to retreat into silence and invisibility. On the other hand, some Albanian young men are involved in sex-work, while many claim to have learnt about homosexuality abroad.

Being homosexual in Albania is an acute drama, both for the individual involved and for his/her family and society. Common reactions range from silence and marginalisation to disgust, open discrimination, maltreatment and abuse. Sexual relations between males were relatively more common in pre-socialist Albanian society, as is testified by several nineteenth-century travel books and ethnographies.[21] However, after the advent of the communist regime in 1944, homosexuality (defined as 'pederasty' by the 1977 Penal Code) became punishable by imprisonment as it constituted a crime against social morality, together with prostitution and pornography. Finally, after a long political struggle and thanks to the intervention of the International Lesbian and Gay Association and the Council of Europe, in 1995 the Albanian Parliament legalised consensual homosexual relations. However, the fact that homosexuality is now recognised in law has not meant the end of harassment and abuse against gays and lesbians, who often face discriminative and abusive behaviour from the police and in Albanian society in general.[22]

Interestingly, the Albanian term which comes close to the western concept of 'gay' is *kurvë*, meaning female prostitute. The symbolic association between the figure of the queer and that of the whore deserves further analysis as it can be seen as consistent with a thoroughly heteropatriarchal socio-cultural context where only 'real' men or, to quote Herzfeld, only men that are really 'being *good at* being a man'[23] are the carriers of honour and respectability and are entitled to administrate power by asserting their predominance and domination on their less

19 See Lewis (2002) and Wilton (1997).

20 Wilton (1997) p 33.

21 Murray (1997).

22 For a detailed account of the current condition of Albanian lesbian women and gay men, see Van der Veur (2001).

23 Herzfeld (1985) p 16 (emphasis in the original).

honourable and masculine others. Within this masculinised moral world, the woman, the whore and the queer share the function of the main constitutive others against which fully legitimate masculine moral selves are reproduced in the social sphere.

In order to grasp the full social and cultural implications of the association of the figure of the whore (the dishonoured woman) with that of the queer (the dishonoured man) within the symbolic and discursive field of Albanian masculinity, it is important to refer to the narrative resources according to which sexual acts between men are experienced and culturally constructed in Albania. Here, Huseyin Tapinc's analysis of the four main models of homosexual relations found in contemporary Turkish society is an important reference point, as Albania was part of the Ottoman Empire for five centuries.[24] In particular, the second model of homosexual relations identified by Tapinc – that between the masculine 'heterosexual' and the feminine 'homosexual' – is the one which best captures the hegemonic way in which 'sexual meanings [... are ...] attached to homosexual behaviour by each participant, along with their assumed gender role' in contemporary Albania.[25] As Tapinc notes in the case of Turkey, and this is true of Albania too, the key aspect of this model is the clear distinction between the masculine, 'active' inserter and the feminine, 'passive' insertee, who regard their sexual/gender identity respectively as heterosexual and homosexual.[26]

Thus, in Albanian culture, 'homosexuality' is constructed around the concept of penetration, as the male *kurvë* (also called *bythqirë*, literally 'fucked arse') is only the person who 'gives' his arse, not the one who penetrates it. However, this performative understanding of the masculine-as-sexually-active co-exists alongside a modern confessional understanding of homosexuality in relation to the subject's sexual choice. This was first introduced via criminalising and pathologising medico-legal discourses in communist times and was subsequently disseminated by foreign media in the form of the Western gay identity discourse. Thus, nowadays in Albania, men who have sex with other men are addressed by different and yet competing regimes of 'subjectification' and various yet normative definitions of masculinity.[27] These originate both from the Albanian historical, social and cultural scenario and from foreign moral and cultural landscapes, whether these are accessed through migration or the media.[28] Although there are many models potentially available, for honourably masculine 'real' men, 'fucking queers' is the widely hegemonic discourse defining sexual relations between Albanian men at home and abroad.

In order to understand how models of male homosexualities available in Albania are implicated in the experience of sex-work abroad, one must analyse

---

24 Tapinc (1992).

25 Tapinc (1992) p 40.

26 Tapinc (1992) p 41.

27 See Rose (1996) *passim*.

28 For a more detailed account of the role of Italian television in the emergence of youth 'migratory' identities in Albania, see Mai (2001b).

how these are harnessed to culturally available practices of knowledge of the self. Oleg Kharkhordin's analysis of the regimes of subjectification at work within Russian civilisation is important here: he shows how the hegemony of performative techniques of knowledge of the self is consistent with a collectivist social and political order based on fixed and moralised codes of public conduct. In such a society, a personal identity cannot be achieved 'through inner light or meditation'. Rather, one 'acquires a self through public deeds which might be said to literally en-person [...], to endow a body with a true self or personality'.[29] In other words, in a socio-cultural context where subjects know themselves by performing for a relevant audience rather than through introspection, one must engage in established 'public deeds' to maintain a viable personal identity.

If we apply these considerations to the hegemonic understanding and experience of the relation between masculinity and homosexuality in Albania, we can identify two main implications of particular relevance. First, the fact that a man may know himself primarily through the public presentation of codified deeds means that his masculine and honourable status depends on the approval by strategic 'constitutive' publics, such as the male peer group and the family. Secondly, the fundamental role of these relevant publics in confirming the permanence of a morally honourable subject means that, if these are absent, moral concerns tend to evaporate. All of these factors are important in sustaining a sense of masculine honourable self in the context of migration and of sex-work and have serious implications for the risk of HIV diffusion.

'Fucking queers' as a strategy of moral and economic resistance abroad

In the context of international emigration, Albanian young men repositioned their gendered identities within a new social, cultural and economic environment. The practice of sex-work abroad is consistent with the hegemonic way in which the relation between masculinities and sexual conducts is negotiated at home. Thus, unsurprisingly, most Albanian male sex-workers referred to their main or collateral occupation as 'fucking queers'. However, sex-work in Italy and Greece is a site of struggle reflecting practices of resistance and domination present in the wider socio-cultural domain. So, the way 'fucking queers' is understood and experienced in the context of emigration reflects new powerful dynamics of social exclusion and exploitation, which are experienced in terms of emasculation and feminisation. So, for Albanian male sex-workers, sharing accounts of 'fucking Italian or Greek queers' in peer talk becomes a way of reappropriating a masculine powerful position by presenting and understanding themselves as sexually dominating their Greek and Italian male dominators.[30]

---

29 Kharkhordin (1997) p 241.

30 For an analysis of these dynamics of discursive resistance with reference to Palestinian men working in Jerusalem, see Bowman (1989).

In public 'peer talk' and when being interviewed for the first time, all Albanian sex-workers described their occupation and their relation to it according to the more 'official' and (hetero)normative 'fucking queers' discourse. Moreover, all of the interviewees insisted that economic necessity and the difficulty of finding a job in the formal and informal labour markets were the only reasons behind their involvement in sex-work. As Beni, 20, explained in his own words in our first meeting in front of two fellow Albanians in Rome:

> Look, it is very simple ... for example tonight it is 8 days since I have last worked and I have got no money at all ... if now a queer comes and offers me 50 Euro I fuck him ... What can I do? I have no money ... When I have money I tell them to fuck off ... when I don't, they give me 50 Euro and in half an hour everything is over.

However, often the very people who defended their masculine status by deploying the 'fucking queers' and 'economic necessity' discourses in peer talk revealed a more complex and ambivalent relation between their gendered identities and their involvement in sex-work. In more private and confidential relational settings, some interviewees voiced their worries about eventually 'becoming queer' by regularly engaging in sex with other men, confessing that memories of sexual encounters with customers had become a regular part of their sexual fantasies. Others conceded being attracted to some of their customers, while a few actually claimed to be 'homosexual' or 'gay'. Although these private 'confessions' seem to contradict the reductive and normative terms set by the 'fucking queers' and the 'economic necessity' discourses, these become the only viable discursive strategies to present morally sustainable masculine selves under the constitutive and evaluating gazes of the peer group.

For both 'gay' and 'straight' Albanian young men, sex-work is a way to reconcile their economic priorities and needs with their understandings of the relation between their gendered selves and their involvement in sexual practices. As we have seen, for Albanian straight men, selling sex can be coherent with their own performative construction of masculinity in penetrative and active terms. For the few interviewees who recognise themselves privately as 'gay', sex-work is a way to earn money as well as to experience previously unknown aspects of, and relations to, their selves: some interviewees had been in a stable relationship with an Italian or a Greek customer and were thus able to 'keep off the street' as long as it lasted. This strategy of economic and moral survival is consistent with the Western confessional experience of 'gay' subjectivity and lifestyle and offers the possibility of breaking away from the performative requirements of the peer group. However, this emancipation is never complete as these relationships are usually temporary and all 'gay' interviewees still have to present themselves to their families as straight honourable men, for fear of being rejected or of jeopardising the family's reputation within the wider Albanian community.

One of the most surprising findings of the research was that nearly all of the interviewees between the ages of 22 and 24 had recently started 'pimping' young women from their own country, as well as from the host and other countries. Since the term 'pimping' indicates a relationship characterised by violent coercion, its adequacy in rendering the complexity of the relationships under examination is questionable. Indeed, the relations between the interviewees and their female partners were characterised by varying degrees of agency and mutual instrumentalisation. Some of these sodalities were undoubtedly abusive for the women involved; more often they were based on a convergence of necessities and priorities and framed and experienced as 'romance' by both subjects involved. In understanding the nature of these relationships, it is important to remember the social profile of the subjects involved. The usual scenario was one in which young women (some of them already selling sex), rejected by or running away from their families, would receive some form of protection and support from male sex-workers willing to 'come clean' of prostitution and sex with other men. This is often a gradual process. In the beginning of the relationship, male sex-workers usually keep selling sex themselves as well as their female partners. In a second stage, especially if the male sex-workers can 'control' more than one woman, he lives off his partner(s), complementing her/their profits with occasional thefts and burglaries.

Although this second stage of independence from direct involvement in sex-work is an ideal objective for most male sex-workers, the majority of them keep selling sex, albeit less regularly, 'to make ends meet'. However, there are other important reasons why young male sex-workers keep selling sex, while having other opportunities for economic survival around them. As explained above, in many cases, the 'official' presentation of the self in masculinised terms does not match the complexity of the relation between Albanian sex-workers' gendered identities and the sexual practices they engage in. In this respect, the 'fucking queers' and the 'economic necessity' discourses were used strategically by many interviewees to silence the anxieties provoked in them by their ambivalent sexual orientations. By experiencing sex with other men exclusively through sex-work and by justifying their involvement in sex-work in terms of economic necessity, most interviewees could keep having sex with other men while avoiding its potential implications for their masculinised public personae and personal identities.

In this respect, the formation of alliances and relationships with female sex-workers should also be seen as part of male sex-workers' strategies of survival as masculine subjects, as it enables them to achieve the necessary economic and symbolic capital to perform their masculinised identities to themselves and in front of their two main 'relevant audiences': the peer group and the family. As far as the peer group is concerned, the ability to control a woman is usually revealed by acts such as the possession of previously unaffordable expensive objects (especially motorcycles and cars) and accounts about hypermasculine sexual performances with their partner(s). As far as the family is concerned, in order to be confirmed as honourable masculine subjects most interviewees had formally to declare their intention to marry their female partners. This is usually their most important moral deed, beside supporting the family unit economically. In this respect, the necessity for Albanian male sex-workers to be seen to be 'having' a woman by their peers and their families in order for their masculine respectability to be confirmed offers their female partners a potential space of resistance against them.

While nearly all Albanian men and women living in Italy and Greece accept low-skilled occupations and exploitative working conditions for the sake of their families, most of the interviewees can be seen as ambivalently reacting against a family-based moral world of individual renunciation and sacrifice. On the one hand, in peer conversation many interviewees publicly ridiculed Albanian migrants who accepted exploitative working conditions and celebrated the fun and leisure-oriented lifestyle they could enjoy by engaging in sex-work. Most had in fact tried working in the informal productive sectors traditionally available to young male migrants (notably construction and agriculture), but refused to return to those occupations, which they perceived as humiliating and unworthy of their free and masculine status. In this respect, resorting to sex-work is not celebrated as a choice, but justified and experienced as the least intolerable strategy of survival among a very restricted range of much worse possibilities, characterised by a higher level of exploitation and considerably less profit. As Altin, 21, put it:

> Look at my hands ... do they look like the hands of a builder … of a farmer to you? They are even smoother than yours ... and these jeans are Levis, this t-shirt is Energie … I am not dressed like a refugee … I don't work 10 hours a day for 50 Euro like the others, no more … if I want I make them in five minutes!

Although in peer talk the 'traditional' figure of the worthy son sacrificing his youth for the survival of his family is often ridiculed, it is never challenged in the eyes of the family. In fact, all interviewees performed their moral selves for their families by conforming to the established canons of appropriate masculine behaviour: by sustaining them economically as worthy male sons and by presenting themselves accompanied by women, who are usually introduced as official, 'proper' fiancées.

Within this socio-cultural context, characterised by an ambivalent relation to the established canons of masculinity and morality and by the refusal of the conditions of exploitation offered to migrant workers in the informal and formal labour markets, sex-work becomes the first of three main strategies of economic survival. These are ordered hierarchically according to the potential threat they are perceived as posing to young men's masculine honour and respectability. The first of these strategies is to engage directly in sex-work by 'fucking queers' and occupies the lowermost position in terms of masculine respectability as it jeopardises the credibility of the male subject. This is especially true, as in Foucault's interpretation of Athenian pederasty, if it extends beyond a certain age or span of time. It is only insofar as the interviewee considers himself and is considered to be a 'man-in-the-making' that his involvement in sex-work is morally sustainable according to the canons of masculine honour and respectability. In fact, the majority of interviewees claimed to intend to stop being involved in sex-work by the age of 22–24, an age when they start feeling and being considered 'too old for that kind of thing'.

It is at this age that the passage to the second survival strategy, relying on the instrumentalisation of female partners, takes place. Although this possibility is relatively more acceptable according to the hegemonic canons of masculine respectability, those involved in these relations are usually considered as 'half-men' by the peer group as they can survive only by depending on women. The third and most honourable strategy of survival is linked to role models such as the pusher, the gangster, the thief, which can be seen as potentially sustaining a sense of superior and omnipotent masculine self through the manipulation and control of other men, women and consistent financial resources. For all of the interviewees, however, this third, more 'honourable' possibility remained only an aspiration, as most were surviving by selling sex either directly and/or through their female partners.

Why me? I am not a sissy!

This final section of the chapter analyses the implications of Albanian male sex-workers' cultural construction of masculinity for the practices of safer sex, focusing on how these impact on HIV/AIDS diffusion. The main observation emerging from the analysis of the interview material is that, for most Albanian male sex-workers, HIV/AIDS is a moral condition associated with 'passive' homosexuality, rather than an infective disease with specific modalities of transmission. In fact, this association was confirmed by a doctor working for an HIV/AIDS clinic in Athens, who reported that the most common reaction of Albanian men after learning that they have become infected was to ask: 'but why me? It is not possible, I am not a sissy!', meaning 'I am not a (passive) homosexual'. This situation is perhaps the inverted version of the logic that Cindy Patton named the 'queer paradigm', whereby people who are HIV positive or living with AIDS 'are constituted as queer'.[31]

The association of AIDS with a morally stigmatised 'homosexual' condition defined by the engagement in 'passive' anal sex impacts heavily on the way condoms are used – and thus on the actual practice of safer sex. Although all of the interviewees reported 'using condoms', the way they did so seemed to reflect their relation to hegemonic cultural constructions of masculinity rather than the modalities of HIV/AIDS transmission. For instance, most reported using condoms only with their male clients and not with women, including their partners, who usually were sex-workers themselves. This is particularly significant since most of the interviewees had occasional sex with many different women as a way of proving to themselves and others that their masculinity was not compromised by their involvement in male sex-work. Furthermore, the few who admitted privately to being available for passive sex used a condom only when penetrated, as if being active (that is, 'real men') would prevent them from being infected. Many simply ignored that condoms had to be used only once, that they must be changed when inserting the penis from one person to another, that one should use water-based lubricants, that condoms deteriorate by exposure to the sun, and other basic information. So, although all of the sex-workers interviewed actually 'used condoms', the way in which they used them did not enable them to be safe from HIV/AIDS and other STDs. Moreover, most of the interviewees were undocumented migrants, and none of them knew that in both Italy and Greece, HIV/AIDS prevention, counselling and therapies are available

31 See Patton (1994) p 19 and Wilton (1997) p 3.

free to everybody. As a consequence, many young people went to the hospital only when it was too late (if they went at all), for fear of expulsion or other legal action.

The mainly performative nature of most Albanian sex-workers' moral worlds prevents the emergence of some form of identity in relation to their sexual orientation or profession. This is another important factor when analysing Albanian young sex-workers' vulnerability to HIV/AIDS infection: because of the lack of a 'professional' or 'sexual' identity, they are unwilling to engage in the outreach projects aimed at sex-workers and gay people in Italy and Greece. In fact, Albanian sex-workers, who do not usually identify themselves as gay and who associate gay people with their despised customers, choose not to seek help from gay-related programmes of social intervention. On the other hand, those projects do not usually target Albanian male sex-workers, since they consider them primarily as migrants, rather than as gay or as sex-workers. As a consequence, nobody, with the exception of a few enlightened clients, is informing this high-risk group about how to keep safe from HIV/AIDS infection.

These dynamics are full of implications for the potential diffusion of HIV/AIDS in Albania. First, the few existing studies of sexual behaviour in Albania show that only about 5% of the sexually active population use condoms, and then not on a regular basis. Whereas men of all age groups tend to refuse the use of condoms, women are insufficiently informed on how to protect themselves from HIV/AIDS and STDs.[32] Moreover, recent research on especially vulnerable young people reveals a high level of sexual risk behaviour as well as poor knowledge of the use of condoms and their protective function. In particular, this research underlines that many young interviewees reported having had unprotected sex with sex-workers and having accepted to have sexual intercourse in exchange for money, drugs or other favours while abroad.[33] Secondly, in Italy and Greece, Albanian women are amongst the largest groups working in the sex industry and are usually in a condition of subjection and isolation which prevents them from being able to negotiate protected sex and from accessing local health services and other forms of assistance. Thirdly, mobility emerges as a key factor in the diffusion of HIV/AIDS since, prior to January 2001, 80% of reported HIV/AIDS cases indicated that they contracted the virus abroad.[34] Most interestingly, over 80% of the 71 cases of HIV/AIDS diagnosed in Albania since 1993 are reported to be amongst young men living as temporary workers in Italy and Greece. This is hardly surprising given the demographic composition and current magnitude of Albanian migration and the fact that before 1991 Albania was one of the most isolated countries in the world. However, there are two main gender-specific and culturally-sited factors enforcing a condition of particular vulnerability to HIV/AIDS infection for Albanian young men and the Albanian population in general. First, the endurance of patriarchal roles and values in Albanian society and a hegemonic cultural construction of masculinity in terms of

32 IOM (2002) p 17.

33 Wong (2002) pp 30–39 and 35.

34 IOM (2003) pp 18 and 21.

moral superiority and dominance strongly hinder the negotiation of safer sex. Secondly, the combination of a performative understanding of masculinity according to the penetrative/masculine vs penetrated/feminine dichotomy with the perception of HIV/AIDS as a disease affecting only 'passive' dishonoured men means that condoms are used, if at all, according to moral rather than scientific criteria.

Bibliography

Barjaba, Kosta, *Ondate Senza Ritorno*, 2002, Rome: IOM Press.

Bowman, Glenn, 'Fucking tourists' (1989) 9:2 *Critique of Anthropology* 77–94.

Faubion, James D., *Modern Greek Lessons*, 1993, Princeton, NJ: Princeton University Press.

Foucault, Michel, *The History of Sexuality, An Introduction (Vol 1)*, 1981, Harmondsworth: Penguin.

Foucault, Michel, *The History of Sexuality, The Use of Pleasure (Vol 2)*, 1990, New York: Vintage Books.

Ghoussoub, Mai and Sinclair-Webb, Emma, *Imagined Masculinities: Male Identity and Culture in the Modern Middle East*, 2000, London: Saqi Books.

Hall, Stuart, 'Introduction: who needs identity?', in Hall, S and Du Gay, P (eds), *Questions of Cultural Identity*, 1996, London: Routledge, pp 1–17.

Hatziprokopiou, Panos, 'Albanian immigrants in Thessaloniki, Greece: processes of economic and social incorporation' (2003) 29:6 *Journal of Ethnic and Migration Studies* 1033–57 (November).

Herzfeld, Michael, *The Poetics of Manhood: Contest and Identity in a Cretan Village*, 1985, Princeton, NJ: Princeton University Press.

IOM (International Organisation for Migration), 'Overview of HIV/AIDS in South Eastern Europe: epidemiological data, vulnerable groups, governmental and non-governmental responses up to January 2002', 2003, Belgrade: UNICEF.

Kharkhordin, Oleg, 'Reveal and dissimulate: a genealogy of private life in Soviet Russia', in Weintraub, J and Kumar, K (eds), *Public and Private in Thought and Practice: Perspectives on a Grand Dichotomy*, 1997, Chicago and London: University of Chicago Press, pp 333–63.

Lambevski, Sasho A, 'Suck my nation – masculinity, ethnicity and the politics of (homo)sex' (1999) 2:4 *Sexualities* 397–419.

Larmour, David *et al* (eds), *Rethinking Sexuality: Foucault and Classical Antiquity*, 1998, Princeton, NJ: Princeton University Press.

Lewis, Jill, 'Mobilising gender issues: report from the Living for Tomorrow project on youth, gender and HIV/AIDS prevention', 2002, Oslo: NIKK.

Mai, Nicola, 'Transforming traditions: a critical analysis of the trafficking and exploitation of Albanian girls in Italy', in King, R (ed), *The Mediterranean Passage: Migration and New Cultural Encounters in Southern Europe*, 2001(a), Liverpool: Liverpool University Press, pp 258–78.

Mai, Nicola, '"Italy is Beautiful": the role of Italian television in the Albanian migratory flow to Italy', in King, R and Wood, R (eds), *Media and Migration: Constructions of Mobility and Difference*, 2001(b), London: Routledge, pp 95–109.

Mai, Nicola, 'Myths and moral panics: Italian identity and the media representation of Albanian immigration', in Grillo, RD and Pratt, J (eds), *The Politics of Recognising Difference: Multiculturalism Italian Style*, 2002, Aldershot: Ashgate, pp 77–95.

Melchionda, Ugo (ed), *Gli Albanesi in Italia. Inserimento lavorativo e sociale*, 2003, Milan: Franco Angeli.

Murray, Stephen, 'Male homosexuality in Ottoman Albania', in Murray, S and Roscoe, W (eds), *Islamic Homosexualities: Culture, History and Literature*, 1997, London: New York University Press, pp 187–96.

Patton, Cindy, *Last Served? Gendering the HIV Pandemic*, 1994, London: Taylor & Francis (Social Aspects of AIDS series).

Peristiany, John George, 'Introduction', in Peristiany, JG (ed), *Honour and Shame: the Values of Mediterranean Society*, 1965, London: Weidenfeld and Nicolson, pp 9–18.

Pitt-Rivers, Julian, 'Honour and social status', in Peristiany, JG (ed), *Honour and Shame: The Values of Mediterranean Society*, 1965, London: Weidenfeld and Nicolson, pp 21–77.

Rose, Nikolas, 'Identity, genealogy, history', in Hall, S and Du Gay, P (eds), *Questions of Cultural Identity*, 1996, London: Sage, pp 128–50.

Tapinc, Huseyin, 'Masculinity, femininity, and Turkish male homosexuality', in Plummer, K (ed), *Modern Homosexualities: Fragments of Lesbian and Gay Experience*, 1992, London: Routledge, pp 39–49.

Triandafyllidou, Anna, 'Greece', in Ter Val, J (ed), *Racism and Cultural Diversity in the Mass Media*, 2002, Vienna: EUMC, pp 149–72.

Van der Veur, Dennis, *Caught Between Fear and Isolation: Lesbian Women and Homosexual Men in Albania*, 2001, Amsterdam: COC Netherlands.

Wilton, Tamsin, *Engendering AIDS: Deconstructing Sex, Text and Epidemic*, 1997, London: Sage.

Wong, Elsie, 'Rapid assessment and response on HIV/AIDS among especially vulnerable young people in South Eastern Europe', 2002, www.unicef.org/albania/finalrar.pdf (last accessed 9 February 2004).

CHAPTER 3

THE SEMANTICS AND POLITICS OF CHILDBEARING AND MOTHERHOOD IN CONTEMPORARY AFRICAN LITERATURE

Nana Wilson-Tagoe

Childbearing and motherhood have paradoxical meanings in African societies. On one hand, they demonstrate women's power in ensuring the survival and continuity of their communities;[1] on the other, they are the source of intense anxiety, conflict and contradiction within the communities themselves. As cultural concepts, they encode notions of sexuality that are continually negotiated from different personal and contradictory situations. Such negotiations have been explored in traditional literature and in the work of male writers, but it is the writing of African women that succeeds most in revealing their complex political and gender ramifications. Because women's art often abolishes divisions between public and domestic spaces, it is able to politicise these concepts in ways that interrogate the very foundations of cultural knowledge. Its struggles with elaborating new meanings and re-inventing language make it the most convenient source for probing issues of gender and politics.

I focus on semantics because it provides a key to the production of meaning and can unravel gaps between the language of culture and the alternative meanings created in imaginative literature. It is through semantics – by which I mean the interaction of words, images, voices and symbolic structures – that cultures organise reality and construct meanings. Language as I deploy it in my notion of semantics means more than words and grammatical rules; it is what Joan Scott has called 'a meaning-constituting system: that is, any system – strictly verbal or other – through which meaning is constructed and cultural practices organized and by which, accordingly, people represent and understand their world […]'.[2] An analysis of language provides insights into how social relations and collective identities are conceived and organised. After all, cultural institutions and phenomena become meaningful only within a set of conventions and assumptions established through language, symbols and myths. These semantic codes do not regulate behaviour so much as create possibilities for particular forms of behaviour.[3] Subjects do not necessarily internalise these codes

---

1 Grace Okereke's (1984) critical analysis of birth songs in Igbo traditional society problematises this power when it identifies its co-existence with forms of coercion, ostracism and ridicule.

2 Scott (1988) p 34.

3 See Culler (1975) p 198 for a fuller discussion of this.

but rather negotiate their various layers, registers, semantics and modes of enunciation. Bakhtin reminds us that 'language is not an abstract system of normative forms but rather a concrete heteroglot conception of the world [...] Each word tastes of the context and contexts in which it has lived its socially charged life'.[4] If all words and forms are populated by intentions, then it is possible to make words our own by appropriating and adapting them to our semantic needs. Language in this regard can construct, deconstruct and transform all kinds of social meanings. This context of adaptation and reformulation is what informs my chapter's general focus on representation. Its premise is that literary representations have the power to extend the limits of the ordinary not simply by modifying existing realities but by inventing and refashioning alternative worlds.

In reading Buchi Emecheta's *The Joys Of Motherhood* (1994) and Yvonne Vera's *Butterfly Burning* (1998) from these perspectives, my aim is to examine the relationship between dominant and normative cultural knowledge and the alternative meanings explored in women's imaginative writing. In both novels, it is this gap that creates a space for potential new meanings in gender, identity and subjectivity. Because such meanings are always shaped by specific locations and histories the contrasting contexts of Emecheta's Nigeria and Vera's Zimbabwe offer comparative perspectives on the inter-relationships of gender, history and narrative. *The Joys of Motherhood* and *Butterfly Burning* are both set in transitional periods in African colonial history but present different narratives of the colonial experience. Spanning a long stretch of colonial history from the early 1900s to the late 1950s, Emecheta's novel straddles the village of Ibuza in Eastern Nigeria and the evolving city of colonial Lagos. Her characters move between village and city and are touched by both worlds as they negotiate new relations to norms of gender in a changing world. Vera's *Butterfly Burning* on the other hand creates a different context of negotiation that reflects the settler history of Zimbabwe. The city of Bulawayo is almost the entire context of Vera's narrative, and the old indigenous Zimbabwe is only a fragile presence in a world completely transformed by the dreams of white settlers. What Vera suggests for this overturned world is a bold reinvention of the frayed 'Word' or language of culture that would include a rethinking of gender relations and values. Accordingly, her narrative works to explore new ways of being in the world and a new language for imagining gender and womanhood in a changed world.

In spite of their different historical contexts, Emecheta and Vera share a similar thematic focus on the struggles of ordinary women as they contest dominant values and reshape their lives in changing worlds. *The Joys of Motherhood*, for instance, appears to structure a world in which everyday life is dominated by the dominant values of a patriarchal world in which women are defined solely in terms of their functions as wives and mothers, yet the semiotic world of the novel is shot through with other languages that undermine such a perspective. The novel's argument rests on the disjunction between characters' perception of their world and the narrative's deployment of new languages and symbols. The protagonist Nnu Ego's view of her failure as a woman is constantly re-interpreted

---

4 Bakhtin (1992) p 293.

in contexts in which 'mother' and 'woman' have other contending meanings and connotations. The story of Nnu Ego's mother, Ona, inscribes a contrasting context in which a woman exercises considerable control over her body. Its narration introduces an eroticism that challenges a purely functional definition of women's bodies solely in terms of their reproductive functions. Ona's belief that Nnu Ego can be a woman, and at the same time 'have a life of her own, a husband if she wants one',[5] suggests a fluidity in definitions of womanhood that contradict any sense of a fixed and homogenous value system. Indeed, the novel itself suggests that a particular tenderness that characterised the art of loving in earlier times has been superceded by new aggressive values that assert male dominance at the expense of women's possibilities. The traditional world itself, the novel suggests, is a world in flux, and its dominant values only appear natural and coherent because they suppress alternative perspectives.

The suggestion that social power is never unified or coherent paves the way for introducing a conceptual language that would resist or reinterpret the ascendant patriarchal values. Emecheta provides this in the powerful figure of the slave girl reborn as Nnu Ego and as her *chi*.[6] The psychological potential of this doubling goes beyond what Florence Stratton sees as 'a female schizophrenic response to male oppression'.[7] It actually enacts the conflicting pulls of insight and regression that move Nnu Ego from blindness to understanding. Contrary to Stratton's assertion that the slave girl responds to oppression with ambivalence, we can actually claim that she disrupts the conceptual hold of traditions and beliefs that have construed masculine desires in universal terms. As a spirit she has the power to control and manipulate events on earth. In refusing to give Nnu Ego children in the traditional village of Ibuza, she not only calls the dominant traditions of motherhood into question but also indirectly exposes their class and gender bias. Her dream messages to Nnu Ego work consistently to subvert constructed notions of motherhood even though Nnu Ego herself constantly misinterprets their meanings. Thus, while Nnu Ego sees only vengefulness in her *chi*'s refusal to hand her the baby she offers, readers see it as merely a hint that the changing world of Lagos, not rural Ibuza, would offer a fertile context for rethinking notions of motherhood. With its colonial power structures and urban context, Lagos holds the potential for forcing a revision of gender, language and worldview. The oppressions of colonial structures raise larger political concerns that intertwine with the cultural and more personal issues of womanhood and motherhood. As a new context, Lagos anticipates several of the novel's own questions: how do normative concepts of manhood, womanhood and motherhood change in situations where men have lost their power base? How do men and women reconstitute identities and shape new languages of legitimation? How do characters, particularly Nnu Ego, negotiate such contexts?

---

5 Emecheta (1994) p 28.

6 Achebe (1975) p 160, gives a useful definition of *chi* in an illuminating article on the concept: '[…] we may visualize a person's *chi* as his other identity in spiritland – his spirit being complementing his terrestrial human being'.

7 Emecheta (1994) p 107.

To trace these negotiations through language and the ideologies it sustains is to discover the contradictions between the new conditions of life in Lagos and the language through which Nnu Ego makes meaning of her experiences. The coded dream messages of her *chi* urge her to grasp her new context and its possibilities for re-thinking cultural meanings. In spite of continually taunting her with backbreaking pregnancies and births, her *chi* challenges her to examine contradictions in the excessive elevation of motherhood and women's isolation and loneliness in childbirth. The contradictions are evident in Nnu Ego's life and in the lives of the women around her. However, it is only when Nnu Ego's last child is born dead that the narrative illuminates them in starkly horrific terms. It dramatises this birth not only as symbolic of a body's depletion but as the epitome of various haunting experiences of birthing in the novel. Significantly, even in this moment of exhaustion and loneliness Nnu Ego is caught in a muddle of feelings and interpretations that blot out the startling implications of her unconscious desires. The fluctuations of her thoughts reveal the semantics of a childbearing culture and calls it into question:

> Nnu Ego knelt in the middle of her room, holding on to the bed post, and, with her teeth dug right into her lower lip to prevent herself from screaming, she gave birth to a baby not bigger than a kitten. She had only lain there for what she thought was a few seconds … but when she woke up, she saw the baby and herself in the pool of blood. The child, a girl, was lifeless. She was dead.[8]

The narrative signals intersections of critique and alternative meanings not only in this horrific picture but also in the conflicting pulls of Nnu Ego's own thoughts, her movement from horror to self-satisfied exultation in her fertility and to the lurking sense that she had actually willed the baby's death:

> She felt like crying, but at the same time she did not want to. She felt the loss of this little piece of humanity, this unfortunate little thing she had carried while climbing up to Zabo market, this thing she knew was probably being hurt as she had bent defiantly down to wash clothes for her sons. 'Oh, poor baby […] I am sorry you are not staying; I am also glad that God has seen fit to take you back. My own reward, the joy of knowing that at this age I can still have children for my husband […]' Then she started to feel guilty. Had she wanted the child to die – was that the interpretation of the slight relief she had experienced when she crawled to the dead child to check what sex it was? That it was a girl had lessened her sense of loss.[9]

Nnu Ego's subconscious wish for her baby's death is an unconscious rejection of traditional assumptions that sanction childbearing even in impoverished conditions. She can entertain this rejection only in the unconscious since it is a nebulous area of experience that is not controlled by the rules of language. Her attempts to obliterate these thoughts only dramatise the struggle between unconscious desire and conscious self-sanctioning that continually stalls her ability to take control of her body. In this struggle, she imagines her father's admonition as a force pulling her, stronger than her will. In submitting to it she bows to its sanctions and condemns herself: 'Could she have so deteriorated into

8 Emecheta (1994) p 194.
9 Emecheta (1994) pp 194–95.

the kind of woman who would not want her own child because she could not afford to feed or clothe her?'[10] However, the ambiguity of this self–reproach suggests an even deeper struggle and repression that threaten a permanent split within her.

What constitutes the subject often resides in hidden depths rather than in transparent surfaces. The hidden depths of the unconscious are the regions from which the slave girl as Nnu Ego's *chi* always transmits dream messages to her. It is not inconceivable then to perceive this struggle as a contest between Nnu Ego's acquiescence in normative values and the slave girl's more radical interrogation of their meanings. This struggle between self and *chi* reflects the constant alternation of radical and regressive thinking that characterises the pattern of Nnu Ego's response to Lagos, for, in spite of new skills and responsibilities that encourage her to interpret old concepts like 'wife' and 'senior wife,' she seems constantly anchored to the epistemological base of traditional culture, especially in its conceptions of childbearing and motherhood. Margaret Daymond makes an important point about Nnu Ego and the pull of the symbolic when she argues that 'her tribal view of motherhood and the importance of male children had been the means of accepting life in Lagos with her potbellied little laundryman husband'.[11] The crucial point, however, is that motherhood is also an institution through which a dominant culture interprets the world and constitutes itself in language. Rituals, symbols and the very language of social intercourse are saturated with assumptions put forth as normative truths. Thus, a woman's infertility is an aberration since it calls a man's manhood into question; a woman who produces no sons fails in her duty to immortalise her husband; a woman without children is a failed and incomplete woman.

The naturalness of these and other concepts are constantly challenged as characters negotiate them in the different conditions of Lagos. The challenge, particularly for Nnu Ego, is to recognise disparities in concept and experience and reformulate or replace old concepts. It involves a slow movement from blindness and contradiction (since as a member of the traditional nobility she is also implicated in its class and gender values) to an understanding of the connection between language and power. The process of interrogation is almost always inspired by personal crisis and trauma, as happens for instance, on the occasion when Nnu Ego recognises how the very notion of a woman's responsibility either as wife or mother could be an avenue for her enslavement.[12] Her thought-processes in this instance are, as always, mediated by radical and conservative strains. Her constant sifting of her thoughts through the values and sanctions of the symbolic (in the figure of her father) is not a challenge but a resignation to its impregnable force. Even the anticipated dialogue with her husband never materialises since he does not return home for three years. However, the very confidence of these correlations and deductions arm Nnu Ego for a much more radical onslaught on the symbolic instigated as always by her *chi*.

---

10 Emecheta (1994) p 195.

11 Daymond (1996) p 282.

12 Emecheta (1994) p 137.

In the course of Nnu Ego's individuation, the birth of daughters (not sons) is always a cause for regret and crisis. For this reason, the radical slave woman constantly provokes her by sending her daughters. The birth of Nnu Ego's last set of twin girls is, for instance, the trigger of her most forceful critique and reformulation of values around motherhood:

> Men – all they were interested in were male babies to to keep their names going. But did not a woman have to bear the woman-child who would later bear the sons? God, when will you create a woman who would be fulfilled on herself, a full human being, not anybody's appendage? [...] Yes, I have many children, but what do I have to feed them on? On my life.[13]

For the first time, Nnu Ego actually revises the epistemological ground of the symbolic. No imagined sanctions from her father mediate this train of thought. They are deduced entirely from measuring received concepts against experiential knowledge. Levi-Strauss has argued that 'language is a condition of culture because the material out of which [it] is built is the same material out of which culture is built: logical relations, oppositions, correlation and the like'.[14] But the language of culture is never static and may be contested when its logical relations and correlations prove illogical by other deductions. It is through the same critical process that Nnu Ego revises the common view that children perpetuate the continuity of the community and are a security for a mother in old age.

Writing on women's relation to language, Nelly Furman argues that 'it is through the medium of language that we define and categorise areas of difference and similarity, which in turn allows us to comprehend the world around us'.[15] For Nnu Ego, this process involves not the creation of a separate language but a critical assessment and re-invention of old concepts on the basis of experience. Such formulations, however, occur only in the recesses of Nnu Ego's mind and are never translated into action. Even her most powerful silence – her refusal to give her souls to her children in death as she had given them her body in life – is left only as a double-edged statement that is perceived in one way by readers and in other ways by her children and community. Critics often write about Nnu Ego as though her inability to act on her thoughts nullifies the value of her experience. They compare her inaction with the radical action of her younger co-wife and see her as having 'sacrificed her human potential to the patriarchal order'.[16] The quality of her individuation, however, provides a far greater range of perceptions on the dynamics of gender, language and power than the one radical move of her co-wife. Her contradictions and failures reveal the psychodynamics of women's relation to culture and provide insights that would later resonate in powerful new dimensions in Yvonne Vera's writing.

In Vera's *Butterfly Burning*, written almost a generation after *The Joys of Motherhood*, the dynamics of women's reconstitution of language becomes part of

13 Emecheta (1994) p 186.
14 Levi-Strauss (1969) p 67.
15 Furman (1978) p 182.
16 See Stratton (1996) p 107.

a wider exploration of their potential and a redefinition of national and cultural space. Vera's wider perspective may be fruitfully compared to what Julia Kristeva identifies as the new agenda of second-generation feminists. Writing in 'Women's time' Kristeva sums up the new feminist perspectives in these terms:

> Essentially interested in the specificity of female psychology and its symbolic realizations, these women seek to give a language to the intrasubjective and corporeal experiences left mute by culture in the past. Either as artists or writers, they have undertaken a veritable exploration of the *dynamics of signs*.[17]

Vera claims a similar agenda but creates a specifically Zimbabwean genealogy to mark the conceptual shift she explores in the Bulawayo of the 1940s. Her protagonist, Phephelaphi, aborts one pregnancy then kills herself when faced with another. Implicitly, the novel asks us to measure her actions in relation to an earlier generation of city women in the 1920s and 1930s who had also negotiated colonial and patriarchal spaces and personal desires.

Phephelaphi's quest for self-definition – a desire for an outline, for self-respect, dignity, balance and a power of her own – collides with her community's notions of motherhood and womanhood, yet the narrative makes its transformative possibilities (its ability to crack open the shell, shatter language and create a new discourse) paradigmatic of the community's own struggle against colonial oppression. In a strategy unprecedented in modern African literature, Vera makes the reorganisation of traditional gender notions a crucial factor in the liberation of the colonised. As in *The Joys of Motherhood*, the urban context (Bulawayo) creates the dynamic for exploring the possibility of conceptual shifts. It is a world transformed by white settlers' dreams yet reinvented in other ways by black people. It is a world of paradoxes and contradictions, one that seems (like Fumbatha, the man who carries the legacy of history and resistance in the novel) constantly suspended between submission and resistance. Its upheaval and newness spawn a new breed of city women, uninhibited and forthright, women who reject their children because they need 'lightness', whose city worlds have no time for a woman raising a child on her own. It is against this background that we should explore the crisis of identity that Vera's protagonist faces over pregnancy and the possibility of motherhood.

In 'Women's time', Kristeva refers to the modern (Western) woman's perception of pregnancy as a 'fundamental challenge to identity', experienced as 'the radical ordeal of the splitting of the subject: redoubling up of the body, separation and coexistence of the self and of an other, of nature and consciousness, of physiology and speech'.[18] Phephelaphi experiences such a crisis of identity but its full meaning must be sought in the larger world of the novel and in the illusions of her relationship with Fumbatha, her lover. Her monumental quest – how to claim a piece of time and make it glitter – sets her in collision with received notions of womanhood that still hold firm even within the upheaval and newness of the city. It is this clash more than the pregnancy itself that overwhelms

---

17 Kristeva (1997) p 202.
18 Kristeva (1977) p 212.

Phephelaphi. What Kristeva calls 'the radical splitting of the subject' is, in the case of Phephelaphi, determined by the apparently impregnable force of the social order. Her struggle is with its various manifestations: notions of womanhood and motherhood, the cultural implications of pregnancy and childbearing, the landscape itself that remains ambivalent (even hostile) to her plight.

Phephelaphi's attempt to recreate the language of culture and seek new ways of being in the world clashes with Fumbatha's dream as a man and a would-be nationalist. The open possibilities of their first meeting do not survive the illusionary nature of their claims on each other. Fumbatha (who never resolves his abandonment of a heritage of resistance) claims Phephelaphi in a new national dream in which her personal dreams would be subsumed in her prescribed role as a woman: 'He needs her even if she stands apart and watches him [...] Only she could bear his children, only then would he dream new dreams and all the children be saved from drowning.'[19] What this dream translates into is the reality of their shack in the township and the intolerable closeness and tenderness of their relationship. Fumbatha believes a man and woman can share a kind of triumph in their solitude but he defines this triumph without reference to Phephelaphi's desires and striving: 'we are happy together. I work. I take care of you. It is not necessary to find something else.'[20]

Phephelaphi's abortion is a rejection of this burden. It is a violent transgression that symbolically displaces the traditional cultural values around fertility and motherhood. Vera dramatises it in the longest chapter of the novel as a journey towards self-understanding and as a lonesome yet self-generating act. In contrast to the sublimation of self and consciousness required of her as a refuge for Fumbatha and a vessel for the nation's children, Phephelaphi is intimately and consciously involved in her self-inflicted torture. Abortion becomes a chance for her own emergence as an individual, freed to claim a piece of time. (The heart beating is hers, her arms, and she is she. She has emerged out of a cracked shell.) Pregnancy is in this sense not an existential dilemma but a specific cultural boulder she must decentre in order to reconstitute a new way of being in the world.

However, the personal quest can become problematic in a closely-knit community like the township. Vera foregrounds its paradoxes in the consequences of Phephelaphi's act. The symbolic order remains ambivalent to her quest. A solid and impregnable part of the landscape yields no sympathy for her act though, paradoxically, a softer more pliant earth welcomes her tears like the rain that could fertilise a new social understanding. Other women judge her quest for self and her rejection of the national burden negatively. The act of self-generation itself splits her consciousness and fragments her being. She is, in this sense, as vulnerable as Emecheta's Nnu Ego who never takes as drastic a step yet recognises how a woman can be trapped in her own body. Nnu Ego's most radical affirmation of a personal destiny ('After all, I was born alone and I shall die alone')

---

19 Vera (1998) p 111.
20 Vera (1998) p 59.

also comes with an awareness of the larger patriarchal forces that prevent a woman (both in life and in death) from being 'fulfilled in herself, a full human being, not anybody's appendage'.[21] Both women transcend these obstacles symbolically in their deaths though each death makes a separate statement in line with its different time and context.

Emecheta's Nnu Ego distances herself enough from her community's childbearing culture to make her personal statement by refusing to grant children to barren women who invoke her spirit. United wholly in spirit with her *chi*, she seems able to understand that the ability to give or withhold children from the living is itself a powerful semantic entry into the symbolic order. She becomes a wicked spirit, judged in the same negative way that she had herself often judged her *chi*, yet 'still [she] did not give children'. Her silence decentres the values of childbearing and motherhood and at the same time marks the independence she had been fearful of expressing while alive. Phephelaphi's death, on the other hand, is a much more self-conscious act of control that asserts a woman's right to selfhood above the social obligation of her womanhood. It affirms the freedom to reject both the imposition of motherhood and the social stigma attached to its rejection. Removing this barrier clears space for the novel's most confident revisions of old concepts. Phephelaphi sets herself on fire, unable to accept a second pregnancy with which Fumbatha has broken her stem.

Her self-immolation is as much an act of courage as her abortion. It initiates a dialectic even as her body burns, 'fearless, and astonishing'. The very act of minutely recording a body's disintegration is a stubborn holding on to consciousness, a way of articulating the significance of her death simultaneously as it happens. For Phephelaphi, this significance is the refusal to be colonised by the egos and dreams of a dominant male-centred discourse. It is the courage to speak and act as an individual and as a woman. It is the right to die in her own storm and rise into her own song.[22] The right to rise into her own song is the right to express different, positive and negative experiences not necessarily contained in or sanctioned by normative concepts of the symbolic. Vera claims this for a woman within the general communal search for a new language of liberation in colonial Zimbabwe.

It would be easy to argue that the deaths of these protagonists do not change the material circumstances in the novels, but, as Dominic La Capra argues persuasively, 'a novel may have transformative effects more through its style or mode of narration than in the concrete image or representation of any desirable society or polity'.[23] In *Butterfly Burning*, Vera moves beyond this level of stylistic transformation to suggest parallel links between Phephelaphi's quest and Zimbabwe's own struggle for decolonisation. This may be a problematic claim since Phephelaphi's quest seems like an individual agenda in a close-knit community where 'dream rubs on dream. Near and close'. However, the images

21 Emecheta (1994) p 186.

22 Vera (1998) p 130.

23 La Capra (1987) p 4.

that define her desires – images of flight, boundless skies, sharp peaks, magnificent wings, butterfly valleys – also abound in the community's own dreams of agency as it lives suspended between submission and resistance. Vera herself suggests this link when she alerts us to the intertwined destinies of all the actors and hints that Fumbatha (and what he represents) would eventually move from his own (strident male song) into Phephelaphi's 'astonishing melody' when all his senses were finally free. If Vera implicates every character and space in a woman's search for a new language of agency, it is because women's struggles for self-realisation have the potential to destabilise and reorganise the cultural foundations of entire communities. By exposing what is often repressed and unsaid, it can reveal a community to itself in new unprecedented ways.

Both Emecheta and Vera expose gaps between the apparently normative language of culture and the contradictory experiences of women. Language is what constructs meaning and relationships of power within the symbolic, and in tackling the social order through language both novelists employ different but complementary strategies. In Emecheta's *The Joys of Motherhood,* the symbolic is very much a visible and impregnable force. Her strategy is to interrogate, deconstruct and reformulate its concepts. In Vera's *Butterfly Burning,* the old world is transformed by the dreams of white settlers and survives only precariously in the new world they create. The urban world is thus entirely the context of the novel. Its upheaval and newness present a chance for recreating the Word. Vera insists that this recreation should be as much about women's transformation as the community's. In both strategies what is needed is, as Vera sums up in *Opening Spaces,* 'an imagination that is plain stubborn, that can invent new gods and banish ineffectual ones'.[24]

Bibliography

Achebe, Chinua, 'Chi in Igbo cosmology', in *Morning Yet on Creation Day: Essays by Chinua Achebe* 1975, London: Heinemann.

Bakhtin, MM, in Holquist, Michael (ed), *The Dialogic Imagination: Four Essays,* 1992, Austin, TX: University of Texas.

Culler, Jonathan, *Structuralist Poetics: Structuralism, Linguistics and the Study of Literature,* 1975, London: Routledge.

Daymond, Margaret, 'Buchi Emecheta, laughter and silence: changes in the concepts of "woman", "wife" and "mother"' in Umeh, Marie (ed), *Emerging Perspectives on Buchi Emecheta,* 1996, Trenton; NJ: Africa World Press, pp 277–88.

Emecheta, Buchi, *The Joys of Motherhood,* 1994, London: Heinemann. (First published by Allison and Busby, 1979, with a second edition in 1988.)

Furman, Nelly, 'The study of women and language: comment' (1978) 3:3 *Signs, Journal of Women in Culture and Society* 182–85.

Kristeva, Julia. 'Women's time', in Belsey, Catherine and Moore, Jane (eds), *The Feminist Reader: Essays in Gender and the Politics of Literary Criticism,* 2nd edn, 1997, Malden, MA: Blackwell, pp 201–16.

24 Vera (1999) p 1.

La Capra, Dominic, *History, Politics and the Novel*, 1987, Ithaca and London: Cornell University Press.

Levi-Strauss, Claude, *Structural Anthropology*; translated by Jacobs, Claire *et al*, 1969, London: Penguin. (First published as *Anthropologie structurale*, 1958, Paris: Plon.)

Okereke, Grace, 'The birth song as a medium for communicating woman's maternal destiny in the traditional community' (1984) 25:3 *Research in African Literature* 19–32.

Scott, Joan W, 'Deconstructing equality-versus-difference: or, the uses of poststructuralist theory for feminism' (1988) 14:1 *Feminist Studies* 30–50.

Stratton, Florence, 'The shallow grave: archetypes of female experience in African fiction,' in Umeh, Marie (ed), *Emerging Perspectives on Buchi Emecheta*, 1996, Trenton; NJ: Africa World Press, pp 159–75.

Vera, Yvonne, *Butterfly Burning*, 1998, Harare: Baobab Press.

Vera, Yvonne, *Opening Spaces: An Anthology of Contemporary Women's Writing*, 1999, London: Heinemann.

CHAPTER 4

WHAT DIFFERENCE DID EMPIRE MAKE? SEX, GENDER AND SANITARY REFORM IN THE BRITISH EMPIRE[1]

Philippa Levine

In the late nineteenth century, colonial contagious diseases laws stretched across the British Empire, designed, as were their British counterparts, to stem a perceived rise in syphilis and gonorrhoea rates by controlling the body of the female prostitute. It has been a common historiographical claim that these ordinances were modelled on the domestic British Contagious Diseases Acts of 1864, 1866 and 1869. In these latter Acts, women in scheduled military and naval districts could be apprehended on suspicion of prostitution, brought before a magistrate and thence a government medical officer, genitally inspected and then either confined in a state-funded hospital for treatment for venereal disease and/or registered as a common prostitute and required thereafter to attend for regular medical inspection.

Not surprisingly, these one-sided and ineffective laws attracted huge controversy. Working class protesters, concerned about the vulnerability of working women, joined ranks with middle class feminists to protest a double standard that blamed women's 'loose' sexuality for disease, but still facilitated men's purchase of female sexual services. By the 1870s, a vigorous and well-orchestrated campaign for repeal was underway in Britain, though it would be 1886 before the movement's objective was fully realised. The campaign, and the Acts themselves, have attracted considerable historical attention; a slew of books since the early 1980s have focused on this legislation as a prime example of the distinctive sexual inequalities of Victorian Britain.

Controversial as this policy was, the considerable array of colonial ordinances which form so much greater a portion of this legislative chapter have been largely neglected by British historians as well as by historians of empire. A few individual case studies discuss such policies in particular colonial settings, but surprisingly little work has been undertaken on these laws as a specifically colonial policy.[2] Moreover, far from being modelled on the allegedly parent legislation of the 'mother' country, colonial legislation around the venereal diseases often pre-dated and differed, in profound ways, from that promulgated in Britain. It is thus that we might ask 'what difference did empire make?', not only with an eye to

---

1 This essay owes much to the research undertaken in the writing of *Prostitution, Race and Politics: Policing Venereal Disease in the British Empire* (2003). Fuller versions of the arguments made here can be found in that volume.

2 See, for example, Kaminsky (1979), Miners (1984), Van Heyningen (1984) and Warren (1990).

righting the historiographical balance, but also to raise broader questions about the centrality of colonialism to understanding domestic British history. Clearly, the relationship between core and periphery is critical here, and this chapter will suggest that the two entities of home and empire form a mutually constitutive and mutually dependent axis, neither operable without its 'other'. This rejection of a traditional linear and top-down approach to empire has significant implications for understanding many of the questions necessarily raised by this legislative moment – questions about gender and sexuality, about sanitary reform and public health, about racial hierarchy and about the politics of imperialism.

Formal contagious diseases legislation was actively pursued in Britain's Asian colonies, some of its African possessions, Labuan and North Borneo in the Malay Archipelago, in the Japanese treaty ports, and in most of Britain's Caribbean and European territories between the 1850s and the late 1880s. Even prior to the 1850s, informal versions of regulated prostitution flourished. The early Australian colonies used the criminal law and the principle of reclamation to control prostitution, though such a policy found far less sympathy in non-white colonies.[3] More commonly there were forms of regulation which tracked and treated infection in female prostitutes without any significant discouragement of the sex trade. In Penang, in the early days of the Straits Settlements, governor Philip Dundas created a red light district early in the 1800s.[4] In the Malay peninsula, a lock hospital (one exclusively for the treatment of sexually transmissible diseases) was established at the start of the nineteenth century at Yogyakarta.[5] In parts of India, lock hospitals funded by the East India Company had begun to appear in the late eighteenth century, and prostitution was regulated, if mostly on an informal and localised basis, by the early 1800s.[6] Since the colonial presence in India was both substantial and well-established by this time, it is likely that the system was better developed there than in small fledgling colonies such as the Straits Settlements, or in white settler colonies such as Australia and Canada, where a domestic and white model of rehabilitation dominated. Lock hospitals were certainly in use in the Madras Presidency by 1805, and in the Bengal Presidency two years later.[7] In 1827, William Burke, inspector general of hospitals for the army in India, outlined best practice for such regulatory systems: a register of prostitutes who agreed to fortnightly examination, certification for the healthy among them, and required hospitalisation for the infected; and punitive measures in the shape of fines and jail time for registered women failing to appear for examination.[8] What Burke described was essentially the system which, some 40 years later, would form the core of the empire-wide system, and which would be heralded – wrongly – as originating in Britain and sent out to the colonies.

---

3 Lewis (1997) p 251.

4 O'Keefe (1997) p 156.

5 Van der Sterren *et al* (1997) p 212.

6 Whitehead (1995) p 47.

7 For Madras, see BL OIOC V/24/3677; Raj (1993) p 23. For Bengal, see BL OIOC P/22/35 (21).

8 BL OIOC F/4/1079.

The earliest of the formal colonial ordinances was Hong Kong's Ordinance No 12 of 1857, which passed into law eight years before the first domestic act of 1864. It required brothels to register with the medical authorities and to ensure that their inmates were regularly examined for signs of venereal infection. Unregistered women engaging in prostitution (which effectively meant those not working within the brothel system) were liable to prosecution, while registered women were confined to the lock hospital if found to be infected. The Ordinance specified brothel locality, limiting brothels serving a European clientele to the East end of the island and those with a Chinese customer base to the West end. This was a shockingly different policy from that in Britain, where such open recognition of brothels as a legal entity was simply unthinkable in the morally upright climate of the mid-Victorian years.

Malta and Corfu followed Hong Kong in formalising legislation in 1861, after two years of experimenting semi-formally with modes of registration and regulation. In 1864, a Cantonment Act (Act XXII) introduced regulation to the military areas of British India; the cities followed suit in 1868 with the Indian Contagious Diseases Act. In 1865, the Canadian provinces of Quebec and Ontario introduced a five-year law and the tiny island of St Helena, sandwiched between South America and Africa, enacted similar legislation. There were new ordinances in 1867 in Ceylon and Jamaica, and a revised one in Hong Kong, in Queensland (Australia), Barbados and Cape Colony in 1868, and in New Zealand and Trinidad in 1869. Between 1870 and 1873, the various Straits Settlements adopted the legislation; in 1877 Labuan; in 1878, Victoria (Australia); and in 1879, in Tasmania, another Australian colony. Domestic campaigns opposing the metropolitan legislation slowed the tide in the 1880s, but Fiji nonetheless enacted an ordinance in 1882 and Cape Colony a new one in 1885.

In almost every instance, colonial ordinances differed in many respects from the metropolitan versions of the law. Perhaps the most striking difference was in how the registration of women was organised. In Britain, registration came about because a woman had been apprehended by a police officer on suspicion of soliciting. It was a police officer's contention that she was a common prostitute that resulted in a woman's appearing before a magistrate and being sent for vaginal examination and subsequent certification. She was thus, by definition, a woman already under the notice of the police. The Queensland Act of 1868, aimed in the first instance at Brisbane's white prostitute population, adopted the same policy.[9] This was a law clearly shaped by the belief that, in such dominantly Christian societies as the white Australian colonies or in Britain, few women would be likely to voluntarily name themselves as prostitutes, given the stigma attached to the trade. Secretive by its nature, prostitution lived in the shadow of shame.

In most non-white settings, by contrast, registration was effected either by the woman herself or by the brothel-keeper who employed her, and not via the actions of the police. While colonial contagious diseases laws differed from one

9 Barclay (1965) p 27.

another in a host of ways, they all stemmed from broadly similar assumptions about the place of prostitution in these societies and about the attitudes of women engaged in the trade. While there was a sense that no white woman, however desperate, would want to identify herself as trading in sex, colonists commonly felt that prostitution carried little shame for women in eastern societies. The assumptions which routinised and normalised prostitution in these settings made self-registration an obvious and an easy option, at least on paper. Colonial law-makers saw little problem in asking colonised women to come forward voluntarily and identify themselves as working in the sex trade.

The policy nonetheless proved endlessly contradictory. The British argued that Asian societies were more sexually open and thus stigmatised prostitution far less than Britain, a clear sign of their immoral inferiority, yet the policies adopted in Chinese-populated colonies such as Hong Kong and the Straits Settlements emphasised the protection of prostitute women who, claimed colonial officials, were kept coercively in the trade by cruel and greedy brothel owners who forced them into long hours of work. The Chinese sex trade was viewed as dominated so completely by pitiless brothel owners that it was on them and not their supposedly terrorised workers that the burden of registration rested. Colonial officials argued that their surveillance of the keepers would help curb their cruelty and thus protect the women from the worst excesses of what was seen as a form of sexual slavery practised on helpless women. While brothel-keepers were required to display at all times a list of inmates and to keep the authorities informed of their health and of their whereabouts, the women themselves remained for the bureaucracy a faceless mass described principally by their squalid anonymity.

The system in British India, on the other hand, was dramatically different. Indian women were expected to register themselves, although the reasons advanced for this choice were as much a condemnation of indigenous morals and mores as were the claims about brothel slavery in other parts of the British Empire. When the Indian Contagious Diseases Act was discussed at the governor-general's council early in 1868, members were appalled at the idea of handing over the power of registration to local police forces. Henry Sumner Maine, the legal member of the council, was convinced that allowing police information to decide a woman's registration 'could not be introduced here without a risk of grievous oppression'.[10] While in Hong Kong and the Malay archipelago exploitative brothel keepers had to be brought under control, in India the alleged untrustworthiness of the local police shaped regulationist policy. The indigenous police force was regarded as a necessarily corrupt body who would use the opportunity offered to bribe women and their worried menfolk. While domestic protest certainly raised the possibility of police corruption in Britain, such wholesale condemnation of a body dedicated to upholding the law did not surface. There was never any serious doubt that in Britain a carefully picked corps of older married police officers could safely work the Acts. In India, by contrast, the very possibility was considered inimical to public safety and peace of mind.

10 BL OIOC V/9/10.

The Indian Contagious Diseases Act thus relied on female volition and rejected the English principle: 'whereas [in England] ... a superior officer of the Police ... lays an information before a Justice of a woman being a prostitute before any compulsory action can be taken in regard to her, the [Indian Contagious Diseases Act] makes it compulsory in the women themselves to come in for registration.'[11] The practice was not singular to the civil law. In a military memorandum on the earlier Cantonment Act of 1864, the same policy was pursued, that 'the onus of demanding to be registered' lay with the women themselves.[12]

Also crucial in distinguishing the colonial from the British variant of these laws was the marked difference in attitudes to street-walking. Street-walking has historically been the definitive mark of sexual commerce in Britain. Indeed, the domestic Contagious Diseases Acts played down the role of brothels in the trade, representing prostitution as the choice of individual women rather than as the institutionalised business it often was. In the theologically-inflected and morally rigorous political climate of the 1860s, it would have been folly for the Acts' architects to attempt formal brothel registration, but such fears evaporated in eastern climes where the reverse was invariably the preferred policy. In colonial environments, the aim was to diminish if not abolish street-walking in favour of the more easily controlled and less offensively visible brothel system. The harshest criticisms of officials were invariably aimed at recalcitrant women who avoided or rejected registration, a group often known as 'clandestines'. Colonial policy was frequently explicit on this topic. An internal Colonial Office memorandum in 1879 classified the Hong Kong ordinances of 1857 and 1867 as dealing 'with *brothels* not with *prostitutes*' (emphasis in original), and saw the same principle at work in the Straits Settlements.[13]

In India, the rules promulgated to facilitate the 1864 Military Act distinguished between 'the prohibition of public prostitution' and that legitimately conducted in the registered brothel.[14] In the 1877 annual report on the lock hospitals in India's Northwest, the surgeon noted that 'registered women are forbidden to solicit publicly'. One of the many conditions of their registration was that business was conducted strictly indoors.[15] In the Madras Presidency the only women eligible to be registered as prostitutes outside the brothel were officers' mistresses and concubines; in short, those who served a wealthier clientele and who would therefore be less likely to solicit trade in public settings.[16] Though Indian women registered themselves and were not seen as bound monetarily or emotionally to the brothel keepers, the brothel in India, as in other colonial settings, was regarded by the authorities as preferable to the street for the conduct of sexual business. In Britain, of course, no politician would have dared entertain such legitimacy for the brothel.

---

11 BL OIOC V/10/29.
12 BL OIOC P/192/38 (70).
13 PRO CO 129/186 (12523).
14 BL OIOC L/MIL/17/5/1828.
15 BL OIOC V/24/2290.
16 Raj (1993) p 38.

On the critically important question of who the Acts were intended to protect, there was, likewise, considerable diversity. Though there was talk of extending the British Acts to the civilian population when a lobbying group was formed for this purpose in 1866, the reach of the domestic Acts remained firmly limited to garrison and seaport towns, funded almost entirely by Admiralty and War Office grants which paid for the lock hospitals as well as for actual policing of the Acts. While military necessity was a potent factor in prompting the use of the legislation in colonial settings, the laws abroad quickly grew beyond an exclusively military purview. The dual legislation in India, separately encompassing the military cantonment and the cities, is a good example. Though Henry Maine claimed that the intent of the 1868 Act was to deal with venereal disease 'in the maritime towns of British India', the law affected a far larger population than just seafarers, military or mercantile.[17] Though the use of registration and compulsory examination of prostitutes in India was certainly more carefully and widely administered in areas of high military presence, the two laws took the principle well beyond exclusively military parameters. The same was so elsewhere in the Empire and, while military demands often swayed the initiation of such legislation (as was the case in South Africa, in Hong Kong and in Queensland, among other places), in very few of these colonies were there permanent large garrisons, and it was rapidly evident that protection was intended for a white clientele regardless of occupation or rank.

The very different strategies, then, by which the attempt to contain prostitution in domestic and in colonial Britain was implemented, suggest that politicians saw these two political and geographic arenas quite differently. Beyond the pragmatic and material issue of what it was possible to do where, another level of social and cultural assumption structured these decisions. In Australia as in Britain, where the white woman was the focal point of the law, the rhetoric of redemption was central. The refuges and asylums intended to reclaim women morally, and to which legislators hoped prostitute women would pass after their lock hospital stays, barely existed in most colonial settings, and nor did colonial contagious diseases enactments write into the legislation a recommendation that they be funded. Indeed, legislators and officials in the colonies spoke directly to why such a costly provision would be useless. Charles Trevelyan contrasted Britain where the Act 'afforded ... unhappy women who had lapsed from virtue' an opportunity of 'shelter [from] which they might recover their place in society', with India where the 'low state of morals' was such that prostitutes, inheriting a long tradition, 'by no means felt degraded'.[18] The colonial surgeon at the Straits Settlements lamented 'the absence of some such home and institutions as abound in the Mother Country, with doors always open for the reception and reclamation of the abandoned, affording an asylum from whence at a fitting time they may be able to return to society, and lead a virtuous and useful life'.[19] His optimism was hopelessly inaccurate. The British magdalene

17 BL OIOC V/9/24.

18 BL OIOC V/9/8.

19 PRO ADM 1/6197.

institutions, dating mostly from the eighteenth century and designed to rehabilitate the allegedly fallen woman, had never been particularly successful in their endeavours; few women embraced the disciplining regime these charitable foundations imposed, and few stayed long within their walls. Still, redemption, whether they chose it or not, was theoretically available to metropolitan women, but seldom to their counterparts in the colonies. This palpable distinction between the possibility of redemption among white women and the apparent lack of shame that characterised prostitute women of colour vividly underlines the critical differences in colonial and domestic policy, shaped by racialised and gendered attitudes which persistently saw Britain as a more morally advanced society.

The contagious diseases legislation visible across the globe of nineteenth-century British colonialism represents an important intersection of law, policy and medicine in the state's effort to reduce the incidence of venereal disease – especially military infection – via controlling prostitution. Other than in divorce proceedings where the contraction of an STD from a marital partner could be grounds for the dissolution of the marriage, the law always saw venereal disease as centrally connected to the sex trade. Only in the twentieth century did policies such as contact notification gradually widen the compass of public health attention beyond prostitution.[20]

This dual management of disease and the sex trade illustrates how the control of sexuality was implemented – if not always terribly successfully – through legislative means. Contagious diseases laws, with their emphasis on the regular examination and involuntary medical detention of female prostitutes, assumed a direct relationship between female sexual activity and efficient disease transmission. The medical reading of the debate was overlain with presumptions about the inevitable and dangerous outcome of promiscuity, and the moral portion was encoded within a new and increasingly technical vocabulary of medical expertise. Over and over in the controversies surrounding contagious diseases legislation, public health is signalled to be the overwhelming dictate, and the control of prostitution on which the laws rested merely a vehicle of effective implementation, almost an afterthought to the over-riding medical necessities of the day. In Queensland, supporters of the law claimed that the proposed measure was medical, not moral.[21] In Hong Kong, the colonial surgeon, Dr Murray, argued that the 'sole object' of the ordinances was to restrict 'the extent of contagion' and cure the disease.[22] Public health measures were proclaimed as modernising progressive measures designed to bring safety and comfort to the population. The Indian quartermaster general's read on the Indian Contagious Diseases Act was that: 'It is not the practice of prostitution that is "legalized" but the attempts to

---

20 Savage (1990). Britain, significantly, was far more squeamish about contact tracing than Australia; see Evans (1992) p 429.

21 *Queensland Parliamentary Debates* (1868) pp 853–85. See also Barclay (1965). Smithurst (1981), vol 1, p 69, points out that the bill's sponsors saw the legislation as public health).

22 PRO CO129/296 (4718).

avert its consequent and accompanying disease.'[23] In this way, the law was, in the words of Sudhir Chandra, 'held up as the harbinger of modernity', its coercive nature justified as necessary means to good health.[24]

Contagious disease laws, centrally concerned with controlling prostitution, were thus offered up as laws in the public interest, concerned above all with the health of the populace but, while public debate may have been focused on the sanitary issues, within ruling circles the emphasis was routinely on the problems associated with the control of so-called public women. The transmission line was clear: the disease passed from women to men, and from women who were sexually active to men whose level of sexual activity was rarely seen as problematic. Promiscuity among women was thus drawn as a radically different entity than promiscuity among men. It was centrally coupled with what was regarded as the promiscuity of prostitution, the selling of sex as a livelihood.

And it was prostitution's illegitimacy that permitted a justification of the coercive and one-way nature of legislation which at no point seriously questioned whether male sexual behaviour might also be harmful. Though officials expressed disdain for the intemperate habits of a working class soldiery from time to time, it is the women who colonial surgeons, magistrates, military officers and others involved in the day-to-day administration of contagious diseases laws found most troublesome. Their lack of discipline, their mendacity, their reluctance to register under the ordinances, their dirtiness, ugliness and greed were endless themes of complaint. Year after year, the Indian lock hospital reports grumbled about the quality of the registered women. 'The classes on the register are the lowest of the low, chiefly old, ugly, broken-down hags, deformed and scarred by disease, and dragging on a miserable existence by the aid of opium, bhang, and liquor.'[25] The fear that lay behind such outbursts was that if the registered women were so unappealing, men would seek out unregistered and perhaps more attractive women whose freedom from examination would disrupt the working of the system, and might spread disease at a rapid rate, and yet, since the same complaints around disease and lack of sanitation were levelled also at the registered women, the lines between these different groups of women, registered and unregistered, were blurred. The message, if subliminal, was that women, sex and disease were in some way intimately linked: this was a public health campaign which veered significantly into gendered and racialised territory in its assumptions about transmission and sexual behaviours. It was, then, despite the public rhetoric, difficult to represent the system of regulation enshrined in contagious diseases law as *purely* concerned with issues of health and sanitation.

Alexander Arbuthnot, a member of the India Council in Whitehall, saw the empire itself as the prime reason for maintaining a system of regulation:

---

23 BL OIOC L/MIL/7/13809.

24 Chandra (1992) p 187.

25 BL OIOC V/24/2290.

> This is essentially a matter of national interest, seriously concerning those classes of the English population from which our soldiers are taken, and demanding grave consideration from all those who regard the health of our population as a question of Imperial importance.[26]

Arbuthnot feared the risk of contamination at the heart of the Empire itself; without a *cordon sanitaire* which kept prostitutes and their associates under control, sex, promiscuity and disease would run rampant. This call to empire was a means of bringing together disparate and clashing interests, of arguing that the larger issues and questions at stake here were of national significance. While the military catalyst often provided the initiative, colonial contagious diseases laws always stressed racial-moral divides, distinctions between the British and those they ruled.

Colonial variants of these laws were thus profoundly different in many and material ways from those promulgated for metropolitan Britain. Far from following the British laws, informal and formal colonial versions pre-dated those passed in Britain, and consistently differed – throughout the nineteenth century – from those operating at home. Both British and colonial officials used this divide as a means to highlight the critical distinctions they regarded as justification for British imperial rule: the greater moral order of temperate Britain, the shame that even women working in the sex trade carried for their own occupation there, the absence of sexual slavery in Britain and, of course, the converse of all of these issues in the licentious, fecund, immoral colonies that Britain ruled. Without the foil of colonial promiscuity and sexual licence, of the backwardness of medical knowledge in colonial settings, and the allegedly increased dangers from tropical versions of STDs, Britain's construction of empire as a bulwark against immorality and medical endangerment would surely have been on a less secure footing.

Bibliography

Primary sources

1 ***British Library, London, Oriental and India Office Collections***:

BL OIOC F/4/1079, *Memorandum on the Health of Europeans, 9 June 1827.*

BL OIOC L/MIL/7/13809, *Quartermaster-General Major-General EB Johnson to HK Burne, Secretary to Government of India, 22 October 1873, sent to the Secretary of State for India by Government of India, 2 January 1874 as an enclosure.*

BL OIOC L/MIL/7/13819, (Note by Sir Alexander J Arbuthnot, 7 May 1888).

BL OIOC L/MIL/17/5/1828, *Special Committee's Exposition of the Lock Hospital Rules, Strachey Committee, 14 August 1865.*

BL OIOC P/22/35 (21), *Bengal Military Consultations, 21 September 1807.*

BL OIOC P/192/38 (70), *India Military Consultations, November 1865.*

BL OIOC V/9/8, *Proceedings of the Council of the Governor-General of India, 1864,* 1865, Calcutta: Military Orphan Press.

26 BL OIOC L/MIL/7/13819.

BL OIOC V/9/10, *Proceedings of the Council of the Governor-General in India, 1868*, 1869, Calcutta: Office of the Superintendent of Government Printing.

BL OIOC V/9/24, *Proceedings of the Council of the Governor-General of India, 1888*, 1888, Calcutta: Office of the Superintendent of Government Printing.

BL OIOC V/10/29, *Annual Report of the Administration of the Bengal Presidency*, 1868, Calcutta: Bengal Secretariat Office.

BL OIOC V/24/2290, *Fourth Annual Report on the Working of the Lock Hospitals in the Northwest Provinces and Oudh for the Year 1877*, 1878, Allahabad: np.

BL OIOC V/24/3677, *Army Sanitary Commission, 4 March 1873*.

2 ***Public Record Office, London, Colonial Office Records*:**

PRO CO 129/186 (12523), *Undated, Unsigned Memo, 1879*.

PRO CO 129/296 (4718), (*Dr Murray, Colonial Surgeon*).

3 ***Public Record Office, London, Admiralty Office Records*:**

PRO ADM 1/6197, Clarke, W.M, *Report on the Working of the Contagious Diseases Act from December 1st 1869 to December 31, 1870*.

4 ***Parliamentary Debates VI, Second Series*, 1868, Brisbane: James C Beal (Government Printer).**

Secondary sources:

Barclay, E, 'Queensland's Contagious Diseases Act, 1868 – 'The Act for the Encouragement of Vice' and some nineteenth century attempts to repeal it: Part 1' (1965) 2:10 *Queensland Heritage* 27–34.

Chandra, S, 'Whose laws? Notes on a legitimising myth of the Colonial Indian State' (1992) 8:2 *Studies in History* 187–211.

Evans, D, 'Tackling the "hidden scourge": the creation of venereal disease treatment centres in early twentieth-century Britain' (1992) 5:3 *Social History of Medicine* 413–433.

Kaminsky, A, 'Morality legislation and British troops in late nineteenth century India' (1979) 43 *Military Affairs* 78–83.

Levine, Philippa, *Prostitution, Race and Politics: Policing Venereal Disease in the British Empire*, 2003, New York: Routledge.

Lewis, M, 'Sexually transmitted diseases in Australia from the late eighteenth to the late twentieth century', in Lewis, M *et al* (eds), *Sex, Disease, and Society: A Comparative History of Sexually Transmitted Diseases and HIV/AIDS in Asia and the Pacific*, 1997, Westport, CT: Greenwood Press.

Miners, N, 'State regulation of prostitution in Hong Kong, 1857 to 1941' (1984) 24 *Journal of the Royal Asiatic Society – Hong Kong Branch* 143–61.

O'Keefe, B, 'Sexually transmitted diseases in Malaysia: a history', in Lewis, M *et al* (eds), *Sex, Disease, and Society: A Comparative History of Sexually Transmitted Diseases and HIV/AIDS in Asia and the Pacific*, 1997, Westport, CT: Greenwood Press.

Raj, MS, *Prostitution in Madras: A Study in Historical Perspective*, 1993, Delhi: Konark Publications PVT Ltd.

Savage, G, '"The wilful communication of a loathsome disease": marital conflict and venereal disease in Victorian England' (1990) 34:1 *Victorian Studies* 35–54.

Smithurst, BA, *Historic and Epidemiologic Review of Venereal Disease in Queensland*, 1981, unpublished MD thesis, University of Queensland.

van der Sterren, A, Murray, A and Hull, T, 'A history of sexually transmitted diseases in the Indian Archipelago', in Lewis, M *et al* (eds), *Sex, Disease, and Society: A Comparative History of Sexually Transmitted Diseases and HIV/AIDS in Asia and the Pacific*, 1997, Westport, CT: Greenwood Press.

Van Heyningen, E, 'The social evil in the Cape Colony 1868–1902: prostitution and the Contagious Diseases Acts' (1984) 10:2 *Journal of Southern African Studies* 170–91.

Warren, J, 'Prostitution and the politics of venereal disease: Singapore, 1870–98' (1990) 21 *Journal of South East Asian Studies* 360–83.

Whitehead, J, 'Bodies clean and unclean: prostitution, sanitary legislation & respectable femininity in Colonial North India' (1995) 7:1 *Gender & History* 41–63.

CHAPTER 5

DANGEROUS BLOOD: MENSTRUATION, MEDICINE AND MYTH IN EARLY MODERN ENGLAND

Margaret Healy

> If the hair of a menstruating woman be taken, and placed under a dung-heap or clod of earth, or where the dung was made during winter or summer, by the virtue of the sun there will be engendered a long and powerful snake.[1]

Symbolic of both creation and corruption, nurture and venom, menstrual blood is frequently enmeshed in a deeply ambivalent and florid web of potent myths and rules; rules which, in some cultural contexts, have a significant impact on the lives of women.[2] Menstrual meanings vary within cultures (between sub-groups),[3] as well as cross-culturally, and taboos range from those relating to the danger and toxicity of the blood itself to those associated ones that forbid menstrual sex, to others that exclude menstruous women from certain places and company, and to yet others that prohibit her from undertaking specific activities such as cooking.[4] Furthermore, in early modern England – as in many cultures around the world today – menstruation and its associated taboos were imagined to have important implications for the health of both sexes and their offspring.

Menstruation was, in fact, fundamental to sex, gender and disease constructs and, in order to grasp the profound significance of the cultural imaginary of 'the menses' between approximately 1400 and 1700, it is essential to gain a familiarity with the interplay of these categories. The only way we can do this, of course, is through recourse to a range of literature that functioned to reflect and, importantly, to shape their socio-cultural understanding. Early modern medical textbooks might seem like the obvious place to focus such a quest for knowledge of the body. This would, however, be an anachronistic and limiting assumption: clear-cut divisions between lay and medical healers were not operative at this time and the majority of interpreters of bodily misfortune were not learned

---

1 'Secrets of women' in Jacquart, and Thomasset (1988) p 76.

2 There are cultures in which menstruation appears to be an unmarked category, considered neither polluting nor propitious and not linked to rules; for example among the Rungus of Borneo (see Appell (1988)). Menstruation continues to have complex, ambivalent meanings in British culture. It is significant that a recent sociological study of menstruation commenced with the words: 'Why do women so often feel uneasy about menstruation? Why is it so thoroughly hidden from public view? Why do young girls still have to learn about it in fear and shame?' See Laws (1990) p 3.

3 For example, in Sri Lanka among Buddhists menstruation is a threat to cosmic purity, whereas among Catholics it is a sign of women's vulnerability to threats from the cosmos; see Winslow (1980).

4 See Stephens (1961).

physicians.[5] Many were illiterate 'wise women' who – sadly, but understandably – left no records for posterity. One notable exception was the highly literate midwife, Jane Sharp, to whose engaging book of her occupation I shall shortly refer. However, for the most part we must rely on a motley bunch of lawyers, clerics, grammar school teachers, 'gentlemen' and a few practising doctors who both translated ancient classical texts and added their own voices to debates about health and disease issues.[6] It was not uncommon, too, for humanist physicians, following the Apollonian example, to pen medical advice in poetic form: thus, for example, the noted Italian physician Fracastoro of Verona wrote a famous epic mythologising the origins of syphilis.[7] Medicine, then, was not a discrete, scientific discourse, and Western humanism understood poetry, like music, as having significant healing properties – a legacy from classical Greece.[8]

Indeed, the authority of ancient Greek, Roman and Hebrew influences was unrivalled in interpreting and constructing the body in European culture. The understanding of 'woman' in the Renaissance was rooted in two ideologies: the Hebraic-Christian tradition of equating Eve with the Fall, and the Aristotelian-Galenic account of her nature and physiology.[9] According to the first, woman's suffering in her menses (her 'curse') and in childbirth was God-given and a consequence of her fatal transgression. In the second, philosophical tradition, 'woman' fared no better: here she was an unfinished or imperfect man. As such, of course, there was always the danger of a woman becoming more manly and, perhaps more terrifying for this intensely patriarchal culture, the danger of a man regressing to his female, unfinished, type. This is how Helkiah Crooke described the formation of the sexes at birth in 1618: 'in males the parts of generation are without the body, in females they lie within because of the weakness of the heat which is not able to thrust them forth [...] the neck of the womb is nothing else but the virile member turned inward and the bottom of the womb nothing but the scrotum or cod inverted.'[10] Lacking sufficient heat at conception, the woman's sexual parts have remained inside her body. Humorally, she is colder and moister than the male, and therein lies the problem of menstrual blood and the diseases associated with it. Whilst men burn off any excesses of the blood humour, women retain it; it is their 'natural disease' which must be purged monthly. Interestingly, *The Midwives Book* by the feisty practising midwife, Jane Sharp, reproduces this authoritative account of woman as inverted man, adding:

> ... so a woman is not so perfect as a Man, because her heat is weaker, but the Man can do nothing without the woman to beget Children, though some idle Coxcombs will needs undertake to shew how children may be had without the use of the woman.[11]

---

5 See Porter and Porter (1988) p 7.

6 Learned physicians were notoriously reluctant to share their knowledge in print.

7 Eatough (1984). For a discussion of the gender politics of this poem, see Healy (2003) pp 22–38.

8 Healy (2001) pp 18–49.

9 See Aughterson (1995) pp 41–66, and Wiesner (1993) pp 44–46.

10 Crooke (1618) pp 270–72.

11 Sharp (1671) p 40.

Women might be less perfect, but it was precisely this lack, Sharp countered, that enabled humans to procreate.

Retained within the body as a potentially polluting and contaminating substance, menstrual fluid was surrounded by taboo, as a wedding sermon published in 1617 reveals. William Whately instructed the newly wedded that:

> ... their nuptial meetings must be seasonable, and at lawful times. There is a season when God and Nature sejoins [separates] man and wife in this respect. The woman is made to be fruitful; and therefore also moist and cold of constitution. Hence it is that their natural heat serves not to turn all their sustenance into their own nourishment; but a quantity redounding is set apart in a convenient place to cherish and nourish the conception, when they shall conceive. Now this redundant humour (called their flowers or terms) hath (if no conception be) its monthly issue or evacuation [... which] always after childbirth [...] is larger and longer [...] Now in all these [...] occasions, it is simply unlawful for a man to company with his own wife. The Lord tells us so. Leviticus 15 vers 19–25; also ch 18 ver 19; also ch 20 ver 18. Of which places it is needful that married persons should take note: to which I send them [...] Where God threatens death to the offender, can the minister be faithful if he do not plainly declare the offence? This fault is by GOD condemned to the punishment of death, Leviticus 20: 18.[12]

As we might expect in Protestant England, the biblical word features prominently in accounts of the prohibitions surrounding menstruation. Leviticus instructed the Hebrew faithful that a woman with an issue should be 'put apart' for seven days and that a man and woman who contravened this law would be 'even both cut off from among their people'.[13] Interestingly, this prohibition was not restricted to the Jews but seems to have been widely observed by ancient and medieval gentile cultures. Dionysius, the third-century Bishop of Alexandria wrote, for example, that 'it was unnecessary to tell menstruating women to keep away from the Eucharist: good Christian women did not need to be reminded of so serious a prohibition'.[14] What is striking, though, is how the glosses of the sixteenth-century Geneva bible (the text deposited in all English churches in the sixteenth century) inserted even more dire warnings than the Jewish original: the Geneva bible urged (Leviticus 15) – in the manner of Whately's sermon – that any man who touched the bed or 'companied with' a menstruating woman 'should die'.[15]

Theology prohibited sexual activities around polluting menstrual blood then, but in the sixteenth and seventeenth centuries, medical ideas often underpinned and reinforced the religious taboo. The popular book, *Aristotle's Master-Piece*, for example, interpreted the biblical injunction in hygienic terms:

> Moses considering, or being so commanded by God, strictly commanded the Hebrew men not to touch a Woman that was unclean of her Blood [...] for by the

12 Aughterson (1995) p 35.

13 Leviticus 20, v 18, in Brown, M (1990) p 45.

14 Brown, P (1990) p 433. Brown describes how this prohibition became normal in the medieval West.

15 Brown, M (1990) p 43.

> violent concussion and motion used in Copulation and evil mixture, the contagion by degrees will seize upon the whole Body, causing the Pox and Leprosy.[16]

Menstrual blood was considered so 'evil' that it could excoriate the penis and cause diseases; it was commonly argued that the new Renaissance disease, syphilis – the Pox – was initially engendered by the unnatural copulation of a menstruating prostitute with a leper.[17] Measles and smallpox, meanwhile, were contracted in the womb and showed themselves in childhood when – as Simon Kellwaye put it – the 'filthy menstruall matter' separated from the 'naturall blood' in a purifying process, when the menstrual matter was 'hoate and slimy' it produced smallpox, if 'dry and subtill, ... the measels'.[18]

According to *Aristotle's Master-Piece*, copulation during menstruation 'violate[d] Nature's Law' so severely that any resultant conception was bound to produce a dull child or a monstrous birth.[19] It relates how the famous physician Levinus Lemnius witnessed this horror. He saw one of his patients (an islander who had married a mariner) give birth to a monster with a crooked back, long round neck, fiery eyes, and a pointed tail. It was very 'nimble footed, for as soon as it came forth it gave the affrighted midwife the slip, and run up and down the Room to seek a hiding place, till at last one woman more courageous than the rest, fell upon it with a Cushion and smothered it'.[20] However, this wasn't the end of the horror: a male child emerged from the womb shortly after the monster but the latter had greedily sucked his blood and eaten his flesh so that the child 'scarcely lived to be Christened'.[21] Such was the outcome of unseasonable, insatiable venery. Curiously, these stories seem particularly to circulate around sailors.[22]

The 'evil' effects of menstrual blood – its negative potency – were imagined to be wide-ranging. According to the tradition of Pliny:

> Contact with it turns new wine sour, crops touched by it become barren, grafts die, seeds in gardens are dried up, the fruit of trees falls off, the edge of steel and the gleam of ivory are dulled, hives of bees die, even bronze and iron are at once seized by rust, and a horrible smell fills the air; to taste it drives dogs mad and infects their bites in an incurable poison ...[23]

It is noteworthy that throughout the twentieth century in Britain and America there were repeated 'scientific' attempts to establish whether or not 'menotoxins', which might cause such effects, were present in menstrual secretions – the jury is still out.[24] Certainly there are persistent 'old wives' tales' that make it

16 Anonymous (1690) pp 46–47.

17 Crawford and Mendelson (1996) p 26, and Healy (2001) pp 132–33. Syphilis emerged in Europe as a virulent, sexually transmitted disease in 1494.

18 Kellwaye (1593) f 39r.

19 Anonymous (1690) p 48.

20 Anonymous (1690) p 48.

21 Anonymous (1690) p 50.

22 Delaney *et al* (1977) p 10.

23 Delaney *et al* (1977) p 7.

24 Buckley and Gottlieb (1988) pp 19–21.

unpropitious to try to bake bread during 'the curse': apparently yeast is rendered inactive and the dough fails to rise.

In early modern England, as we have heard, menstrual blood proved that women's bodies were inefficient, less perfect than men's and potentially hazardous. Lacking sufficient natural heat they simply could not burn up humoral surpluses or purify their blood. *Aristotle's Master-Piece* cites this as evidence that women were not so strong, wise, prudent or reasonable as men: *her* 'faculties' were hindered in operation because of this lack.[25] Her inferior nature was thus the legacy of her unfinished bodily model and this understanding justified male dominance and female subjugation. In a fascinating aside in *The Sicke Woman's Private Looking-Glasse,* John Sadler makes exception of one type of woman 'the Amozonites, who being active, and alwayes in motion, had ther fluxions very little, or not at all.'[26] In most women, however, the excess, impure matter had to be shed regularly, but as *Aristotle's Book of Problems* warns: 'when the Flowers do run from a Woman, then a most venemous Air is dissolved in them which doth ascend into the woman's head'. The evil vapours multiply when they reach the eyes and seek passage through 'insensible holes' or pores. This is how a menstruating woman's glance tarnishes a mirror. In the way that she transmits 'evil' she resembles that 'venemous and infected' beast, the Basilisk.[27]

However, things did not get better – as we might assume – in periods of amenorrhoea or post-menopause: then, the poisonous matter simply accumulated as 'black and dark Smoke' in the brain.[28] Women who suffered 'stoppages' of their 'terms' became subject to a range of illnesses: 'frenzy of the womb' and melancholy, madness, hysterical fits, breaking out in sores;[29] or worse – they might become murderous. Let me remind you of Shakespeare's Lady Macbeth's spine-chilling invocation of the powers of darkness:

> Come, you spirits
> That tend on mortal thoughts, unsex me here,
> And fill me from the crown to the toe, top-full
> Of direst cruelty. Make thick my blood,
> Stop up th'access and passage to remorse,
> That no compunctious visitings of nature
> Shake my fell purpose. (I v 39–45)[30]

The transformation that she desires is simultaneously physical, emotional and moral. Blood that was 'thick' was commonly associated with 'stoppages' and the word 'passage' was often used as a synonym for the cervix. 'Visitings of nature' was an early modern euphemism for menstruation. In Lady Macbeth's belief system (one possibly shared by many in the original audiences) 'stoppages' led to

---

25 Anonymous (1690) p 5.

26 Sadler (1636) p 13.

27 Anonymous (1764) p 15.

28 Lemnius (1667) p 268.

29 Crawford and Mendelson (1996) pp 23–25.

30 Shakespeare (1988) p 980. I am grateful to Dominic Harman for drawing this passage to my attention.

moral fog, mystical mischief and dire bloody acts – a perverse inversion of maternal nurturing behaviour.

Paradoxically, health required women to undergo their natural 'disease' at regular intervals – if not, finances permitting, they had to be artificially bled by a surgeon. Post-menopausal women – their brains bulging with toxic smoke – were imagined to be particularly venomous: the glance of an old lady, or the vapours emitted from her mouth, could dry up a nursing mother's milk, cause animals and children to sicken, and even kill a baby in its cradle. It is not difficult to see how it was most commonly women, and frequently 'old beldames', who were implicated in witchcraft. Indeed, as Stuart Clark describes in *Thinking With Demons*, one famous commentator, Pierre Crespet, argued 'for a general affinity between the hideousness of old women and the repulsiveness of the demonic', suggesting that bewitching was the direct result of the 'predomination' of menstrual blood as evil fumes in the head.[31]

So far I have concentrated almost entirely on the dangerous, defiling effects of menstrual blood. What do these lurid myths tell us about the culture which produced them? Given the seminal work of anthropologists in this field – especially Mary Douglas – it would be impossible not to ascribe a social meaning to these cultural constructions of polluting menstrual blood.[32] Menstrual taboos are usually understood as suppressive of women, signifying a general debasement of the female sphere: they suggest a society in which men are more highly valued than women and exert the greater agency.[33] This interpretation certainly seems apposite in relation to patriarchal early modern England, yet this is not the whole of the story and, as the anthropologists Buckley and Gottlieb caution in their seminal study, *Blood Magic*, it is overly reductionist to attribute one meaning to menstrual blood in any culture. As even Pliny acknowledged, menstrual blood was linked to a range of positive as well as negative effects: it encouraged the fertility of wheat fields and it was used to treat gout, goitre, haemorrhages, puerperal fever, worms, headache and hydrophobia.[34] It was an ambivalent signifier, then, but in ancient Rome, as in early modern England, it was certainly construed as powerful. It is time to consider this issue in relation to another set of myths and indeed, facts, about the potency of 'flowers'.

In *The Late Lancashire Witches*, a play written in 1634 and based on a true case of witchcraft, there is an interesting episode that can be brought to bear on this discussion.[35] Lancashire had a pronounced reputation as a hotbed of ritualistic Roman Catholicism, of pagan superstitions and, of course, of witches. This Protestant play, written by Thomas Heywood and Richard Brome, portrays a small unsuspecting rural community turned upside down by an epidemic of supernatural occurrences: it shows family relationships inverted, hunts spoilt,

31 Clark (1997) p 113.

32 Douglas (1984) and Douglas (1996).

33 Hammond and Jablow (1976) p 7, and Laws (1990) pp 18–19.

34 Buckley and Gottlieb (1988) pp 21 and 26–47.

35 Barber (1979) p 100. Barber notes that in *Hierarchie of the Blessed Angels*, Heywood, the playwright, tells us that he believes in witches and disapproves of them.

men rendered impotent, and wedding feasts spirited away. Four women and their familiars are implicated in all this devilish confusion – Gooddy Dickison, Mal, Meg and Mrs Generous. The latter, as her name implies, is married to the most likeable, generous and gullible well-to-do man in the neighbourhood. Three quarters of the way through the play we encounter Mr Generous shocked and baffled having just discovered that his trusted partner of many years is a witch. In the most lengthy soliloquy of the play he laments what 'Man is loath to entertaine' (l 1604), that is, that his wife, whom he had never before had reason to rebuke – indeed in her youth 'she was taken for a seeming Saint' (l 1611) – whose loyalty he had never doubted, had turned out to be – indisputably – in league with the Devil. But how has he made this discovery? His soliloquy seems particularly concerned to detail this mechanism for audience consumption:

> The Gentile fashion sometimes we observe
> To sunder beds; but most in these hot monthes
> *June, July, August*, so we did last night.
> Now *I* (as ever tender of her health)
> And therefore rising early as I use,
> Entring her Chamber to bestow on her
> A custom'd Visite; finde the Pillow swell'd
> Unbruis'd with any weight, the sheets unruffled. (ll 1617–24)

While the couple have been sleeping in separate chambers, according to the 'Gentile' custom, Mrs Generous has been taking advantage of the situation – and of Mr Generous – regularly leaving the house and disappearing on his horse, flying through the night to consort with her familiar and participate in witches' feasts and pranks.

Married couples were most likely to sunder beds, as we have seen, for the duration of the woman's 'flowers'. We might infer then that for Mrs Generous a 'seeming' godly practice has been perverted to the service of the devil in an extremely fortuitous way: menstrual blood was imagined to be greedily devoured by the devil and a key ingredient of witches potions, playing a powerful role in magic, especially love magic.[36] Could there be a warning here that sundering beds in 'the Gentile fashion' (there is a pun on gentle and the biblical Gentile here) gave rather too much opportunity for mischief to wayward womankind? Mrs Generous was certainly enjoying her freedom. Indeed, there does seem to be some male anxiety circulating in this play around the issue of female space and it is noteworthy that, in some cultures around the world today, menstrual seclusion is seen as bringing women sexual autonomy and opportunities for illicit love affairs.[37]

Furthermore, there are strong indications that not all Protestants thought the Levitical laws worthy of observance; indeed, some thought them downright dangerous. Radical dissenters like William Barrow railed against them, associating Old Testament Jewish taboos with the bad old ways of Roman

---

36 Crooke (1618) p 289.

37 For example, among the Djuka of Dutch Guiana, the Warao of Venezuela and the Kaska of western Canada, in Buckley and Gottlieb (1988) p 13.

ritualism. Barrow dismissed as idolatrous such practices as 'the weoman's monethlie restraint and separation from your church, her comming after that just tyme wympeled, vealed, with her gosips and neighbours following her, her kneeling downe before and offring unto the priest, the prieste's churching, praying over her, blessing her from sonne and moone, delivering her in the end to her former vocation'.[38] In *A Briefe Discoverie of the False Church*, he went further, declaring, 'Is not all this absolutely Jewish? Though in deed the prieste's part savor more of poperie [...] This trumperie is so grosse, as it deserveth no refutation, but a doung forke to cast it out'.[39] However, as Gail McMurray Gibson has observed in her excellent essay on churching, Barrow's main grouse seems to be the privileging of women's bodies that he locates in these practices: 'why should women have this prerogative?', he rails.[40] What his writing suggests is that women might actually have valued the opportunity for private female space and for female dominated rituals surrounding their fecundity: in post-Reformation England women voluntarily and steadfastly maintained the practice of churching. Far from being a signifier of shame, blood from the womb might have been associated with pride because it symbolised fertility and potency: in fact it was a sign of something that men could not achieve and might even envy.

At least one Northern European physician, Cornelius Agrippa, writing in Latin in 1529 (*De nobilitate et praecellentia sexus foeminei*), argued that women were superior to men because they could produce milk which nourishes human life, and only they had a natural process to rid the body of poisons.[41] Others, like the physician Thomas Raynold, lambasted the shameful lies and slander told about menstrual blood:

> Is it to be thought that nature wold feade the tender and delicate infant in the mothers womb, with the refuse of the blud, or not rather with the purist of it [...] Yet much more are to be detested and abhorred the shamefull lyes and slaunders that Plynie, Albertus Magnus de secretes Mulierum and dyvers othermore have wrytten, of the venemous and daungorous infectyve nature of the womans flowers or termes: The which al be but dreames and playne dotage; to reherse [...] here were but losse of ynke and paper.[42]

Raynold's book was extremely popular undergoing 13 editions between 1540 and 1634. He was referring to the kind of 'lies' characterised by the epigraph to this chapter and to those found in Pliny's *Natural History*. In actual fact we probably learn most about such troubling myths in treatises which sought to undermine them. For example, in Reginald Scot's famous treatise, *The Discoverie of Witchcraft*, the author ridiculed the assertion that 'old [...] bowed women' were often found to be witches because of their evil humours and 'venomous exhalations' which

---

38 Carson (1966) p 72.

39 Carson (1962) p 463.

40 Carson (1962) p 464, and Gibson (1996) pp 139–54. In the Roman Church, 'churching' of women after childbirth was a public ritual in which the priest gave the woman a blessing for her fruitfulness, sprinkling her with holy water and reciting the 23rd Psalm.

41 Agrippa, Cornelius, *'De nobilitate et praecellentia sexus foeminei'*, 1529, in *Opera*, 1970, vol 2, p 533, Heldesheim: Olms; cited in cited in Wiesner (1970) p 9.

42 Raynold (1545) f 44v.

caused them to 'belch up a certaine breath, wherewith they bewitch whomsoever they list'.[43] In Scot's view, this was all arrant nonsense.

So it *is* possible to find sceptics who refuted the venomous aspects of menstrual blood; it is equally possible to find exponents of the view that taboos surrounding menstruation were so much hocus pocus, Romish ritualism. Furthermore, it is possible to find writings which are wholly positive about the pure and creative menstrual flux. Perhaps, however, the commonest type of outpouring on the matter is that to be found in such works as the treatise by the physician, John Sadler, which simply articulates the contradictions in the medical and popular understanding of menstrual blood, and tries to account for them. Sadler argues that the 'monthly flux of excrementous and profitable bloud' must be 'pure and incorrupt, like unto the bloud in the veins' because it is for:

> ... the propagation and conservation of mankinde [...] the child whilst it is in the matrice is nourished with this bloud [...] being out of the womb, it is still nourished with the same; for the milke is nothing but the menstruous bloud made white in the breasts; and I am sure woman's milke is not thought to be venomous, but of a nutritive quality [...] It may be objected, if the bloud bee not of a hurtfull quality, how can it cause such venomous effects, as if the same fall upon trees and herbs it maketh the one barren, and mortifies the other. And Averroes writes, that if a man accompany with a menstruous woman, if she conceive, she shall bring forth a Lepar. I answer, this malignity is contracted in the wombe; for the woman wanting native heat to digest this superfluity, sends it to the matrice, where seating it selfe untill the mouth of the wombe be dilated, it becomes corrupt and venomous, which may easily be, considering the heat and moisture of the place. This bloud therefore being out of his vessels, offends in quality.[44]

So, menstrual blood is 'matter out of place':[45] excrementous, corrupt and venomous, leaving disease and disaster in its wake; yet it is also pure, profitable and nourishing. Sadler manages to accommodate these binaries and paradoxes in his confusing and contradictory medical constructions of female physiology.

It seems appropriate to draw this chapter to a close amidst Sadler's confusion. In early modern England, the symbolic voicings and valences of menstrual blood were variable, often compendious and ambivalent and very one-sided: with the exception of Jane Sharp, women were virtually silent in print about menstruation. In the absence of more female voices, it would simply be adding to the inevitable androcentric focus this encourages, to assume that men always inscribe the cultural production and women simply and unquestioningly perform their allotted roles within it. I have tried to suggest that prohibitions surrounding menstrual blood might not have been experienced by women as totally negative: to assume that prohibiting men from having sexual contact with their wives is a form of suppressive discrimination against women is, after all, rather limited. We should recall, too, Jane Sharp's jibe at 'coxcombs' in relation to female anatomy – women might be lesser men but only they could bear children. Associated with

---

43 Scot (1584) pp 278–79.

44 Sadler (1636) pp 8–10.

45 Douglas (1984) pp 36 and 41.

fertility and thus with positive potency, it is conceivable that many women experienced menstruation as desirable and therefore traumatic to lose. Additionally, the male inscriptions from this period about women's 'flowers' speak volumes about the intense anxiety generated by the social contradiction of which menstrual blood was the marker – that is, the undeniable potency and creativity of the – culturally constructed – weaker sex.[46]

Perhaps I am putting too much of a positive gloss on things; after all, fears about the polluting effects of menstrual blood do seem to intensify in the sixteenth century, especially around the issue of monstrous births. This observation might, however, cause us to pause and ask another really vital question about menstrual prohibitions. Whom do they seek to protect: the man, the woman, or any offspring which might emerge from unlawful sex? Males do not, it seems, have the sole prerogative in this respect: indeed, the heightened pollution anxieties in this period seem to cluster around discussions of offspring. There is a tendency to explain pollution taboos today almost exclusively in social or psychological terms but might a biological event be just as – if not more – implicated here? The arrival in Europe in the 1490s of the new disease – syphilis – with which these defilement myths are closely associated did give rise to a sharp increase in the birth of sickly, mentally impaired and deformed children in the sixteenth century. Undoubtedly, this disease event contributed to a general climate of anxiety surrounding unlawful copulation and about the negative effects of witchcraft too.

To conclude then, I have tried to illustrate the multivalency of menstrual symbolism in early modern England and to resist the temptation to interpret pollution taboos in this profoundly patriarchal culture monocausally, as simply debasing of women. The social construction of menstrual blood in all cultures needs to be far more complexly understood and necessitates an interdisciplinary approach. A combination of ideological, psychological, social and biological factors were undoubtedly operative in shaping the meanings of menstrual blood in this culture, and the taboos associated with it may have functioned in the management of male – *and female* – anxiety and health, as well as in social organisation.

Bibliography

Anonymous, *Aristotle's Book of Problems*, 1764, London: JW.

Anonymous, *Aristotle's Master-Piece: Or, The Secrets of Generation Display'd in all the Parts thereof*, 1690, London: np.

Appell, Laura WR, 'Menstruation among the Rungus of Borneo: an unmarked category', in Buckley, Thomas and Gottlieb, Alma (eds), *Blood Magic: The Anthropology of Menstruation*, 1988, Berkeley, CA: University of California Press, pp 94–112.

46 As Buckley and Gottlieb (1988) pp 30–34 point out, Mary Douglas linked menstrual pollution taboos with particular societies in which there was structural ambiguity surrounding women.

Aughterson, Kate, 'Physiology', in Augherson, Kate (ed), *Renaissance Woman: A Source Book. Constructions of Femininity in England*, 1995, London: Routledge, pp 41–66.

Barber, Laird H (ed), *An Edition of The Late Lancashire Witches*, 1979, New York and London: Garland Publishing, Inc.

Brown, Michael H (ed), *The Geneva Bible: A Facsimile of the 1599 Edition with Undated Sternhold & Hopkins Psalms/with an Introduction by Michael H Brown* 1990, Ozark, MO: LL Brown Publishing.

Brown, Peter, *The Body and Society: Men, Women and Sexual Renunciation in Early Christianity*, 1990, New York: Columbia University Press.

Buckley, Thomas and Gottlieb, Alma (eds), *Blood Magic: The Anthropology of Menstruation*, 1988, Berkeley: CA: University of California Press.

Carson, Leland Henry, 'The writings of Henry Barrow, 1587–1590', in Carson, LH (ed), *Elizabethan Nonconformist Texts*, vol 3, 1962, London: Allen and Unwin, for the Sir Halley Stewart Trust.

Carson, Leland Henry, 'The writings of Henry Barrow, 1590–1591', in Carson, LH (ed), *Elizabethan Nonconformist Texts*, vol 5, 1966, London: Allen and Unwin, for the Sir Halley Stewart Trust.

Clark, Stuart, *Thinking With Demons: The Idea of Witchcraft in Early Modern Europe*, 1997, Oxford: Oxford University Press.

Crawford, Patricia and Mendelson, Sara, *Women in Early Modern England 1550–1720*, 1996, Oxford: Clarendon.

Crooke, Helkiah, *Microcosmographia*, 1618, London: np.

Delaney, Janice *et al*, *The Curse: A Cultural History of Menstruation*, 1977, New York: Mentor.

Douglas, Mary, *Purity and Danger: An Analysis of the Concept of Pollution and Taboo (1966)*, 1984, London: Routledge.

Douglas, Mary, *Natural Symbols: Explorations in Cosmology (1970)*, 1996, London: Routledge.

Eatough, Geoffrey (trans), *Fracastoro's 'Syphilis' (1530)*, 1984, Liverpool: Francis Cairns.

Gibson, Gail McMurray, 'Blessing from sun and moon: churching as women's theater', in Hanawalt, BA and Wallace, D (eds), *Bodies and Disciplines: Intersections of Literature and History in Fifteenth-Century England*, 1996, Minneapolis, MN: University of Minnesota Press, pp 139–54.

Hammond, Dorothy and Jablow, Alta, *Women in Cultures of the World*, 1976, Menlo Park, CA: Benjamin Cummings.

Healy, Margaret, 'The Humoral-Paracelsan body' in Healy, Margaret, *Fictions of Disease in Early Modern England: Bodies, Plagues and Politics*, 2001, Basingstoke: Palgrave, pp 18–49.

Healy, Margaret, 'Anxious and fatal contacts: taming the contagious touch', in Harvey, Elizabeth D (ed), *Sensible Flesh: On Touch in Early Modern Culture*, 2003, Philadelphia, PA: University of Pennsylvania Press, pp 22–38.

Jacquart, Danielle and Thomasset, Claude, *Sexuality and Medicine in the Middle Ages*, 1988, Cambridge: Polity Press.

Kellwaye, Simon, *A Defensative against the Plague*, 1593, London: np.

Laws, Sophie, *Issues of Blood: The Politics of Menstruation*, 1990, Basingstoke: Macmillan.

Lemnius, Levinus, *A Discourse touching Generation*, 1667, London: np.

Porter, Roy and Porter, Dorothy, *In Sickness and in Health: The British Experience, 1650–1850*, 1988, London: Fourth Estate.

Raynold, Thomas, *The Byrth of Mankynde, Otherwise Named the Womans Booke*, 1545, f 44v, London: np.

Sadler, John, *The Sicke Woman's Private Looking-Glasse*, 1636, London: np.

Scot, Reginald, *The Discoverie of Witchcraft*, 1584, London: np.

Shakespeare, William, 'Macbeth', in Wells, S, and Taylor, G (eds), *The Oxford Shakespeare: The Complete Works*, compact edition, 1988, Oxford: Clarendon, pp 975–99.

Sharp, Jane, *The Midwives Book*, 1671, London.

Stephens, William N, 'A cross-cultural study of menstrual taboos' (1961) 64 *Genetic Psychology Monographs* 385–416.

Wiesner, Merry E, *Women and Gender in Early Modern Europe*, 1993, Cambridge: Cambridge University Press.

Winslow, Deborah, 'Rituals of first menstruation in Sri Lanka' (1980) 15 *Man* 603–25.

PART II
THE REPRESENTATION OF SICKNESS AND HEALTH

CHAPTER 6

REMEMBRANCE OF HEALTH LOST: DIS/FIGURING AFRICA IN EUROPEAN AIDS WRITING

James N Agar

In this chapter I discuss some of the interactions, contradictions and conflicts within and between European and African AIDS discourses, especially in relation to differing narratives of gender and sexuality. Against this background, I situate a reading of two pieces of European fiction in order to analyse how they figure and disfigure, appropriate and interpellate (or give a stabilising identity to) 'Africa' within their own representations of AIDS. These readings of fiction suggest that 'literature' can, and indeed must, contribute to what is understood as 'AIDS'. Moreover, reading fiction can provide for a reflective and critical space wherein reading (as a critical and cultural practise) is mobilised to provide a space for interrogation and speculation. Reading fictions about and of AIDS then allows for a critical re-reading of some of the seemingly dominant and stereotyped issues inherent in AIDS discourse.

Susan Sontag has convincingly made the case that discourses and representations of AIDS are inextricably linked to a narrative of both origination and expulsion, testifying to 'the need to make a dreaded disease foreign'.[1] Common, so Sontag asserts, to the cultural construction of a range of plagues, different cultures construct AIDS as though it is a foreign condition, a viral threat from abroad to the boundaries of the domestic space. As such, AIDS is, particularly in North America and Western Europe, both culturally specific and nationally configured, constructed and disseminated in ways which betray the desire to protect the ideological boundary of the nation from invasion and infection by a foreign body. The supposed purity of the homeland is threatened with contamination and one discursive move which either supposedly harnesses resistance to such a threat, or alternatively dismisses the domestic danger of the threat, is to locate the origin of this threat in a mystified foreign land, at once expelling the origination of the contamination from the domestic space. The threat comes from elsewhere, from (an) outside(r). One supposed example of the danger of this discursive trajectory is given by Frédéric Martel in his discussion of the emergence of AIDS policies in early 1980s France.[2] Recounting (in perhaps implicitly homophobic ways) what he sees as the characteristic silence and denial

---

1 Sontag (1991) p 133.

2 Martel (1996). In many ways an important and landmark study, Martel's work has been criticised as an act of self-promotion in which much of the argument is supported by potentially homophobic anecdote which aims to counter forms of militancy which advocate homosexual visibility.

of the gay French response to AIDS in the early to mid-1980s, Martel remembers how French author Pierre Kneip had suggested that HIV and AIDS were seen as being quintessentially American concerns. Martel maintains that this notion was central to French discourses on AIDS despite the crucial French role in the discovery of HIV (an episode itself coloured by US-French competition and national rivalry).[3] Kneip is quoted by Martel as suggesting that the virus would have been taken more seriously in France had its socio-cultural and politico-economic associations been with Cuba or the USSR rather than North America. The basis for this belief, Martel suggests, was the penchant of the French left (and AIDS activists in the mid-1980s) for an anti-American and anti-capitalist strain in their thought. This strain of thought helped its proponents mystify North America as a puritanical and reactionary society based on values which they believed were not as central in France, Cuba or the USSR.[4] The implication here is clear: as the virus is the concern of an other (in this instance the USA) it need not unduly concern the self (in this instance France). Such complacency facilitates the silent, unacknowledged spread of the virus among 'us' while simultaneously allowing for the solidification of the myth of (ideologically framed discourses of) homeland purity and overseas degeneration.

This discursive trajectory, which has been so central to the (Western) national and international construction of the AIDS epidemic, is replicated within the rhetorical framing of discourses which construct AIDS as a global pandemic. In this global situation which is constantly changing and developing with growing hotspots of epidemiological catastrophe in Eastern Europe, Asia and China, a similar discursive strategy of origination and expulsion is, and always has been, at work. The narrative is by no means set in stone; it is a narrative which has shifted and changed over time (from Africa to Haiti and back to Africa, for example) and is equally a narrative which has been filtered through a range of changing sexualised and gendered narrative lines, themselves filtered through the issues of cultural difference and misrepresentation. 'Africa', the 'dark continent', a mysterious entity presented as a kind of cultural, linguistic, geographic, religious and social homogeneity, has long been seen in Western Europe and North America (two further presumed homogeneities) as the starting point of the AIDS pandemic.[5] Such a narrative is based on racist stereotypes of a Third World Africa, figuring Africa (from a Western and Eurocentric position of supposed superiority) as an overpopulated, primitive land marked by animalistic sexual licence. This narrative is itself, as Cindy Patton observes, linked to 'colonialist mystifications' of the nineteenth century which posited Africa as primitive, wild and natural, a space yet to be 'modernised' (and economically exploited) by the

3 AIDS (Acquired Immune Deficiency Syndrome) is not a disease as such, but a condition which is marked by a severely weakened immune system. The immune system is attacked and weakened by the work of the virus known as HIV (Human Immuno-deficiency Virus). A Person With AIDS (PWA) suffers from a range of diseases and infections which the immune system is no longer strong enough to fight against.

4 Martel (1996) pp 238–42.

5 Sontag (1991) p 137.

presumed grandeur of European civilisation.[6] A discursive violence which presents a fantasised 'African culture' as 'other' is mobilised within Western AIDS discourse such that 'pretended cultural sensitivity' (towards 'Africa') is translated into 'the conceptual categories of the modern, Western *episteme*'.[7] The presentation of the self to and by the self is achieved through an incorporation of, and a discursive sovereignty over, an other which is always/already a fantasy and scapegoat created by and for the self. Nowhere has this situation had more dire consequences than in the realm of science and medicine in relation to HIV/AIDS in Africa. The models adopted in Europe and North America for antibody testing, for example, produced a distorted image of HIV prevalence within Africa since the antibody tests used were based on definitions of pathogens which made clinical (and ideological) sense in North America and Europe.[8] The antibody tests used in the mid-1980s in Africa were, however, incapable of distinguishing between HIV antibodies and antibodies to malaria.[9] There is, then, little surprise that the picture quickly emerged, in popular media as well as medical research papers, of a continent both ravaged by HIV and beyond redemption. A continent, moreover, crying out for vaccine trials which were more dangerous than those conducted in either Europe or North America (but deemed to be 'compassionate' given the catastrophic situation in Africa), trials which would reap much greater benefit to Europe and North America than they would to Africa itself. One further illustration of the ways in which a European and North American assumed model has been imposed onto AIDS in Africa is in the realm of the gendering and sexualisation of the epidemic in Europe, North America *and* Africa. In short, the discursive presentation of the relationship between Western AIDS and African AIDS has been based on an opposition of the homosexual/gay plague of Europe and North America to the heterosexual plague of AIDS in Sub-Saharan Africa where far greater numbers of women (and children) have been infected with the virus. A conjunction of the policing of sexuality and desire and an acute racism attempt to explain this situation away. Active (white) gay men in Western Europe and North America, so the hypothesis goes, passed the virus to passive gay men through anal intercourse (this model itself rests on a reductive schematisation of active/passive roles in gay sex while equally insisting on the centrality of anal penetration within gay sexual activity). In Africa, however, and amongst prostitutes and blacks in the USA and Europe, the practice of anal intercourse with women resulted in the virus being transmitted to heterosexual men. A bizarre conjunction of a range of gendered and sexualised stereotypes are at play here. As Cindy Patton observes: 'The collision of homophobia and racism provided the anus with a curious but pivotal gender: the female anus was thought

---

6 See Patton (1990) pp 77–97. For an interesting and insightful discussion of the kind of 'colonial mystifications', which abound in European literature and thought, see Harrison (2003).

7 Patton (1990) p 77.

8 A 'pathogen' is a micro-organism which causes disease in the body.

9 The most widely used HIV test is the Elisa test (developed in France) which detects the presence of antibodies to HIV rather than the actual presence of HIV itself. In the logic of the Elisa test, the former is taken to imply the latter.

capable of doing what the male anus was not.'[10] The centrality of anal intercourse in this scheme of things signals a Western concern, not to say fascination, with the presence of (a symbolic and synecdochal image of) homosexuality, that of the active gay male penetrator who infects his passive recipient. The discourse equally assumes that if heterosexual activity might allow for anal intercourse, it is here the active male penetrator who becomes infected by the female passive recipient. The active partner in anal penetration is exonerated from being an agent of infection if his receiver is a woman, but not if his receiver is a man. Within and between Western Europe, North America and Africa, then, there is a policing of a sexual act (anal penetration) which is marked by prejudices related to sexuality and desire masquerading as (possibly altruistic) social and medical research. While sexual acts may be the same the world over, their organisation and cultural meaning in relation to identity and social bonding may differ hugely. Rather than imposing a problematic model from Europe and North America on the huge diversity of Africa, a greater sensitivity to a non-judgmental economy of pleasures and sexual activities is required. Sexual and gendered identity complicate and falsify the understanding of sexual acts (in relation to modes of viral transmission) in Europe, North America *and* Africa. A *supposed* sensitivity to expressions of alternative sexual identity does little to increase freedom of thought or sexual activity and possibly inhibits the successful fighting of a virus. What is required is a more nuanced understanding of the interrelation between a range of sexual activities and the actors who indulge in them, regardless of gender or sexuality. The introduction of the issues of gender and sexuality into the activity of anal penetration, for example, has led less to an understanding of the position, importance and risks associated with this activity for gay and straight men and women alike, and more to a prejudiced schematisation which is at pains to identify and vilify gay men and loose women in order to allow the activity and identity of active straight men to remain unquestioned and unquestionable.

Time and countless 'accidents of history' (Patton's term for incidences of infection)[11] continue to disrupt and complicate the reductive (and possibly reassuring because reductive) picture of gay AIDS in Europe and North America as opposed to straight African AIDS. In the UK, HIV infections are currently increasing more quickly amongst young straight individuals than within the so-called gay community.[12] In South Africa, for example (predominantly in and around Cape Town, home to South Africa's largest commercial gay scene and an increasingly popular holiday destination for gay travellers), a constellation of gay organisations and self-help groupings are beginning to emerge in the post-Apartheid Rainbow Nation. These organisations are asserting a visible and audible presence (of alternative modes of sexuality and of HIV/AIDS) which was absent from South Africa prior to November 1993.[13] In the coming years the role

10 Patton (1990) p 91.

11 Patton (1990) p 96.

12 A hypothesis supported by figures released by the UK's Health Protection Agency (HPA) in November 2003. For details of these figures see: www.hpa.org.uk/hpa/news/articles/press_releases/2003/031124_wad.htm (last accessed 15 July 2004).

13 The apartheid constitution ceased to exist from 9am on 18 November 1993.

played within South Africa of this emerging 'gay community' in relation to AIDS may well become a crucial one. There certainly seems to be a discursive vacuum, aside from the issue of drug patents, given President Mbeki's shying away from his previous position which, while possibly seeming ridiculous, at least managed to keep the debate about HIV/AIDS centre stage.[14] Uganda has made great advances in its education programme in relation to HIV/AIDS and has, seemingly against all odds, managed to dramatically slow the rate of HIV infection in recent years.[15] Time, political changes and the assertion of political will, new drug treatments and the constantly fluctuating epidemiological trends of the transmission of the virus all feed into and constantly modify the narratives which HIV/AIDS offer up. Sontag's plague narrative, where this chapter began, is also linked to an inexorable move toward death. Some, such as Andrew Sullivan, have (perhaps prematurely) celebrated the end of the pariah plague culture (and narrative) asserting that, with triple combination therapies, the plague is over.[16] It is, however, a tragic reminder of the imbrication of politics, big business and money within the realm of AIDS that such therapies remain unavailable in many parts of the African continent. Equally, it is often overlooked that such treatments (which often lead to health-threatening side effects) do not work for all HIV positive patients in the West. Combination therapy, while undoubtedly a positive development, may not be the 'saviour' which some would like to think it is. All narratives of AIDS, whether in the realm of film, fiction or medical research, are, then, historically bound and culturally specific. However, the majority of Western fictional portrayals of AIDS situate themselves within a broad schematisation of AIDS linked to (gay) sexuality, either at the level of the author or the characters and, in some cases, both. The sexuality in question is predominantly male gay sexuality and it is striking how such narratives (in film and prose fiction) present an extremely narrow, highly codified and stereotyped depiction of women. Female characters, often framed as supportive friends or mothers, are normally used either as a backcloth to highlight issues of masculinity rather than femininity, or as screens on to which are projected the concerns of the (male, gay) protagonist/s.

Furthermore, writing about AIDS enforces a range of important ethical questions on both writer and reader alike, and this especially in the case of written texts whose authors have now died from AIDS-related conditions. In a sense, the

---

14 President Thabo Mbeki caused widespread controversy in 1999 by seeming to cast doubt over the orthodox medical view that HIV is the viral agent which leads to AIDS. Mbeki had sought the opinions of a range of medical professionals including numerous 'AIDS dissidents', notably Professor Peter Duesberg, in order to frame South African policies on AIDS. The 'AIDS dissidents' cast doubt over the importance of HIV as a viral agent leading to AIDS: see Epstein (2000). The controversy and the reactions it caused in South Africa can be traced in Cherry (2000a, 2000b, 2000c).

15 A report prepared for the United States Agency for International Development (USAID) describes Uganda as 'a model for curbing the epidemic in the developing world'. From 1992–99, Uganda managed to reduce its HIV prevalence by 50%: see TvT Associates (2002).

16 Sullivan (1999) pp 3–7.

weight of testimony, as Ross Chambers has convincingly argued,[17] passes from the author through the text and lands on the shoulders of the reader. For the text to work as testimony, it falls to the reader to carry the weight of the act of witnessing. This is a personal situation for each and every reader to confront. In relation to HIV/AIDS, which have become such mobile signifiers of a range of issues within culture (fractured and constituted, as AIDS discourse is, by and through issues related to gender, sexuality, lifestyle, religion, politics, etc), reading (AIDS narratives) places the text and the reader him/herself both within and outside the immanence of the text as self-sufficient object. Both text and reader come to be immersed within and infected by the discourses which surround the discursive construction of AIDS. Literature ceases to be simply a reflection of another situation (AIDS) which is separate from and outside of literature (I would argue this basic case for the representational function of all literature). Rather, through language and narrative construction, literature contributes to the very essence of what AIDS is, what we understand by it, and *how we live (with or without) it*. Fictional texts cease to be simply cultural inventions, while reading itself becomes a form of cultural (and political) intervention into the very reality of what positively constitutes our world.

How then do some examples of fiction writing from Europe interpellate and appropriate 'Africa'? I want, first, to discuss 'Slim', a short story by Adam Mars-Jones,[18] before moving on to the novel *Paradise* (*Le Paradis*) by French writer and photographer Hervé Guibert.[19] Both of these texts address AIDS in a somewhat oblique fashion, but in different ways and for different reasons. Mars-Jones's story is an attempt, at a fairly early stage of the entry of discourses of AIDS into (his) writings of fiction, to come to terms with *how* to talk about and write about AIDS without succumbing to the defining and restricting definitions of science and medicine (figured in the story through the inventive relexicalisation of medical acronyms) which were gaining currency in the mid-1980s. Guibert's novel, published posthumously at a time when AIDS had saturated his writings from the early 1990s, attempts, on the other hand, to *stop* talking *about* AIDS, to escape the potential internalisation of AIDS language and identity which his earlier work had dramatised and which Mars-Jones's piece begins, at an earlier juncture in the history of AIDS (in fiction), to resist. While both texts also appropriate a highly stereotypical image of Africa in a seemingly negative way (potentially racist and Eurocentric in their interpellating/hailing of 'Africa' as a poor, disease-ridden, wild and exotic entity), both texts also allow for an undoing of their own appropriation of Africa. Both texts thus allow the reader to recognise the stereotype as stereotype, at once suggesting its inauthenticity as a reflection of the real Africa while, at the same time, deploying its usefulness for fiction as a trope which reveals its own fictionality. In this way, both texts suggest the dangers to (reading) health of taking the trope as fact, of not recognising the fictionality of the trope. The texts achieve this to differing extents. The reasons for this are several,

---

17 Chambers (1998).

18 Mars-Jones (1992) pp 9–18.

19 Guibert (1992); translated by James Kirkup, published as *Paradise* (1996).

including first of all the different dates of composition of the two pieces. Written some five years after Mars-Jones's story, Guibert's novel can inventively allude more to AIDS without recourse to a discourse *about* or *of* AIDS since the official language of AIDS was more widely known when Guibert wrote *Paradise* than was the case when Mars-Jones composed 'Slim'. Secondly, the different generic conventions within which the texts operate limit and differentiate the extent to which they can overplay a stereotype in order to undermine it. The concision traditionally required of the short story to enforce a unity of impression lessens the extent to which Mars-Jones's story can develop this strategy. As such, the single, dominant impression of 'Slim' is the dramatisation of the isolation of the protagonist and narrator as he attempts to come to terms with his altered health status and self-image. With a wider scope and more space for narrative development, Guibert's novel can develop to a much greater extent the strategy of presenting the stereotype in order to undermine it. Helping Guibert in this endeavour is the fact that, given the time of the composition of *Paradise*, the stereotype he is dealing with (of Africa) was more solidified and recognisable than when Mars-Jones wrote 'Slim'.

In 'Slim' the nameless narrator describes the changes in his daily routine in the home. The physical setting is exclusively the domestic space, since the narrator never leaves his London flat. An extended emotional domesticity is invoked through reflections on relations with parents and family. This extension of the domestic space is foregrounded through the ways in which a nameless volunteer from 'the Trust' helps with domestic chores and aims to keep up the narrator's spirits. The term 'AIDS' never once appears in the story. The story plays here on the positive senses for Anglophone readers of (being) 'slim' as opposed to (having) 'Slim' referring to (having) AIDS within an African context. 'AIDS' is, however, strongly evoked in the opening lines since these lines make it clear that (having) 'Slim' is not to be understood as (being) 'slim': 'I don't use that word. I've heard it enough. So I've taken it out of circulation, just here, just at home. I say Slim instead, *and Buddy understands.* I have got Slim' (my emphasis).[20] '[T]hat word', though never mentioned, is clearly 'AIDS'. Written in 1986, the story provides enough clues to indicate that the absent present, the suppressed signifier, is indeed AIDS. There are a range of linguistic inventions within the story: AIDS becomes 'Slim', KS lesions become 'blackcurrants',[21] the companion becomes the character 'Buddy' (as he is sent to carry out the act of buddying); the narrator ironically comments that he himself has come to be apostrophed: 'apparently in Trustspeak I'm a string of letters, which I don't remember except the first one's P and stands for person. Apparently they have to remind themselves.'[22] Clearly, the absent acronym of identification here is PWA (Person With AIDS). What is interesting is the way in which the title for the story is appropriated from the Ugandan condition of 'slim disease', which was much in evidence in the popular

20 Mars-Jones (1992) p 9.

21 *Kaposi's Sarcoma* (KS) is a (normally) uncommon form of skin cancer which PWAs sometimes suffer from.

22 Mars-Jones (1992) p 10. Mars-Jones makes extensive use of such (humorous) linguistic play in his work, particularly in relation to (medically associated) acronyms.

press and TV media in the mid-1980s. Africa is further appropriated within the story for the purposes of domesticating the condition which the narrator lives with. Commenting on his own linguistic inventiveness, and possibly ironically highlighting the domestic enclosure of the story, the narrator says: 'Illness is making me quite the internationalist: an African infection and some dated American slang.'[23] A conjunction, then, is presented to the reader: the origination for the infection is stated as being Africa, an infection which is linguistically presented through the optic of American slang (through the reference to 'Buddy'). It is an interesting conjunction that the English/London setting plays with: it is as though the world of the flat is forever separate(d) from the life of the city. The flat is an outsider cell within the body of the city, a tiny space of foreign infection wherein the disease that dare not speak its name is ever more insidiously present due to its evident linguistic absence. The narrator rationalises his own condition by imagining that he has been adopted by an African family: 'I think that maybe I've been adopted by an African family, that – poor as they are – they are sending me what they can spare from their tainted food, their poisoned water, their little lifespans.'[24] AIDS, then, is domesticated by and for the narrator but is equally desocialised and desexualised: the narrator is out of contact with his real family and friends and never leaves his flat. This desocialisation and desexualisation is achieved through reducing Africa from its own multiple specificity into a mystified and stabilising entity (as uniformly 'poor' and 'tainted'). Africa is presented as the origin of disease, as 'tainted', 'poor' and 'poisoned', while the story supposes that the family structure in 'Africa' can be understood through, and thus transferred to, the family structure within a European context. The same process is at work with the usage of 'Slim' as both title and name for the medical condition which the narrator lives with. Denying the specificity (as did scientists with Ugandan 'slim disease') of the local usage in Africa of 'slim' (to designate a particular disease within a Ugandan context) the narrator maps 'slim' against what the European reader sees as AIDS. Through its own absence as graphic signifier, AIDS imposes itself as the European model through which 'slim' can, in this story, be understood. The same thing happened in medical reality as the very concept of 'slim disease' was outlawed in favour of the imposed category of 'AIDS', Western science once again imposing its own standards and denying the specificity and cultural meaning of local terms.[25] The strength and 'usefulness' of the story as fiction is that it reveals this process at work through performing the process in fiction. As such, despite its stereotypical and possibly racist homogenising of 'Africa', the story allows the reader to consider the nature and indeed ethics of communication and human interaction (on a small scale) in the light of AIDS. 'Kid gloves are better than surgical gloves', remarks the narrator toward the end of the story.[26] The story thus tentatively broaches the issues of how we might begin to talk about, represent and come to terms with a new and, at least in 1986, life-threatening disease.

---

23 Mars-Jones (1992) p 10.
24 Mars-Jones (1992) p 10.
25 See Patton (1990) p 79.
26 Mars-Jones (1992) p 17.

Hervé Guibert died in December 1991. An openly gay man, though by no means a spokesperson for gay politics in any conventional sense, his output comprises in excess of 25 creative works across a wide range of genres and media: novel, diary, journalism, short story, theatre, autobiography, video diary, photography. *Paradise* was published posthumously in 1992 and is Guibert's last published novel. Guibert rose to fame and notoriety after the 1990 publication of *To The Friend Who Did Not Save My Life* (*A l'ami qui ne m'a pas sauvé la vie*), his first work to explicitly and extensively focus on AIDS as a trope of his fiction and fictionalised autobiography.[27] The final two years of his life were marked by a voracious outpouring of writings, all of which to differing extents are either *about* AIDS or, as in the case of *Paradise*, 'simply' write AIDS. The novel is remarkable in Guibert's corpus as it involves an indepth recounting of a love affair of the narrator (Hervé Guibert) which, on the surface at least, is a straight love affair. A range of intertextual references, in fact, open the potential for seeing this straight love affair rather as a gay romp. The interest here, however, lies in an openly gay writer with AIDS figuring Africa and a straight love affair within a text which is stalked by AIDS and the distant rumblings of the narrator's and writer's death agony.

The notion of *paradise* evoked by the novel's title is, as is common with titles of many of Guibert's works, somewhat misleading. A kind of travelogue *manqué*, in the novel the reader visits Zurich, Washington, Martinique, Bora-Bora and Africa (Mali, specifically Bamako and Ségou). These places are without exception associated and directly linked in the novel to boredom, a painful and ultimately futile MRI brainscan (since the results defy reading), death, disappearance and erasure, disease and madness. Guibert has used the concept of *paradise* in previous (pre-AIDS) works, notably in *Blindsight* (*Des Aveugles*) where it is the name of a stinking pet shop where a character buys mice in order to torture them, and is also the sinister name which the blind people of this novel use for their belated entry into the world of the sighted when due to their advanced age the Blind Institute throws them out and sends them to old people's homes.[28] The chronology in *Paradise*, though the use of flashback techniques is evident, is impossible to reconstruct; it is unclear whether the narration is in or about Bora-Bora, before or after Africa, if indeed either, and individual incidents might happen in one or the other and possibly neither. The principal character, apart from the narrator, Hervé Guibert, is Jayne Heinz (a distant relative of the inventor of ketchup!) who is found dead on the opening page of the novel only to be subsequently resuscitated by the fiction (through flashback). Approximately 20 pages into the novel the reader learns that Jayne probably never existed, police identity checks show that no such person has existed in the past 200 years, her diaries (which the narrator has repeatedly seen Jayne writing) are filled with blank pages and the CDs which she has repeatedly listened to render no sounds. All the markers of what the

27 Guibert (1991). This is also the first book (a semi-fictionalised autobiographical novel) in which Guibert begins to appropriate a discourse about Africa in relation to AIDS, linking the latter to African 'witch doctors' and 'evil spells', see Guibert (1996) p 9.

28 Guibert (1995) p 34.

narrator might see posthumously of Jayne's character and personality turn out to be empty vessels. *Paradise* is infuriatingly slippery (the usual markers which allow one to get a hold on a novel, time and chronology, setting, character, etc, in this case do not help), at once tragic and yet curiously amusing, disturbing and yet deeply moving.

For what it is worth, Guibert did travel to Bamako and Ségou in early 1991, purportedly (according to his biographer, François Buot)[29] as both an escape and the only possible way to continue writing. While the oppressive stinking heat and chlamydia-ridden sex which takes place in Mali might present what one critic has described as 'Africa ... as a kind of postmodern black hole reflected by post-colonial French culture',[30] the novel presents such an unbelievably contradictory inventory of judgment on Africa as to suggest (and ultimately state) that 'Africa' as such does not exist. In the closing 25 pages of the novel, where madness, exhaustion and narrative breakdown begin to take over, the reader encounters a range of contradictory declarations: he went to Africa to find forgetfulness and to forget himself; he no longer knows how he got from Martinique to Africa; a psychiatrist's report claims the journey to Africa followed a family bereavement; the narrator returned from Africa covered in red pustules; the narrator went to Africa in search of eternity, no longer knows exactly when he left, but may have met God in Africa; the narrator no longer believes that he was ever in Africa and yet has, as proof that he was there, African banknotes on his desk, despite then declaring that he has no proof that he was ever there. Such confusion continues to the declaration very close to the end of the novel that 'Africa does not exist'.[31]

The exoticism of Africa as a potential earthly paradise is clearly debunked, and yet this is equally not any form of realist writing based on the experience of travelling to Africa in order to document the lived reality of a part of equatorial Africa. Reading about Africa and looking at photographs of it, the narrator tells his reader, also taught him nothing about the reality of the place. The reality of Guibert's 'Africa' lies elsewhere. It is an imaginary and fantasised entity, his own mystified foreign land as site of both relation to and escape from infection, European conventions of identity, sexuality and logic.[32] It both does not exist and yet must exist in Guibert's dreams (and writing) as narrator and, I think, writer. As the book stumbles to its end, the attempts to sustain the narrative of Guibert and Jayne become ever more futile and, though the narrator declares that an HIV test proffers a negative result, AIDS continues to stalk the last third of the novel. A mourning this text may well be; for Jayne, for Vincent (a gay lover of Guibert's who recurs in numerous works), for Guibert's Aunt Suzanne (in his real life and in the novel); textual and intertextual references could support any and all of these

29 Buot (1999) p 281. Much of the evidence cited in Buot's biography is taken from Guibert's own published works and the then unpublished diary of Guibert. I am somewhat sceptical of the extent to which Guibert's own writing should be seen as reliable evidence of Guibert's own real life, even if much of his writing is about (a textually represented) 'Guibert'.

30 Boulé (1999) p 256. For an interesting critical reading of the novel, see Sarkonak (2000).

31 Guibert (1996) pp 97, 102, 104, 105, 106, 107, 108, 119.

32 See Pratt (1997).

hypotheses. Africa is, however, both figured and fabulously disfigured as a mental, imaginative space into which the narrator, writer (and reader) might attempt one last time to escape. A mourning of the previously imagined death of the self (figured in many previous works, especially *To The Friend Who Did Not Save My Life*), a death which is ever closing in on narrator and writer, the novel is also for a short time a clinging to life, a writing of life, an act of creation which, however momentarily, defies death. 'Every fiction is a mystification' writes Guibert in his diary;[33] in mystifying Africa and the stalking of death, the fiction necessarily ends when the writing off of AIDS can no longer be sustained.

Despite their very different temporal (in relation to the AIDS pandemic) and cultural contexts of production, both Mars-Jones's and Guibert's texts appropriate 'Africa' into their own representations of AIDS. Rather than simply reproducing stereotyped set narratives, however, both texts manage to mobilise fiction as a speculative space of (self-)interrogation and creation. Both texts suggest that the reader question presumptions and supposedly authoritative versions of 'African AIDS', especially in relation to the dominant discourses of AIDS which exist(ed) in the cultures from which the texts emerge(d). By thus dis/figuring Africa, each text strongly suggests that any discourse of (or about) AIDS should not, simply, be taken as read.

Bibliography

Boulé, Jean-Pierre, *Hervé Guibert: Voices of the Self*, 1999, Liverpool: Liverpool University Press.

Buot, François, *Hervé Guibert: le jeune homme et la mort*, 1999, Paris: Grasset.

Chambers, Ross, *Facing It: AIDS Diaries and the Death of the Author*, 1998, Ann Arbor, MI: University of Michigan Press.

Cherry, Michael, 'Letter fuels South Africa's AIDS furore' (2000a) 404 *Nature* 911 (27 April).

Cherry, Michael, 'South Africa turns to research in the hope of settling AIDS policy ...' (2000b) 405 *Nature* 105–06 (11 May).

Cherry, Michael, 'The Durban Declaration' (2000c) 406 *Nature* 1, 3, 15–16 (5 July).

Epstein, Helen, 'The mystery of AIDS in South Africa' (2000) 47:12 *The New York Review of Books* (11 June), www.nybooks.com/articles/9 (accessed 28 January 2004).

Guibert, Hervé, *Des Aveugles*, 1985, Paris: Gallimard, Folio edition. (Translated by Kirkup, James, as *Blindsight*, 1995, London: Quartet Books.)

Guibert, Hervé, *Fou de Vincent*, 1989, Paris: Minuit.

Guibert, Hervé, *A l'ami qui ne m'a pas sauvé la vie*, 1990, Paris: Gallimard, Folio edition. (Translated by Coverdale, Linda, as *To The Friend Who Did Not Save My Life*, 1991, London: Quartet Books.)

Guibert, Hervé, *Le Paradis*, 1992, Paris: Gallimard, Folio edition. (Translated by Kirkup, James, as *Paradise*, 1996, London: Quartet Books.)

33 Guibert (2001) p 556 (my translation).

Guibert, Hervé, *Le mausolée des amants: journal 1976–1991*, 2001, Paris: Gallimard, Folio edition.

Harrison, Nicholas, *Postcolonial Criticism: History, Theory and the Work of Fiction*, 2003, Cambridge: Polity Press.

Mars-Jones, Adam, 'Slim' in *The Monopolies of Loss*, 1992, London: Faber and Faber, pp 9–18. (First published in *Granta* (1986), issue 19.)

Martel, Frédéric, *Le rose et le noir: Les homosexuels en France depuis 1968*, 1996, Paris: Seuil. (Translated by Todd, Jane Marle, as *The Pink and the Black: Homosexuals in France since 1968*, 1999, Palo Alto, CA: Stanford University Press.)

Patton, Cindy, 'Inventing "African AIDS"', in *Inventing AIDS*, 1990, London: Routledge, pp 77–97.

Pratt, Murray, 'Imagining positive geographies: French AIDS writing in the 1990s as refusing and destabilising the psycho-social untouchable body' (1997) 1:3 *Mots Pluriels*, www.arts.uwa.edu.au/MotsPluriels/MP397mupr.html (accessed 12 December 2003).

Sarkonak, Ralph, *Angelic Echoes: Hervé Guibert and Company*, 2000, Toronto, ON: University of Toronto Press.

Sontag, Susan, *Illness as Metaphor: AIDS and its Metaphors*, 1991, London: Penguin.

Sullivan, Andrew, *Love Undetectable: Reflections on Friendship, Sex and Survival*, 1999, London: Vintage.

TvT Associates under The Synergy Project, 'HIV/AIDS in Uganda. A USAID Brief', prepared for USAID (2002): http://63.107.122.20/summaries.asp#africa (accessed 9 June 2003).

CHAPTER 7

VULNERABLE MARGINS: THE ICONOGRAPHY OF BLOOD, DIRT AND DISEASE IN THE EARLY TWENTIETH-CENTURY SOUTH AFRICAN SETTLER NOVEL

Lynda Morgan

In her biography of Doris Lessing, Carole Klein refers to Lessing's 'painful sense of not belonging',[1] and a childhood in which 'family life revolved around English values and customs that had little meaning to a girl who roamed the African veld'.[2] These words provide a paradigmatic starting point for discussion of the lives and literary representations of English-speaking South African settlers. They inhabited an in-between state, their mental landscapes deeply divided between the marginalised land of settlement and the imagined community of the original homeland – a mythologised connection that appealed even to settlers who were born in South Africa and had never visited so-called 'home'. It was sufficiently noteworthy for Patricia Pifer, an American newly settled in the little town of Nigel, south of Johannesburg, to mention it in a letter to her mother-in-law in 1933: 'All we have heard about here is England and the Prince of Wales – always something about him.'[3] However, the England of idealised origin was also the England that utilised colonies to dispose of its human excess, and many settlers of English descent were disowned by the homeland before they had set foot in Africa. They were for the most part members of the working classes for whom colonisation was an answer to unemployment. Sarah Gertrude Millin describes the 1820 settlers as 'humble people mostly',[4] and 'bound to be chiefly those who have little to lose by going away'.[5] The colonies continued to tempt those who saw little opportunity in their country of birth. According to Drury Pifer, Patricia's son: 'The Africa of 1932 promised an outside chance to marginal people, those willing to hock everything and borrow to pay their passage, those willing to bet everything on a letter or a rumor.'[6] A particular attraction was that marginality in the homeland could be transformed into superiority in the colonies. John X Merriman, Prime Minister of the Cape Colony, remarked in 1908 that white workmen who had been located in the lower classes in Europe were 'delighted on arrival here to find themselves in a position of an aristocracy of colour',[7] yet

---

1 Klein (2000) p 1.
2 Klein (2000) p 2.
3 Pifer (1994) p 50.
4 Millin (1941) p 9.
5 Millin (1941) p 11.
6 Pifer (1994) p 10.
7 Ranger (1983) p 213.

marginalisation was not so easily escaped as Merriman's comment might suggest. The colonies were always regarded as peripheral, and Ann Laura Stoler identifies a shift in thinking in the early twentieth century that 'focuses not only on the Otherness of the colonized but also on the Otherness of colonials themselves'.[8] The South African settler is clearly not African, but is not authentically European either. This uncertain identity finds particular representation in English language settler fiction of the late nineteenth and early twentieth centuries through metaphoric concern with bodily coherence and integrity, expressed through obsessive attention to miscegenation and the associated imagery of disease.

In this chapter I mobilise several discourses in order to suggest that images of disease intersect with those of blood, semen and dirt in representations of sexual exchange to construct a hierarchised system of racialised, class-inflected and gendered bodies, and to reveal considerable anxiety at the level of unconscious fantasy about the breaching of the European, middle class, settler body. The first is the work of Joseph Arthur Comte de Gobineau on mixed-race sex, and his ideas about the draining away of what he calls 'the blood of the civilizing race' which is, he says, 'parcelled out among the peoples that are conquered or annexed'.[9] His imagery of increasing weakness is strikingly like that associated in the nineteenth century with the draining away of semen through masturbation or excessive sexual intercourse, and a metaphorical figuring of blood-as-semen and semen-as-blood is central to settler novels about miscegenation, where blood and semen become bonded in a complex racial exchange that carries messages of both loathing and desire, and where the notion of the weakening and infecting of the 'pure white' bloodline is narrated in terms dependent on the imagery of venereal disease. I also employ Mary Douglas's anthropological work of 1966, *Purity and Danger*, to bring dirt into the equation. She emphasises the symbolic roots of attitudes to dirt and rituals of purity. Cleaning is a way of establishing order, 'a positive effort to organise the environment'.[10] Rituals of purity are thus connected with the identity and beliefs of societies, and bear 'a symbolic load'.[11] Central to such rituals is the human body, which is, she argues, specially vulnerable at its margins, its vulnerability symbolised by 'marginal stuff of the most obvious kind. Spittle, blood, milk, urine, faeces or tears by simply issuing forth have traversed the boundary of the body. So also have bodily parings, skin, nail, hair clippings and sweat'.[12] How this 'marginal stuff' is dealt with is central to the integrity of the body's boundaries. Julia Kristeva develops this into a psychoanalytic reading of the ways in which such symbolic systems are constructed by, and function in response to, psychological needs. She connects dirt and bodily waste fluids with the border separating self from non-self, and in particular separating self from the ever-present threat of the engulfing mother: 'There I am at the border of my condition as a living being. My body extricates itself, as being alive, from that

8 Stoler (2002) p 66.
9 Gobineau (1915) p 33.
10 Douglas (1984) p 2.
11 Douglas (1984) p 3.
12 Douglas (1984) p 121.

border. Such wastes drop so that I might live.'[13] Thus, dirt and margins establish identity, identity relies on boundaries not being transgressed, and anything that symbolises a threat to boundaries must be abjected. This is particularly relevant to literary representations of miscegenation, in which the threat to subjectivity through the *breaching* of the body's boundaries is symbolised through the pervasive and interconnected iconography of blood, semen, dirt and disease.

Given the prevalence of infectious diseases in the nineteenth century, and inadequate means of controlling them, it is not surprising that the notion of their hidden corruption takes on a powerful metaphoric resonance, and, post-Darwin, carries with it the omnipresent terror of fall from white, middle class grace. In his 1886 study of disease, J Milner Fothergill employed Darwinian terminology to define disease as 'the undoing of evolution', and 'a species of degradation or reversion [...] or in other words, a dissolution, or return to more primitive and lower forms of life'.[14] Prevalent diseases that were never far from the nineteenth-century mind were, of course, syphilis and gonorrhoea, but tuberculosis was another threatening and secretive disease, in which bodily fluid transgressed corporeal margins, and it too was believed to be associated with sexual excess.[15] Thus, sexual desire and activity came to be figured as insidious impurity.

In order to relate this adequately to *settler* society it is necessary to recognise that in Western culture sex and sexual disease typically coalesce in the figure of the non-white body. Indeed, a particularly virulent form of venereal disease was incorrectly associated with non-Europeans, as demonstrated in Bracebridge Hemyng's essay 'Prostitution in London': 'the disease communicated by the Malays, Lascars, and Orientals generally, is said to be the most frightful form of lues to be met with in Europe'.[16] Sander L Gilman, for example, has pointed to the long history of the connection, stating: '[t]he association of the black with concupiscence reaches back into the Middle Ages.'[17] By the eighteenth century, both male and female blacks have become in the visual arts 'an icon for deviant sexuality in general'.[18] Then, well-established ideas of women as sources of corruption intersect with such perceptions of blackness to turn the black *woman* into a particularly potent symbol of debased sexuality and infection. Thereby she becomes the threatening locus of interrelated anxieties about the moral corruption of sex and of female sexuality in particular, the insidious corruption of disease, and the otherness of the racialised body. As Gilman says: 'Miscegenation was a fear (and a word) from the late nineteenth-century vocabulary of sexuality. It was a fear not merely of interracial sexuality but of its results, the decline of population.'[19] Mixed-race sex is dominantly presented in the settler novel as introducing metaphoric degenerative 'disease' into the blood of the resulting

---

13 Kristeva (1982) p 3.
14 Fothergill (1886) p 11.
15 See, for example, Motion (1997) p 500.
16 Hemyng, in Mayhew (1985) p 485.
17 Gilman (1985) p 79.
18 Gilman (1985) p 81.
19 Gilman (1985) p 256.

mixed-race offspring. What is at stake here is the promotion and preservation of a 'pure' white ruling group.

I also employ contemporary relational theory, and in particular the work of Jessica Benjamin, in order to connect the iconography of blood, dirt and disease already outlined to unconscious fantasies of otherness. Benjamin's position is arrived at through DW Winnicott's work, notably his contention that there is no such thing as a baby, only the mother-baby dyad. Although operating within a different conceptual framework from Kristeva, Winnicott too is concerned with boundaries between mother and child. He holds that in the earliest stages of the baby's life the mother is experienced by the baby as part of itself, and goes on to argue that as the baby develops it has to separate out from the mother and reach a point at which 'the mother becomes objectively perceived'.[20] Building on Winnicott's work, Benjamin claims that the developing child experiences a 'crisis' in recognising the mother as an independent subject.[21] This means that the child will find it difficult to achieve the *objective* perceptions of the mother that Winnicott refers to, and will therefore inevitably construct its own *subjective* view of her. For normal development the child must eventually achieve an objective view of the mother, but Benjamin argues that the objective view will never entirely replace the subjective fantasy, even in adult life. The two will co-exist and interact throughout.

According to this theory the relationship with the mother is paradigmatic of all later relationships. The mother is the original other/Other, and all subsequent others will engender reactions that replicate the primal 'crisis' of separation from her, generating relationships that are both intra-psychic (meaning that the subject takes into him/herself the other as a subjective fantasised Other), and inter-subjective (meaning that the subject recognises the other objectively as 'an equivalent but different center of existence').[22] The most interesting and complex cultural analyses are likely to concern intra-psychic relationships rather than inter-subjective ones, or at least to be aware of fluid shifting between the two. When an intra-psychic rather than inter-subjective relation is dominant, 'the subject [...] fills the position of the other [...] not with an outside, differentiated being but with the self's disowned, unconscious experience, which appears as a threatening Other'.[23] In this case the other becomes Other, an internalised object of fantasy, in a defensive process called projective identification. The greater the degree of perceived difference, the less likely the other is to be regarded objectively as an equivalent centre of self, and the more likely to be experienced as an internalised object of fantasy.

This theoretical perspective can usefully be applied to the history of black subordination. For the white coloniser the black races function as the fantasy M/Other, their existence as equivalent centres of self denied, which results in an

20 Winnicott (1966) p 131.
21 Benjamin (1995) p 38.
22 Benjamin (1995) p 6.
23 Benjamin (1995) p 18.

intra-psychic relationship in which black people become the split-off and disowned parts of the subordinating subject and thus a locus of threatening Otherness. Such fantasy relationships between whites and black are typically present in settler literature, and this psychological paradigm can be connected with the discourses of blood, dirt and disease already mobilised, to suggest that in novels about miscegenation the threatening internalised object is often represented at the level of unconscious metaphor through blood pollution, mixed-race pregnancies, and pregnancies experienced as disease or poison.

That cleanliness was a major concern in settler society can be deduced from the number of advertisements devoted to cleaning products of various kinds. On 6 March 1929, for example, the East London *Daily Dispatch* includes advertisements for *Pepsodent*, which provides 'Film-Free Teeth' that are 'white and sparkling'; for *Sunlight Soap*; for *Amami* shampoos; and for *Ronuk* floor polish, that not only 'Polishes' and 'Preserves', but, significantly, 'Purifies', and is described as 'The Sanitary Floor Polish'. Furthermore, there are numerous advertisements concerned with health products of various kinds. For example, *Rose's Lime Juice* is described as 'The Meal Time Health Drink', and 'Wholesome';[24] *Waverley Blankets* are promoted, since 'Healthy covering at night is *vital* to your health'; *Rumford Baking Powder* is known for its 'healthful properties', and it 'actually adds *real food value* to all baked foods'; an instant drink called *Postum* is advertised as being 'genuinely good for you', and the reader is encouraged to try it for the next thirty days 'and see how much better you feel'; while *Symington's Pea Flour* makes soups and stews 'more nourishing'.[25] Stoler points out that '[d]isease and lethargy were deemed a threat to all Europeans, but children were thought particularly vulnerable',[26] so it is not surprising that there is a particular emphasis on baby foods and supplements. For example, *Virol* is recommended to mothers to enable them to 'Take special care of your *boy* baby'. The advertisement explains that boys are often more delicate than girls, and concludes: 'Many a strong man to-day has to thank a childhood diet of *Virol* for the splendid constitution that has remained with him throughout his life.'[27] Clearly, the health of the settler is at a premium, and with the barely disguised suggestion of 'virility' in the name *Virol*, successful settler reproduction is also being promoted. Health, hygiene and strength combine in these advertisements to protect and mark off settler society at its boundaries.

Of particular threat to the white settler body, which needs the protection of all these products if it is to retain its (precarious) integrity, is the black African body. In her autobiographical work *Oh, Miss Maginty!*, which records her time spent living on the diamond diggings of the Orange River, the novelist Thirza Nash makes considerable use of dirt as a marker of racial/social boundaries. She describes her maid, Annie, in terms of both dirt and impropriety of dress, so that dirt functions as an implicit marker of sexual corruption:

---

24 *Daily Dispatch*, Wednesday 15 October 1924, front page.

25 *Daily Dispatch*, Wednesday 6 March 1929, 'Eve's Corner' page.

26 Stoler (2002) p 35.

27 *Daily Dispatch*, Wednesday 15 October 1924, front page.

> She is so dirty – she trails about in voluminous, long print skirts and leaves the back of her scanty blouse (the only above-waist garment she has on) all open and unsecured so that when she bends it falls down in front of her in such an immodest way. She is always chewing – when she peels the potatoes she drops the peel on the floor and eats scraps of it. When she cleans the plates and pots she employs her forefinger before she applies the clout, and licks it. She asked me for a 'pruimpje,' that is a plug of tobacco, and she chews *that*. And spits – all over – or rather she did until I told her to stop it. And her kid chews all day long too.[28]

In fact, as we learn later, Annie is hungry and short on life's pleasures, so it is small wonder that she scrapes the remains from the plates and begs tobacco. At the level of the symbolic rather than the real, however, dirt and implications of immodesty combine to construct the inferior and threatening Other. Referring to another servant, Anna, Nash explicitly establishes the boundaries between Anna's body and her own by her description of Anna's dirt, and her own responsive washing ritual. She gives Anna a gift of sugar: 'when she realised she was getting so much sugar for nothing, awe came into her face. She took my hand and kissed it. I stood it. Poor soul, had no one ever given her a gift in her life? Then I came away and washed my hand hard.'[29]

Clearly, any kind of contact with the black body poses a threat to the white settler, but the greatest danger lies in miscegenation, when the boundaries of the white body are literally breached by the sexual act. This threat is obsessively revisited in settler fiction that attempts to encode taboos around sexual behaviour through the cultural imaginary of disease. It is a highly voyeuristic writing, in which the colonial gaze focuses on black bodies in an act of surveillance, functioning to police the boundaries between black and white through oppositions based on dirt and disease, but sexual relationships are in fact revealed to be a contested exchange, exposing fractures in European identity through transgressed and infected bodily boundaries. At the centre of the sexual threat are the bodies of women, both black and white, since they are typically the locus of metaphors of infection, even in the novels written by women. Men's bodies do deteriorate as a result of miscegenation, but descriptions of them tend to focus on the exterior: bodies become dirty, hair becomes unkempt, clothes become filthy and shabby. In contrast, the woman's body is conceived of in terms of its interior; it is envisaged as *housing* infection. Women's bodies are ambivalent sites in this fiction: white bodies are hallowed temples of the maternity that settler dreams of a dominant white race in South Africa rely on, yet they also exhibit unruly signs of excess, of which, ironically, childbirth itself is one, since it often results in monstrous, mixed-race progeny; black bodies are degenerate and repellent, but are also erotically irresistible.

'I have a feeling about colour as if it were a catching disease', says Miriam, a character in Sarah Gertrude Millin's *Adam's Rest*.[30] Her words reveal the

---

28 Nash (1920) p 101.

29 Nash (1920) p 161.

30 Millin (1922) p 35.

importance of metaphors of disease as markers of degenerate and essentialised racial types. The psychoanalytic theory already discussed can be used to develop this beyond the literary strategy of metaphor, however, to show that this figuring functions as an indicator of profound psychological anxiety. In Millin's *Dark River*, the white John Oliver lives with Annie, a black woman, and fathers four children. The metaphorical conjunction of dirt and degradation is made explicit in a description of Annie's effect on John: 'In time he even became accustomed – or, at least, indifferent – to her habitual unsavouriness. He lost his sense of delicacy – his plunge in the river ceased to be a daily habit.'[31] Eventually John leaves his black family and marries his white love, Hester, but while Hester is pregnant she discovers his past. So contaminating is the sexual contact with a black woman that Hester's pregnancy becomes figured as, in effect, a sexual disease. She says: 'I hope I may die before I bear a child to you. I hope the child may die before it is born. I can never be clean again – never. You have degraded me to the level of that coloured woman. She and I have both borne you children.'[32] Later, speaking to her sister Alma about her desire to kill herself, Hester's dialogue connects the existing metaphorical complex of dirt, degradation and venereal disease with the sexual suggestiveness and blood-threat of vampirism: 'How else can I be free of him while his child is getting life from my body. I sound [...] like a stage character, but that is how I feel. As if a vampire were sucking my blood.'[33] Thus, the influence of ideas about race purity, expressed by theorists such as Gobineau, come into powerful conjunction with the need of an emerging settler society to connect its sexuality with its building of a national identity as white South Africans. Furthermore, the pregnancy functions as a persecutory object. The racial Other is so potent in intra-psychic fantasy that it infects Hester with the terror of engulfment, even though her contact with it is an indirect one. And through her *own* pregnancy, which is *not* the result of miscegenation, Hester symbolically bears the excessive and monstrous products of inter-racial sex in her own body, even though she is innocent of sexual transgression herself.

Millin's *God's Stepchildren* reveals the typical construction of black women as sexually excessive. Silla, a seventeen-year-old Hottentot girl, provocatively tries to teach the English missionary, the Reverend Flood, to pronounce the 'Hottentot click': 'She would open her mouth and show him her red tongue achieving the correct effect.'[34] Like the incompletely expelled mother theorised by Kristeva, she threatens to engulf Flood in her open mouth. His decision to marry her is preceded by a description of his own deterioration into a dirty, neglected and unwholesome man, and the suggestion of degeneration caused by his association with Silla is emphasised by the fact that Mr Burtwell, a fellow missionary, attributes Flood's decision to 'mental sickness'.[35] Thus, the white man is symbolically infected by the engulfing black female, and his subjectivity is

---

31 Millin (1920) p 72.
32 Millin (1920) p 219.
33 Millin (1920) p 223.
34 Millin (1924) p 37.
35 Millin (1924) p 51.

seriously under threat, no longer protected by rituals of cleanliness. Millin's narrative figures the black woman not as a subject in reality but as a fantasised intra-psychic object consuming Flood, and functioning at the projective level as both loathsome and desired. Notions of consumption, dirt and infection are thus brought into connection with the sexual theme at the level of fantasy. Embedded in this text, as in so many others, is the settler's masochistic imagining of loss of subjectivity and engulfment by the 'primitive', and blood functions as the internalised persecutory object in the mixed-race children produced, staining them forever with the otherness that haunts and terrifies the settler.

In Ethelreda Lewis's *The Harp*, Andrew Falconer marries Dora who, unknown to him, is already pregnant and intends to pass the child off as his. When Charlie is born, however, it is obvious that Andrew cannot be his father. A young nurse looks closely at the child, and then 'runs shivering' to her room. Her recognition that Charlie is of mixed race remains unspoken, but the silence suggests it to the reader. The shock of the young nurse stands for the future reactions of South African society. She is 'shaken with cold nausea' and she 'cries her heart out as she lies on the bed'.[36] She weeps for the innocent young man who was so easily tricked, but she also weeps 'for her father and mother, for her little white room at home, for quiet, safe voices under the small roof'.[37] In other words, she weeps for white blood purity that has been corrupted. At an unconscious level she may also weep for the loss of her own sexual innocence, since the appearance of a mixed-race baby draws particular attention to the sexual act that precedes its birth. Placed against the white body of his mother, Charlie is a reminder of the black or coloured body that engaged in sexual intercourse to sire him. The narrative prepares for its horrific revelation that Dora's relationship with her child's coloured father was consensual rather than, as Andrew has always assumed, a rape, by connecting Dora with flagrant behaviour that is suggestive of a 'primitive' sexuality. When she breast-feeds her second child, Andrew's 'pure white' son Olaf, she is: '[s]hameless as a savage [...] almost flaunting her tigerish duties until the day when Andrew ordered her to her own room.'[38] Andrew's discomfort at the sight of his son 'feeding at her breast' is described as 'something stronger than an outrage to his delicate boyish instinct'.[39] This suggests that it is not simply the act of overt breast-feeding in general that disturbs him, but the specific feeding of his pure-blooded child by her. Implicit is Dora's metaphorical contamination through her previous sexual contact with a man who was not white, and through her bearing of his mixed-race child, a contamination that still stains her body and the milk she produces. While *blood* functions as the threatening internalised object in Millin's novel, here it is the mixed-race *child* Dora has carried in her womb that represents the internalised fantasy Other: an Other that corrupts Dora's expelled bodily fluids. What Andrew wants hidden from his sight is his son's physical contact with this defiled woman, particularly

---

36 Lewis (1925) p 126.
37 Lewis (1925) p 127.
38 Lewis (1925) p 155.
39 Lewis (1925) p 156.

as breast-feeding replicates the sexual act, an aspect emphasised by Dora's 'tigerish' pleasure. Even though Andrew's son is not of mixed race, at a symbolic level he ingests with Dora's milk the (venereal) infection of blackness that has grown in her body.

The notion of infection is developed later in *The Harp* when Charlie, the mixed-race boy, becomes ill, and we are told that this is an 'infectious' case.[40] Andrew's son Olaf is forbidden to enter Charlie's room, but Dora goes out leaving the boys alone. Hearing his brother call, Olaf goes to him. He becomes infected and subsequently dies, symbolically wiped out by Charlie's impurity. Thus, Charlie's disease is a marker of the corrupting nature of miscegenation that defiles the white race. Millin's *God's Stepchildren* functions through repeated sexual acts, making the narrative's figurative dependence on the imagery of venereal disease obvious. In Lewis's novel the dependence is less direct, but the representation of Charlie as a tainted presence at the heart of the family is similarly suggestive of a domestic/sexual corruption that cannot be evaded.

In an interesting variation, leprosy also functions in colonial writing as an image of (sexual) contamination associated with black bodies. There are many examples, but I select Dorothea Fairbridge's short story 'Pamela' (1911) since its reference to penetration and blood makes plain the way in which representations of racial infection are haunted by the idea of venereal disease:

> Her father died of the sickness before her. He took it from a native who doctored him for a thorn in his foot, and bound up the wound with a strip torn from his own rags. So he drew the poison into his blood for a legacy to his children's children. God help them![41]

Numerous novels could have been used to illustrate these points, but it is also important to acknowledge that there are some novels that suggest the *attractions* of black/white relationships. For example, Perceval Gibbon's *Margaret Harding* presents a positive view of a friendship between the eponymous white heroine and a black doctor, Kamis, returned to South Africa from training in England, yet even here disease plays a significant role. The relationship is presented as a friendship rather than an overtly sexual liaison, but at the level of metaphor a sexual relationship is surely indicated. Margaret suffers from that *other* 'sexual' disease, tuberculosis, and at one point has a haemorrhage. Only Kamis can save her, but, as a black man, he is not allowed to enter her bedroom. Instead Ford, a suitor to Margaret, has to treat her by following Kamis's instructions. As Kamis's proxy he goes into her bedroom and injects her on Kamis's behalf. The scene is clearly suggestive of sexual consummation, with Ford a conduit for Kamis's forbidden desire. Margaret's excessively desiring body pours out blood from her lungs, in a metaphoric mirroring of the expulsion of menstrual blood and babies. It seems that the discourse of infection is, even in this more ambiguous representation, still a potent one for a writer addressing miscegenation.

---

40 Lewis (1925) p 205.

41 Fairbridge (1998) p 359.

This chapter has concentrated on black and white bodies in English language settler fiction, and although it is beyond its scope to do more than that, it should at least be mentioned that race relations in South Africa were more complex than a simple black/white binary opposition. As Robert Thornton points out:

> Westerners in southern Africa did not see themselves as a homogenous group uniformly representative of self-evident European power and culture. The field was not so neatly structured and the ways that cultural understandings emerged were not so orderly. The reality of southern African history and the identities and attributes of the contending parties were much too messy to sustain any neat tale of White vs Black, Intruder vs Indigene, the West vs Africa.[42]

For writers who obsessively revisited the topic of miscegenation, the tale *was* one of 'White vs Black'. However, Thirza Nash was unusual amongst settler novelists in not writing about mixed-race sex, and for her the debate sharpened into a class-inflected one concerned with 'qualities' of whiteness, and, as her novels demonstrate, the 'quality' of white bourgeois identity required more complex modes of identification than skin colour alone. Poor whites and the Trekboer replace Africans in her fiction as the inferior Other, embodying the ever-present threat of degeneration from an assumed state of superiority that is perceived to lie not just in whiteness *per se*, but in *middle class* whiteness. Significantly, the metaphors of blood, dirt and disease already discussed as constructing discourses of race are the strategic tools she uses for her exclusions of certain white people from middle class identity. Degeneration of the white settler body is a concept so terrifying that her final novel, *For Passion is Darkness*, debates extensively the issue of eugenics for the 'poor demented diseased wretch'[43] who typifies the poor whites in the novel. The most sympathetic characters are against eugenics, yet the depiction of dirt and disease amongst these people, and the extended debates on the topic, render the novel's conclusions ambivalent. It must have struck a fearful chord with many of Nash's middle class readers, who felt threatened by increasing numbers of poor whites and black Africans. The story also concerns the passing on of madness through a family's bloodline, so that even in a novel that is not directly about miscegenation, blood, dirt and disease coalesce as connected metaphors for white, middle class, settler sanctity, and function to suggest the ever-present psychological threat of the intra-psychic persecutory Other.

The novels discussed here can be seen fruitfully as frontier narratives, generated by settlers for whom margins and boundaries were inevitably significant. The history of settlement in South Africa is one of continual pressure by white settlers on the edges of their territory, and the gradual acquisition of more land. The 'boundaries' of the body may well be experienced as under particular pressure when the 'boundaries' of land dominate existence, and images of blood, dirt and disease intersect in this fiction to articulate powerful fantasies of otherness, and anxieties about the integrity of the white settler body.

---

42 Thornton (1995) p 194.

43 Nash (1951) p 106.

Bibliography

Benjamin, Jessica, *Like Subjects, Love Objects: Essays on Recognition and Sexual Difference*, 1995, New Haven, CT and London: Yale University Press.

Daily Dispatch, East London, 15 October 1924 and 6 March 1929.

Douglas, Mary, *Purity and Danger: An Analysis of the Concepts of Pollution and Taboo*, 1984, London and New York: Routledge. (First published, 1966, London: Routledge and Kegan Paul.)

Fairbridge, Dorothea, 'Pamela', in Boehmer, Elleke (ed), *Empire Writing: An Anthology of Colonial Literature 1870–1918*, 1998, Oxford and New York: Oxford University Press, pp 349–60.

Fothergill, J Milner, *Disease: A Study*, 1886, London: Baillière, Tindall & Cox.

Gibbon, Perceval, *Margaret Harding*, 1911, London: Methuen.

Gilman, Sander L, *Difference and Pathology: Stereotypes of Sexuality, Race, and Madness*, 1985, Ithaca, NY and London: Cornell University Press.

Gobineau, Joseph Arthur Comte de, *The Inequality of Human Races*, vol 1 (1854) 1915, London: William Heinemann.

Hemyng, Bracebridge, 'Prostitution in London', in Mayhew, Henry, *London Labour and the London Poor*, selections made and introduced by Victor Neuburg, 1985, Harmondsworth: Penguin, pp 473–91.

Klein, Carole, *Doris Lessing*, 2000, London: Duckworth.

Kristeva, Julia, *Powers of Horror: An Essay on Abjection*,1982, New York: Columbia University Press.

Lewis, Ethelreda, *The Harp*, 1925, New York: George H Doran.

Millin, Sarah Gertrude, *Dark River*, 1920, London: W Collins Sons and Co.

Millin, Sarah Gertrude, *Adam's Rest*, 1922, London: W Collins Sons and Co.

Millin, Sarah Gertrude, *God's Stepchildren*, 1924, USA: Grosset & Dunlap.

Millin, Sarah Gertrude, *South Africa*, 1941, London: William Collins. This later edition has the publisher as William Collins.

Motion, Andrew, *Keats*, 1997, London: Faber and Faber.

Nash, Thirza, *Oh, Miss Maginty!*, 1920, London: Hodder and Stoughton.

Nash, Thirza, *For Passion is Darkness*, 1951, London: Cassell and Company.

Pifer, Drury, *Innocents in Africa*, 1994, London: Granta Books.

Ranger, Terence, 'The invention of tradition in colonial Africa', in Hobsbawm, Eric and Ranger, Terence (eds), *The Invention of Tradition*, 1983, Cambridge: Cambridge University Press, pp 211–62.

Stoler, Ann Laura, *Carnal Knowledge and Imperial Power: Race and the Intimate in Colonial Rule*, 2002, Berkeley, CA, Los Angeles, CA, and London: University of California Press.

Thornton, Robert, 'The colonial, the imperial, and the creation of the "European" in Southern Africa', in Carrier, James G (ed), *Occidentalism: Images of the West*, 1995, Oxford: Clarendon, pp 192–217.

Winnicott, Donald W, 'The Child in the Family Group', 1966, in *Home is Where We Start From*, 1990, Harmondsworth: Penguin, pp 129–41.

CHAPTER 8

SEX IN A HOT CLIMATE: MORAL DEGENERACY AND EROTIC EXCESS IN *THE STORY OF JAN DARAA*

Rachel Harrison

> The reason I wrote Jan Daraa was because I thought I was in the last throes of my life. Thinking I was close to death, I wanted to put everything I had into writing my masterpiece. That's what my body was telling me to do, so I went with my gut instinct.[1]

> Jan Daraa – that's my name. So let me introduce myself as the owner of this, the strangest of stories, since we'll be spending quite some time together from now. That is, as long as nothing happens to me along the way. For at least two things could happen. Yes, I could go mad. Or I could die.[2]

Introduction

In 1964, Utsanaa Phloengtham's *The Story of Jan Daraa (Reuang khorng Jan Daraa)* was serialised in *Sayaam Rat Weekly*, the newspaper where he worked as a senior journalist.[3] The novel's focus on the sexual adventure and misadventure of its hero Jan Daraa (literally 'Jan the Accursed') was initially greeted with uproar from readers, who found it obscene (*ujaat*) and immoral (*anaajaan*).[4] According to one commentator, most viewed the work as pornographic, disgusting, or at best a

---

1 Utsanaa Phloengtham, in reference to *The Story of Jan Daraa*, written in 1964, 24 years before his death in 1988, following a protracted illness; see Utsanaa (1985). Marcel Barang, editor of the English translation of *The Story of Jan Daraa*, notes Utsanaa's long history of bad health, induced by heavy drinking. According to Barang, the author was plagued since his mid-thirties with stomach ulcers, had a third of his stomach removed in 1959, underwent further surgery between 1970 and 1973, and was frequently hospitalised in the years prior to his death: Barang (1994) p 291.

2 Utsanaa Phloengtham, *The Story of Jan Daraa* (1964): see Utsanaa (2000) p 13.

3 Utsanaa Phloengtham is the pseudonym of Pramoon Unhathoop (1920–88). Utsanaa is primarily regarded as a short story writer and translator of fiction into Thai, most particularly of Steinbeck's *Tortilla Flat* (*Lokiiyachon*) and of DH Lawrence's short story *The Woman Who Rode Away* (*Lon khii maa khorng khao pai*). *Reuang khorng Jan Daraa* is the author's only novel.

4 See Katsamaa (2001) p 13. Katsamaa quotes the response to the novel, that it was deemed *po nai radap ujaat anaajaan* (pornographic to the level of obscenity and immorality), but does not provide the source of this comment.

The novel continued to be serialised due to the support of Khukrit Pramoj, editor of Sayaam Rat. Khukrit dispelled criticism of the work with the simple statement, *phom chorp* ('I like it'). The publication of *Jan Daraa* was also commended by fellow erotic novelist Rong Wongsawan, who proclaimed it to be 'a novel about sexual desire which makes a most daring appearance in the world of books'; see Khomnai (1987) p 90.

lesson on the nature of sexual perversion.[5] Even the author himself alluded to his sense in writing the piece, of 'treading the very thin line which divides art from immorality'.[6] For, despite the common construction of Thailand in the Western imagination as a site of sexual liberation (based on the widespread availability of commercial sex) that has held fast since at least the time of the Vietnam War, sexuality is in fact viewed with disapproval and is seldom a topic deemed appropriate for Thai public discourse.[7]

This cultural sensitivity is captured in the words of the contemporary female novelist Anchan, that 'sex is an issue rarely raised and little understood' in a Thai society she characterises as 'essentially conservative'.[8] Penny Van Esterik confirms this in her observation that: 'Talking about sexual matters, particularly in mixed groups is not polite (*phit kalathesa*)',[9] while Sutham Thammrongwit labels this 'culture of silence' surrounding discussion of sexuality in Thailand as the consequence of predominant distaste for overt expressions of sexuality:[10]

> The topic of sex is taboo in many societies where it is linked to notions of danger, destructiveness and the darker powers that be. Here sex is a great sin, associated with the negative values of craving (*kilet*), passion (*tanhaa*) and lust (*raakha*), and precipitates the downfall of the individual, and hence society at large.[11]

As Peter Jackson demonstrates with reference to Thailand's culture of silence on sexual matters, 'while this regime of dissimulating power may not interfere in private sexual practice, it is far from benign. It is a form of power that permits all manner of consensual sexual acts but forcefully silences and invisibilises public representations'.[12] Jackson's point is deeply pertinent to the staging of sexuality that enters the public sphere through discussions in Thai fiction given that the contradictions he argues to exist between private sexual practice and the invisibility of sexuality in the public domain produce 'psychic tensions among those who live under the Thai regime of power'.[13] Nowhere better are these psychic tensions expressed through literature than in *The Story of Jan Daraa*.[14]

---

5 Khomnai (1987) p 88.

6 See Katsamaa (2001) p 14.

7 For a further discussion of the construction of Thailand as a site of unrestrained sexuality in the Western imagination, see Harrison (2001). For discussions of the relationship between sexuality and public discourse in Thailand with particular reference to homosexuality, see Jackson (1999).

8 See Anonymous (2003)

9 Van Esterik (2000) p 212.

10 Sutham (2001) p 125.

11 Sutham (2001) p 120.

12 Jackson (2003).

13 Jackson (2003) p 12.

14 As Penny Van Esterik appositely observes, the consequence of placing sexuality in the public domain is that, 'In Thailand, as in other parts of the world, exposing what should be private to the public gaze entails a loss of face'; see Van Esterik (2000) p 219. Jackson further contextualises this in his specific study of Thai sanctions against masculine homoeroticism at the level of discourse, when he writes: 'In a culture which places great significance on preserving face (*naa*) and constructing and maintaining positive images (*phaap-phot*) of the self, innuendo, gossips, and other forms of criticism are extremely strong forces of ensuring conformity [...]'; see Jackson (1999) p 239.

The aim of this chapter is therefore to examine the multi-layered tensions and contradictions that appear to co-exist within Thai attitudes to sexuality as evinced on the pages of this literary text, a work now considered a modern Thai classic despite, or perhaps because of, the controversy surrounding its erotic content.[15] Its further purpose is to suggest how such apparent contradictions significantly complicate widespread popular Occidental imaginings, fantasies and simplistic constructions of Thailand as a site of sexual excess.[16] The following analysis of the novel not only underscores the complex interconnections that exist between Thai beliefs concerning gender, sexuality, physical and psychological ill health, but also serves to indicate that these features cannot be reduced to Western paradigms and instead oblige a reading that is cognisant of local patterns of meaning.

Psychological frailty, sexual over-indulgence and physical decay in *The Story of Jan Daraa*

The Story of Jan Daraa functions at a number of differing, and apparently contradictory, interpretative levels, making reference to sexuality in a variety of different tones. In certain scenes sex is connoted as mindless but healthy fun, yet raucous and devoid of the aesthetic sense it acquires at other moments in the novel. In contrast to this, it is alternatively and frequently portrayed in a deeply moralising and puritanical tone that draws its inspiration from a Buddhist distaste for the corporeal blended with a quasi-Victorian belief in the evils of sexual desire. Moreover, these multi-layered and often seemingly incongruous attitudes to sexuality reveal more than merely the personal tastes and attitudes of its author, Utsanaa Phloengtham; they reflect more broadly the various belief systems at play with regard to sexuality in Thai society at large. As a result, this text further serves to question assumptions grounded in Western literary studies that fictional texts bear little relationship to wider social truths. Instead it confirms critical observations that close links exist between writers and society in Thailand, as elsewhere in South East Asia.[17] Given their close involvement with the professions of teaching and journalism, modern Thai authors frequently envisage

---

15 To date, the novel is in its seventh edition (rendering it a well-established work by Thai publishing standards). It has been canonised as one of the 20 best novels of Thailand by the widely-researched project of Marcel Barang (1994) (although it does not appear on the list compiled in 1998 by Thai academic Witthayakorn Chiangkul as one of 'the hundred works that Thais should read' (*rooi lem thii khon thai khuan aan*)) and has consequently been translated into English under the same project; see Utsanaa (1995). *The Story of Jan Daraa* also appears in two film versions, the most recent of which was directed and produced by Nonzee Nimibutr in 2001.

16 Notions of Thailand as a site of excess are also to be found in academic studies. Anthropologist Rosalind C Morris (1994, 2002), for example, frequently regards it as a place of multiple 'excesses', especially sexual excesses. Jackson (forthcoming) warns, however, that with regard to this tendency in Western analysis 'the full implications of Thailand's excesses are not developed, namely, that the empirical "excessiveness" of cultural forms that defy delimitation within Western theory is a sign that this theory needs to be rethought'.

17 See, for example, Manas (1982); Salleh (1977); Anderson and Mendiones (1985); Braginsky (2001); and Harrison (2000).

a similar didactic and/or socially and politically committed purpose for their fiction.[18]

Set for the most part in a minor palace compound in Bangkok, *The Story of Jan Daraa* is a self-confessional tale, narrated in *skaz* style in a direct address by the 40-year-old Jan to his readers. Jan introduces himself with a statement expressing the possibility that he might either go mad or die before relating the full story of his life, whereupon he muses on the topic of suicide, on the various causes of death and on spontaneous rebirth. Buddhist notions of cyclical birth, death and rebirth are thus placed centre stage in the narrative, reiterated by Jan's subsequent discussion of the tragic circumstances of his arrival in the world, at which his mother died in labour, poignantly transforming the delivery room into a mortuary. Consequently, Jan's so-called father – *Khun Luang* ('His Lordship') – vows a hatred for his 'son' that comes to bind the two characters together in inseparable psychological pain.

In childhood, Jan longs with utter loneliness for the dead mother he feels responsible for having killed:

> I knew that the reason my mother had died was because she had given birth to me. Oh yes, I knew it all right, because my father never stopped chiding me over it. He thought it was all my fault – and he made me admit that I was totally to blame. [...] Everyone knew I had no mother because she had died giving birth to me. So even at that tender age I had to accept I was in the wrong. I knew how terribly wicked I had been and, although I had never heard of the crime of matricide, I knew how bad I was. For nothing could be more vicious than to murder your own mother. And I knew that if you did something wrong, you deserved punishment for it.[19]

Herein lies the root of Jan's psychological trauma and unstable sense of self, mental disorders which present themselves pathologically in the novel in the form of insatiable carnal desires, and which are compounded by Jan's early realisation that His Lordship cannot be his real father. Issues of guilt, retribution and lack of clear origins are placed to the fore in the narrative and bound into the theme of sexuality. Jan explains to the reader that the obsession with breasts he develops in adult life comes from having been deprived of the maternal breast and instead reared on Glaxo baby milk: 'My desires were for really big breasts, the bigger the better. Had they been big enough to reach the skies, I'd have been in my seventh heaven.'[20] The boy seeks maternal affection in his mother's country cousin, Aunt Waat, with whom he has his first sexual experience, at the age of 10, unintentionally ejaculating after she permits him to suckle at her breast for comfort. Although Jan does not know exactly what is happening in his body, he nevertheless confesses to the reader an instinctive awareness that 'my sheer contentment (*kasem jai*) and delight (*khwaam prii prem*) was coloured by a sense of

---

18 Writers in Thailand are rarely able to earn a living from the publication of fictional works alone and of the additional professions they practice, journalism and teaching are among the most common.

19 Utsanaa (2000) pp 19–20.

20 Utsanaa (2000) p 40.

shame (*khwaam ot suu*) and evil (*maan*)'.[21] Utsanaa's choice of the word *maan* to allude to Jan's feelings of disgrace is a potent one, derived from Mara, the Buddhist figure of demonic temptation. As such, it clearly connotes the ambivalent attitude to sexuality which, as this chapter argues, is entirely typical of the novel and representative of widely-held socio-cultural views.

Prefiguring the novel's standpoint that lust and desire form both the very *raison d'être* and the precise demise of his existence, Jan recalls his very first memory as a child, from the age of four, as a sexual one: he wakes at night in bed next to Aunt Waat to find her submitting to the sexual attentions of Khun Luang. The man continues unabashed and Jan repeatedly returns in the novel to the hatred that this event instils in him for his 'father', for putting Aunt Waat through such dishonour before a witness. In a style typical of Utsanaa's depiction of sexuality as shameful crime, Jan relates the scene with quasi-simulated distaste:

> ... What the hell was going on!
>
> Two adults, naked, in the state of children taking a bath, were lying together in such a naughty way they deserved a good thrashing. I had never witnessed, nor ever expected to witness such a thing happening before my very eyes, and when I did I felt instantly feverish and sickened to the bone.[22]

Here sex is depicted as base (*khorng tam*), reprehensible and fully capable of triggering ill health.

As a teenager, Jan develops his sexual experiences with the maidservants in the palace compound, all members of the extensive harem of Khun Luang, a man whose philandering is referred to with constant moral distaste. Both Jan and his best friend Khein engage in 'heavenly pursuits' (*tham wimaan*) with these girls, who are depicted as little more than low class 'slappers', knowing no sexual bounds. Intercourse with them is an entirely earthy experience, as Jan reveals in his remarks on the unsanitary state of Khein's bed, where the action takes place:

> Whenever I think of Khein and his bed I always think of a pig wallowing in filth – seemingly content enough, as if its body were only a matter of its surface skin (*pleuak nork*). For however much filth it had been rolling in, nothing could penetrate it to the core, or touch its real essence, which was a mere tiny spot concealed deep within. Khein always slept soundly on his mat, soiled with the stains of his own promiscuity.[23]

Relationships with two different women which Jan strikes up in his later teens provide for an expansion in his categorisation of the opposite sex and a splitting between love and lust that underscores the novel's morality throughout. Firstly, Jan meets Hyacinth, a modest and reserved schoolgirl whom he demurely accompanies home at the end of classes, whom he deeply loves and respects 'as one would one's own mother', and with whom he has no physical relationship.

21 Utsanaa (2000) p 39.

22 Utsanaa (2000) p 50.

23 Utsanaa (2000) pp 94–95.

Hyacinth is, in Jan's view, 'purification for the mind', his soul mate and the woman he hopes to marry, but she dies of typhoid before he is able to do so.

In stark contrast to Hyacinth, the second woman he encounters in his late teens is Khun Luang's former wife, the seductive noblewoman Mrs Bunleuang (alias Mrs B):

> Among Mrs Bunleuang's most singular features were her enormous and voluptuous breasts, the like of which I had never laid eyes on in my life. Nor had she ever felt obliged to conceal their majestic curves, unlike most women of her day. Not only did she fail to conceal them, but she also wore the most revealing of low cut blouses. And rarely did she have a bra on underneath. Not only that, she often went around completely bare breasted at home, so that she became, in my mind, a figure of worship and contemplation for my regular wet dreams.[24]

Mrs B's subsequent affair with Jan forms the major erotic focus of the novel, described in highly aestheticised terms through reference to the symbols and metaphors of classical Thai literary works. In contrast to the squalid setting of Jan's escapades with the servant girls, sexual exchanges with Mrs B are conducted in the beautiful surroundings of her quarters, among furniture, books and accessories imported from abroad. Their relationship is one perpetuated not only by erotic desire, but by the finer things of life.

As the result of a conspiracy against him by Khun Luang's obnoxious daughter Kaew, Jan is expelled from the compound and comes to learn of his true origins, as the child conceived following the gang-rape of his mother on a visit to the countryside. Once again, sex is linked in the work to acts of brutality and shame.

Jan returns to the compound several years later to perform the honourable duty of marrying the 15-year-old Kaew, who has been made pregnant by her half-brother Khajorn. He agrees to the marriage on the condition that the palace become his own. Gradually he follows in Khun Luang's footsteps, becoming a precise mirror image of the very man he hates. He returns to an intermittent relationship with Mrs B, together with seducing most of the servants and women in the harem Khun Luang is no longer physically capable of servicing himself, for Khun Luang's sexual excesses have been punished with impotence, the novel's 'scientific' explanation for which lies in a comparison of males to guns: 'We all start off with a supply of 5000 bullets', Jan explains:

> ... and the more we squander them, the faster our stocks are depleted. And once we've exhausted our allocation, there's not a supply unit in the world that can re-equip us with new provisions, be it in the form of monkey glands or hormones of any brand.[25]

Khun Luang's surfeit of desire has resulted in premature aging, the fermented traces of lust having clearly bled into his skin, which has yellowed like a foetus preserved in formaldehyde. As Jan remarks:

---

24 Utsanaa (2000) p 68.
25 Utsanaa (2000) pp 107–08.

> Although he had never been ill before, his health was clearly failing (*ruang roi*), the powerful cravings (*kilet*) that drove his intoxicating carnal desires (*kaam khun*) having sucked the juices from his body, eaten away at his flesh and shrivelled him up before his time.[26]

In keeping with the novel's quasi-puritanical stand on profligacy, Jan's conclusions regarding Khun Luang's declining health lead him to understand one significant truth, 'which is that lust tempts all men to feed on their own flesh and blood'. Here sexuality is viewed not only as morally reprehensible, but it is also frequently referred to as an attack on both the physical and spiritual self.

As retribution for the incestuous relationship between Kaew and Khunjorn, their child, Prii Daraa ('Prii the Despicable'), is born handicapped. Moreover, Jan's worst suspicions are confirmed when he discovers Mrs B and Kaew engaged in a lesbian affair. While this episode is inevitably included in the novel as yet another possible source of titillation, Utsanaa also depicts it with disgust, moral outrage and fear of the threat it poses to male sexual prowess:

> I was aroused by the sight of two pale, naked bodies, despite the indistinctness of the image in the darkness. [...] But when I saw exactly what was going on, there was no way it could have excited in me the thrusts of carnal desire (*ranjuan*) that instinct might normally have dictated. Instead I was cast into a terrible abyss of turmoil, shock and horror. For what did I see before me but two women, so different in age as to be mother and daughter, encoiled in each other's lascivious and tender embrace in an expression of lust so obscene (*u-laamok*), bizarre (*utri*) and misgendered (*phit phet*) that they deserved to be struck down by lightening.[27]

Jan is relieved, however, to discover that, unlike Kaew, whose 'condition' or 'ailment' (*aakaan*) as a lesbian 'is sadly and quite hopelessly incurable',[28] Mrs B proves retrievable from the ills of homosexuality.[29]

Perhaps as an attack on her lesbianism, Jan rapes Kaew with the intention of siring a child of his own. He explains her lack of sexual response to the rape in the same way as he justifies her hatred of motherhood – as perverse, homosexual abnormality:

---

26 Utsanaa (2000) p 106.

27 Utsanaa (2000) p 3. Nevertheless, the author is unable to resist the opportunity for an aside, furnishing the reader with the prejudiced opinion that a fully satisfying lesbian affair could only be conducted with the use of equipment 'ordered confidentially from abroad'; see Utsanaa (1995) p 243. This corresponds with his attitudes to autonomous female sexual pleasure exhibited through his squeamishness over female masturbation: 'I had the well-known outlet of my five fingers to release my pent-up feelings – how about her then? Women must have their own ways of coping with the problem. How do they do it? How would I know? I didn't – not for sure anyway. Better leave the matter alone, then'; Utsanaa (1995) p 173. While Utsanaa is inclined to add a scene of lesbian encounter to his novel, his imagination does not draw him to expand upon the details of female masturbation. It would appear that for a Thai, largely male readership, the former plays to stereotypical (and cross-cultural) heterosexual male fantasy, while the latter holds far less potential for titillation and erotic intrigue.

28 Utsanaa (2000) p 364.

29 The concept of homosexuality as mental illness in Thailand is further discussed in Jackson (2003).

> Had she been an ordinary woman she'd have been thrilled all over as her inner flesh secreted the precious milk lubricating my way and sped me up to the final salute, but she deflected any climatic feeling by uttering words full of resentment. 'If I ever get pregnant, you'll never get the child.'[30]

The baby is stillborn – further retribution.

At the close of the novel, Khun Luang suffers a seizure and is paralysed as a result of glimpsing Jan bedding Mrs B. Soon after, in similar punishment for sexual excess, Jan himself becomes impotent, an affliction precisely mirroring that of his 'father' in that it is coupled with intense lust and desire, so depriving his existence of all meaning.

Such is the excuse that Jan provides in the novel's closing pages for having related the story of his life, as a remedy prescribed by his doctor for impotence, in the hope that expressing his pent-up carnal desires might serve therapeutically to dispel his mental disorders, and hence improve his level of sexual performance!

Exploring multiple attitudes to sexuality though mental and physical ill health

An analysis of *The Story of Jan Daraa* clearly reveals how the novel stands, at least in part, as a tale of erotic adventure, with the express intention of tantalising a voyeuristic audience with a panoply of sexual intrigue. In one sense, sex is deemed as an entertaining pastime of clean, healthy fun, one in which Utsanaa follows the bawdier traditions of local folk culture, depicting intercourse in humourous tones, as, for example, 'a game of athletics', 'an entry into battle' and 'a digging for the ancient treasures promised by the clues of a woman's body'.[31]

In a further layering, sex is, on occasion, aestheticised in the text, within a framework of references to the classical literary tradition of the elite and its poetic '*bot atsajan*' or erotic interludes (literally 'miraculous episodes'). Here, classical metaphors stand in for the detail of sensual experience, allowing for sensitive renditions of such experiences as hurried penetration and premature ejaculation through the long-standing symbolism of the boat that enters the gulf and overturns!

At the same time, however, *The Story of Jan Daraa* addresses themes that are seemingly opposed to its presentation of sexual exchange as sheer unsullied pleasure, for Utsanaa's concerns are also distinctly moral ones, his novel conveying an altogether darker message of degeneracy and carnal excess, couched in a display of psychological fragility, mental disorder, physical decay, sexual impotence, paralysis and death. In this frame of reference, sex stands in for ultimate moral depravity, hence meriting punishment in both physical and psychological form.

---

30 Utsanaa (1995) p 235.

31 Utsanaa (1995) p 61.

The roots of this equation between carnal desire (*kilet*) and sin (*baap*) in the Thai psyche derive from Buddhist beliefs in the denial of the body and the close attachment to the material world it represents. The novel's view of sexuality as physical over-indulgence is directed by a Buddhist rejection of excess. Its related espousal of notions of *karma,* retribution and the endless cycle of birth, death and rebirth drives the construction of a mirrored image between Jan and his 'father' Khun Luang. It also accounts for the visitation of physical and mental handicap on Prii Daraa and likewise provides an explanation for Jan's own terrible existence, pathologically reducing his presence in the world to 'the chance outcome of a seminal chemical reaction', resulting from the gang-rape of his mother by a band of criminals.[32] Thai religious views on physical contamination and the prurience of bodily functions further inform the squalid portrayals of Khein as all physical body and no spiritual centre, and the morbid images of Khun Luang's physical decay, complete with their focus on bodily fluids as filth.[33]

With such a view of sexuality offered in *The Story of Jan Daraa,* it is hardly surprising that one critic classified the work not as an erotic classic, but as a Buddhist treatise: 'Once I had read it,' he proclaimed, 'I was touched by a sense of pity and made fully aware of the meaning of justice. And I placed this book on the shelf with all my other books on religion.'[34]

Cognisant of the various contributions from Thai folk culture, elitist classical tradition and Buddhist religious views discernible in *The Story of Jan Daraa,* this chapter therefore seeks to argue that the novel's apparently incompatible views on sexuality in fact result from a multiple layering of diverse attitudes to sexuality that have evolved over a lengthy period of Thai history and across different social classes.

Commentators on Thai gender history discern the forms which this evolution has taken, Rosalind C Morris remarking that:

> ... a history of sex/gender systems must always be an analysis of the changes in politico-economic order. I do not, however, mean to suggest a linear progression from one system to the other. While they emerge in sequence, there is no necessary telos of integration and rationalization. Both exist in the present and vie for hegemony in a society that is deeply influenced by but not fully determined by transnational forces and ideologies.[35]

---

32 Utsanaa (1995) p 106.

33 In certain rural areas of Thailand, Buddhist monks are noted to practise meditation through the use of photographs of mutilated corpses or through exposure to the smell of real decaying corpses as an aid to focusing the mind on the rejection of corporeality. An ability to deny the physical impact of this experience is considered to increase spirituality. However, the regular display of gruesome photographic images of the victims of murders or fatal accidents in Thai tabloid-style newspapers and crime magazines points less to a widespread quest for spirituality than it does a popular and somewhat morbid interest in the macabre. See also Harrison (1995) for a discussion of the use and significance of macabre images in Thai short story writing of the 1970s. In the detailed descriptions of disease and decay in *The Story of Jan Daraa,* both trends may be present.

34 Khomnai (1987) p 88.

35 Morris (1994) p 17.

Penny Van Esterik's concept of palimpsests also operates as a useful paradigm here for understanding the substance of Thai gender relations and, in particular, the various and often seemingly inconsistent roles prescribed for Thai women. Referring to McKinley's view of South East Asia as a region in which the ideologies and meanings of each new age are always engaged in a dialogue with earlier ideologies,[36] Van Esterik goes on to argue that:

> Past ideologies reoccur and influence later ideologies by adding layers of new meanings, new interpretations which then become commentaries on these changes. [...] I refer to these layers of images and meanings as palimpsests. [...] I find this image intriguing because it suggests layers of representations from the past that have never been completely erased – inscriptions and representations that can be read, however, faintly and incompletely, even in the latest, most contemporary versions.[37]

In illustration of her terminology, Van Esterik provides an example of the multi-layering of gendered culture that occurred when the feudal kingdom of Ayutthaya (1351–1767) destroyed the egalitarianism inherited from the Sukhothai era (mid-thirteenth to mid-fifteenth centuries) by imposing Khmer hierarchical laws onto the traditional rights of Thai women.[38]

Most importantly, Jackson contends,[39] through reference to the work of Nidhi Aeusrivongse and of Sutham Thammrongwit,[40] that current Thai views on sexuality were significantly influenced by the cultural values of Victorian England, disseminated via the Thai elite who studied abroad from the reign of King Rama V (1868–1910). As a result, issues of sexuality were transferred from the public domain to that of the private, in an elitist bid to create an outer surface (*pleuak*) of civilisation (in the image of the imperial West) that would serve to conceal the so-called 'barbarity' (*khwaam paa theuan*) of the Siamese in the eyes of the colonial powers.[41] The squeamishness regarding overt sexuality that took hold among the upper and middle classes was then disseminated to the lower classes, so alienating people from their own indigenous cultural values, in which sexual relations were viewed as a simple, ordinary matter, one which local people could use as a basis for bawdy jokes.[42]

Such historical processes that Jackson describes for Thailand confirm the production of multi-layered attitudes to sexuality, elements of which are

---

36 McKinley (1979) pp 307–08.

37 Van Esterik (2000) pp 41–42.

38 Van Esterik (2000) p 44.

39 Jackson (2003).

40 Nidhi (1998) and Sutham (2001) p 123.

41 Thailand's past concern for a 'civilised' presentation of itself to the European gaze is reiterated in Van Esterik (2000) p 120, and discussed at length in Thongchai (2000) and Peleggi (2002) continues to play out in the present: when the feature film *Jan Dara* was shown at the London Film Festival in November 2001, Thai members of the audience expressed concern that 'foreigners' might infer from it an unseemly Thai obsession with sexuality that they felt the film implied when screened in an overseas context.

42 Sutham (2001) p 123.

concealed behind new veneers but remain at the level of trace, as Van Esterik's concept of palimpsests encapsulates.

A pertinent literary example of this process is provided by the fifteenth-century epic, *Lilit Phra Lor*, the story of a handsome prince who deserts consort and kingdom to pursue the sexual favours of two beautiful princesses from a neighbouring enemy realm. The unrestrained passions of the key protagonists end in misfortune as they are murdered by a vengeful relative. With its roots in Northern Thai folk legend, this romantic tragedy was reconstructed by elite literary culture, transmuting it into a didactic text for kings, in which the Buddhist evil of excessive pleasures of the flesh results in punishment by death.[43]

Similar layers of meaning are discernible in *The Story of Jan Daraa*, manifested in particular through the differing perspectives of sexuality in relationship to social class in the novel. For Utsanaa, sex among the lower classes – as represented by Khein and the servant girls – is portrayed as a mindless, bawdy (*sapadon*), yet largely harmless indulgence of the physical senses, devoid of Buddhist spirituality and the aesthetic sensibilities of the elite. Utsanaa's own complex positioning vis à vis social class reflects in part an empathy with characters such as Khein (based on a close childhood friend of the author), his source of inspiration having been what he had heard 'through the keyhole' as a child growing up in a house that backed onto the kitchen of the minor palace compound of Wang Thewet – tales of upper class masters divulged by the servants to the cook.[44] By contrast, education and the interest in literature he developed would also have drawn Utsanaa to the aesthetic traditions of courtly culture.

Male members of the elite in the novel therefore provide a vehicle for the portrayal of sexuality akin to that of the classical work of *Lilit Phra Lor*, in the sense that for them sex is either aestheticised or punishable in Buddhist terms through its association with lust. Among the upper class females, Mrs B represents the only character for whom sexuality is not only aestheticised but dissociated from impurity and retribution. On the contrary, intercourse is essential to her good health. In contrast to Khun Luang, she does not experience physical decay as a result of her frequent sexual encounters, but instead remains ever-young:

> The distressing signs of aging showed only in the form of some wrinkles on her face, and nowhere else – from the swell of her breasts to the spring of her toes, age had no hold on her. I can guarantee this because I've explored every inch of her body for so long, including in the evening of her life, when her beauty shines through under the moonlight.[45]

---

43 For a full discussion of the various sources of the *Phra Lor* story and the persistent appearance of transformation versions in the twentieth century, see Soison Sakolrak (2003).

44 Utsanaa (1985) p 33. The palace compound of Wang Thewet was home to two well-known writers, Dorkmaai Sot and her half-sister Bunleua Khunjorn Thephayasuwan. The implied attack on such public figures that Utsanaa's novel may be argued to represent has implications for its wider message as covert criticism of the Thai elite in general and specific criticism, made at a time of strict censorship, of Prime Minister Sarit Thanarat (1958–63), a confirmed womaniser.

45 Utsanaa (1995) p 244.

Two explanations for this are possible: one is that Mrs B has escaped the puritanical and the bawdy belief systems at play for Thais in the novel as a result of the combination of her origins as both high born and 'foreign'– she hails from a merchant family in Penang, or Songkhlaa, in the extreme south of Thailand; another is that as a woman she simply fails to carry weight within a Buddhist system of thought that concerns itself with male spirituality, asceticism and denial of the flesh but which, at least at the level of popular religious belief, associates women firmly with the physical world.[46]

As a result of this nuanced portrayal, Mrs B comes to represent the only female character in the novel who triggers the combined sentiments of sexual desire and love in Jan Daraa, emotions that remain otherwise pathologically dissociated in the novel, as a reflection of Utsanaa's own tendencies to disconnect them. Speaking in an interview Utsanaa recorded:

> I used to be madly idealistic and totally strict about not mixing love and lust (*khwaam khrai*) and I'd be furious with people that did. Because I thought that love was love, and it was there to be used with respect. If you were going to write about sex (*kaamaarom*), then that was a different subject, which had nothing to do with love. I would write about both – but definitely not together, at the same time. But then I realized I was wrong to think this way. Maybe I changed my mind when I got married. I used to be so strict about keeping love and sex separate that I didn't used to believe in sex before marriage. I even wondered if I should sleep with my wife after we had married.[47]

Echoing this youthful 'idealism', Utsanaa's only option in *The Story of Jan Daraa* is to have Hyacinth die an early death, before Jan is faced with the psychological crisis of a sexual liaison with her that his separation of women into the 'pure' and the 'impure' would instil in him. In consequence of her prompt removal from the plot, Hyacinth therefore remains the only woman whom Jan really loves, and one of the very few he does not bed and so debase through sexual contact. As Jan himself states, his purpose is to place Hyacinth on a level of worship one would one's own mother, a position that cannot, therefore, include the possibilities of sexual congress. 'Isn't it possible for a man to have one woman he can think about in a nice way (*thaang thii dii*), and not think of sleeping (*khit lap khit norn*) with her?'[48] Utsanaa's choice of her name echoes a deep-rooted connection in Thai tradition between (ideal) women and flowers, mirrored in Jan's musings in her company: 'I had caught a whiff of her natural scent, like the sweet fragrance of *saiyut* flowers that drifted by on the mornings.'[49] The significance of this is explained by Jan's proclamation: 'What was rising quietly and deeply inside me was unlike any feeling I had ever experienced. It was like the mood conjured up

---

46 See Van Esterik (1982).

47 Utsanaa (1985) p 33. The anger Utsanaa talks of feeling in this interview for those who do not understand the distinction he is making between love and sex is reflected in his novel in the irritation Jan shows for Khein on this subject; see Utsanaa (1995) pp 55–57.

48 Utsanaa (2000) p 85. The Thai term used here, *khit lap khit norn*, is an extremely bland one, indicating thinking of literally 'sleeping' with someone and lacking any of the sexual overtones that pepper Utsanaa's use of language in other contexts.

49 Utsanaa (1995) p 50.

by the fragrance of flowers, not the craving triggered by the musk of hair follicles all over one's body.'[50]

Jan's idealisation of Hyacinth in the image of his highly revered (white-skinned, delicate, dead) mother reflects a continuum between mother and wife in the Thai male stereotyping of women that consequently excludes the sexual and in some senses mirrors Judaeo-Christian divisions of women into the categories of Madonna, mother and whore.[51] Jan wants Hyacinth not for the pleasures of her flesh, but for what he sees as the 'valid' reason of intercourse – the higher task of procreation. This cultural reluctance to link motherhood to sexual pleasure manifests itself in Jan's disenchantment at the connection between female promiscuity and pregnancy, which draws him to the distasteful realisation that 'bad' women can become mothers.[52] An alternative portrayal of this 'phenomenon' is provided in the character of Kaew the lesbian, and her 'unnatural' abhorrence of motherhood.

The overstated emphasis on the distinction between mothers and lovers underscores the Oedipal tones of the novel, further illustrated by a loathing for his (adopted) father that is notably incited by Jan's witnessing of the primal scene between Khun Luang and the mother-figure of Aunt Waat. Although Thailand has its own equivalent of the Oedipus myth – in the form of the Phra Phatom Chedi legend of 'Phyaa Kong and Phyaa Phaan' – much of Utsanaa's affection for notions of psychology in the novel derives from his interest in Western thought. It may, in particular, have originated from his love of DH Lawrence, a writer who (by his own admission) exerted the single most powerful influence on his approach to fiction, and earned him the title among local literary circles as the *DH Lawrence of Thailand* – despite the discernible differences in the approach to sexuality that exist between the two authors.

As one of the first Thai literary works to deal with notions of psychology, it is perhaps not surprising that they are only partially digested and incompletely followed through: deprivation of the maternal breast is, in reality, unlikely to result in an obsession with breasts in adolescence; witnessing the primal scene at a tender age does not lead Jan into a life tormented by nightmares, as it did in Freud's classic case of the Wolf Man. Consequently, Buddhist thought and Western psychological explanations sit uncomfortably side by side as justification for Jan's mental frailties and obsessive sexual practices.

The incorporation of Western philosophical accretions to this already complex text adds a further tool for the interpretation of its diverse attitudes to sexuality, for Utsanaa is influenced not only by folk culture, high classics, Buddhist thought and Western psychology, but also by Western literature, of which he was an established translator. This is illustrated in *The Story of Jan Daraa* by numerous references to international writers and their works, from Rider Haggard, Boccacio,

---

50 Utsanaa (1995) p 49.

51 See Harrison (1999).

52 See Harrison (1997).

Balzac, Maupassant and Joseph Heller to Grimm's fairy tales, *Jack and the Beanstalk*, *The Arabian Nights* and Norman Lindsay's 1932 novel, *The Cautious Amorist*. These texts receive their mention alongside Thai literary classics such as *Lilit Siiwichai Chaadok*, *Khun Chang Khun Phaen*, *Sangthorng* and *Saao Khreua Faa* (itself an adaptation of *Madama Butterfly*). It is in this context that we come to appreciate the description of Aunt Waat as a hybrid form of Ursula Andress and Naang Laweng, a heroine of Sri Lankan origin from the well-known Thai epic, *Phra Aphaimanii*.[53]

Conclusion

The Story of Jan Daraa transgressed against the Thai taboo of placing representations of sexuality in the public domain, a taboo which had held firm throughout the period of modern literature, dating from the close of the nineteenth century. To legitimise its subject matter, Utsanaa referred back to Thai classical works and the erotic episodes of its highly aestheticised poetic conventions. This he combined with a more ribald and humourous approach to sexual relations that has its basis in Thai folk tradition and non-elite culture. Further, seemingly incongruous, layers of meaning are discernible in the novel in its commitment to a morality informed by Buddhist ethics, one in which sex transmutes from being good, clean fun to a degenerate and filthy practice, meriting punishment in this life or the next. For Utsanaa, such punishment is also disguised with various forms of psychological suffering, mental disorder, physical decay, impotence and paralysis. A shadow of mortality casts itself over the text, the work of an author who was in constant ill health and felt himself in 'the last throes of life', penned in his early forties, the mirror-image of his 'hero', Jan Daraa's age. A clearly expressed link is established between (sexual) excess, ill health and imminent death, and which is played out in the novel through the character of Jan. Jan counters his own frail sense of self through an obsessive commitment to sexual encounter, which confirms his existence in the world. His actions are in part explained through references to (Western) psychology, adding yet a further layer of cultural eclecticism to the text. The multiple attitudes to sexuality which manifest themselves in the novel reflect the complexity of views held in Thai society at large, a matrix of apparently paradoxical positions which can only be elucidated through an awareness of the evolution and multi-layering of Thai cultural beliefs. *The Story of Jan Daraa* is therefore particularly important because it illuminates the intricacy of Thai attitudes to sexuality that are commonly overlooked or erased in popular Occidental imaginings of the Thai sexual landscape.

---

53 The character of Naang Laweng is herself of curious ethnic origin, often described as a *farang* (ie Westerner) because of her pale complexion and reddish hair. Although she is in fact South Asian, Naang Laweng appears to stand as a broad, ethnic 'other'.

Bibliography

Anderson, Benedict and Mendiones, Ruchira, *In the Mirror: Literature and Politics in Siam in the American Era*, 1985, Bangkok: Editions Duang Kamol.

Anonymous, 'Behind sexual desire' (2003) *Bangkok Post*, 17 May.

Barang, Marcel, *The Twenty Best Novels of Thailand*, 1994, Bangkok: Thai Modern Classics.

Braginksy, Vladimir I, *The Comparative Study of Traditional Asian Literatures: From Reflective Traditionalism to Neo-Traditionalism*, 2001, Richmond: Curzon.

Harrison, Rachel, 'Birth, death and identity in the short story writing of Sidaoru'ang', in Chitakasem, Manas (ed), *Thai Literary Traditions*, 1995, Bangkok: Chulalongkorn University Press, pp 87–117.

Harrison, Rachel, 'The good, the bad and the pregnant: why the Thai prostitute can't be seen to give birth', in Somswasdi, V and Theobald, S (eds), *Women, Gender Relations and Development in Thai Society*, 1997, Chiangmai: Women's Studies Centre, Chiangmai University Press, pp 323–48.

Harrison, Rachel, 'The madonna and the whore: self/"Other" tensions in the characterization of the prostitute by Thai female authors', in Jackson, P and Cook, N (eds), *Genders and Sexualities in Modern Thailand*, 1999, Chiangmai: Silkworm Books, pp 168–90.

Harrison, Rachel, 'Looking forward, looking back: towards a comparative study of the interaction between the traditional and the modern in contemporary South East Asia' (2000) 42 *Tenggara* 19–47.

Harrison, Rachel, 'Prostitution, politics and power. Issues of "foreigness" in Western television documentaries of female sex workers in Thailand', in Munshi, S (ed), *Images of the 'Modern Woman' in Asia*, 2001, London: Curzon, pp 138–68.

Harrison, Rachel, '"A Hundred Loves", "A Thousand Lovers": portrayals of sexuality in the work of Thidaa Bunnaak' (2002) 33:3 *Journal of South East Asian Studies* 451–70.

Jackson, Peter, 'Tolerant but unaccepting: the myth of a Thai "gay paradise"', in Jackson, P and Cook, N (eds), *Genders and Sexualities in Modern Thailand*, 1999, Chiangmai: Silkworm Books, pp 226–42.

Jackson, Peter, 'Performative genders, perverse desires: a bio-history of Thailand's same-sex and transgender cultures' (2003) 9 *Intersections* http://wwwsshe.murdoch.edu.au/intersections/issue9/jackson.html (accessed 4 February 2004).

Jackson, Peter, 'Translation and poststructuralism in Thai Studies' (unpublished manuscript), London: School of Oriental and African Studies.

Katsamaa Satayaahurak, '*Siang kong jaak khwaam song jam: theung thii maa khorng Jan Daraa*' ('The echo of memories of the origins of Jan Daraa'), in *Jan Daraa – sanwaat naatakam bon jor ngoen (Sexual Drama on the Silver Screen)*, 2001, Bangkok: Samnakphim Rawaang banthat (Between the Lines Publishing).

Khomnai Tunlajit, '*Reun jarung klin tham nai heun khao haeng kamaa*' ('The enticing smell of virtue within the stench of sexual craving') (1987) 4:9 *Thanon nangseu* ('Book Road') 88–92.

Manas Chitakasem, 'The development of political and social consciousness in Thai short stories', in Davidson, J H and Cordell, H (eds), *The Short Story in South East Asia*, 1982, London: School of Oriental and African Studies, pp 63–100.

McKinley, Robert, 'Zaman dan Masa, Eras and Periods: religious evolution and the permanence of epistemological ages in malay culture', in Becker, A and Yengoyan, A (eds), *The Imagination of Reality: Essays in Southeast Asian Coherence Systems*, 1979, Norwood, NJ: Ablex, pp 303–24.

Morris, Rosalind C, 'Three sexes and four sexualities: redressing the discourses on gender and sexuality in contemporary Thailand' (1994) 2:1 *Positions* 15–43 (Spring).

Morris, Rosalind C, *In the Place of Origins*, 2000, Durham, NC and London: Duke University Press.

Morris, Rosalind C, 'Failures of domestication: speculations on globality, economy, and the sex of excess in Thailand' (2002) 13:1 *Differences* 45–76.

Nidhi Aeusrivongse, *Watthanatham khwaam jon ('The Culture of Poverty')*, 1998, Bangkok: Phraew Samnakphim.

Peleggi, Maurizio, *Lords of Things*, 2002, Hawaii: University of Honolulu Press.

Salleh, Mohammad Haji, *Tradition and Change in Contemporary Malay-Indonesian Poetry*, 1977, Kuala Lumpur: Universiti Kebangsan Malaysia.

Soison Sakolrak, 'Thai literary transformation: an analytical study of the modernisation of *Lilit Phra Lor*', 2003, PhD dissertation, London: School of Oriental and African Studies.

Sutham Thammrongwit, *'Khwaam ngiap' kap 'kaan phuut': Khwaam dat jarit reuang phet nai sangkhom thai'* ('"Silence" and "voice": sexual dissimulation in Thai society'), in *Jan Daraa – sanwaat naatakam bon jor ngoen ('Sexual Drama on the Silver Screen')*, 2001, Bangkok: Samnakphim Rawaang banthat (Between the Lines Publishing), pp 116–27.

Thongchai Winichakul, 'The quest for "Siwilai": a geographical discourse of civilizational thinking in the late nineteenth- and early twentieth-century Siam' (2000) 59 *Journal of Asian Studies* 528–49 (August).

Utsanaa Phloengtham, *'Poet thep samphaat Utsanaa Phloengtham'* ('A Taped interview with Utsanaa Phloengtham') (1985) 3:3 *Thanon nangseu* ('Book Road') 28–34 (September).

Utsanaa Phloengtham, *The Story of Jan Daraa*, translated by Phongdeit Jiangphatthanarkit; edited by Barang, M, 1995, Bangkok: Thai Modern Classics.

Utsanaa Phloengtham, *Reuang khong Jan Daraa ('The Story of Jan Daraa')*, 2000, Bangkok: Phraew Publishing.

Van Esterik, Penny, 'Laywomen in Theravada Buddhism', in Van Esterik, Penny (ed), *Women of Southeast Asia: Occasional Paper, Number 9*, 1982, DeKalb, IL: Northern Illinois University, Centre for Southeast Asian Studies, pp 55–78.

Van Esterik, Penny, *Materializing Thailand*, 2000, Oxford and New York: Berg.

CHAPTER 9

SOME FUNDAMENTAL RIDDLES OF CHOLERA: SEX, SODOMY AND REPRESENTATIONS OF THE FUNDAMENT

George S Rousseau[1]

> Dear mudlarks! my brethren!
> Of all scents and degrees,
> (Yourselves and your shes)
> Forswear all cabal, lads,
> Wakes, unions, and rows,
> Hot dreams, and cold salads
> And don't pig in sties that would suffocate sows!
> Quit Cobbet's, O'Connell's, and Beelzebub's banners,
> And whitewash at once bowels, rooms, hands, and manners![2]

> We had not realised that what the public really loathes in homosexuality is not the thing itself but having to think about it. If it could be slipped into our midst unnoticed, or legalised overnight by a decree in small print, there would be few protests. Unfortunately it can only be legalised by Parliament, and Members of Parliament are obliged to think or to appear to think.[3]

It is easy to forget that diseases in human history have always been mentalised and conceptualised before they can be diagnosed for cure and internalised for their human meaning. The mind selectively interprets aspects of the malady and – through a set of complex processes based on preconception and association – builds up a picture assumed to be more or less reliable and stable. Hence consumptives and tuberculars in history are imagined by combining images of defective pulmonary cavities with the types of air they breathe and the way their lungs process this loosely imagined oxygen through the vessels of the body. Likewise those in the gout, who are pictured as having arthritic joints, crumbling bones, swollen bones and a bodily regimen compromised in this way as a consequence of loose living and too much port. So it is with all maladies, whether these or cancer and AIDS.

Cholera, however, like its cousin dysentery and all those fatal diseases arising from diarrhoea, displays a difference: its selective part of the anatomy can barely be named. Except in medical schools where anatomical terms have been used

---

1 Some of the research presented here was supported by Leverhulme Trust Grant F793A, and I am indebted to Dr Caroline Warman for her translations from the French.

2 Coleridge (1997), *Cholera Cured Before Hand*, p 414. The lines were enclosed in a letter of 26 July 1832 to Joseph Henry Green.

3 Forster (1971) pp 240–41.

(sphincter, rectum, organ producing motions), polite society has been unable to name the part. The toll this has taken has not been fatal for cholera but it has resulted in a different historical pathway than almost all other maladies, certainly different from those where the 'fundament' does not play a principal role. The matter is not merely lexical – that the word cannot be uttered in polite society – but visual as well: it has been too painful for most people to imagine a disease that deranges the lower bowel and rectum to such a degree that its already filthy streams are polluted beyond imagining. Cholera, whatever else it has been in medical history and human memory, has always been the condition of speed-of-lightning dehydration in which the body's fluids are emptied through a polluting rectum acting as the guarantor of the body's entire reservoir of filth. No other disease condition presented this heightened drama of putrid rivers rampaging through the body, recklessly and swiftly depleting its fluids – pure and impure – until the creature is brought down. In no other illness was the rectum so palpably implicated, or so it was popularly thought.

This matter of the anatomical place of primacy – the fundament in cholera – would be of minor interest were it not that another condition *also* exists in which the same bodily region plays a lion's share: sodomy, the sin of male penetration, or so it was imagined until the twentieth century in both Western and Eastern civilisations. The claim was not that the rectal hemispheres actually determined the pathway of *both* maladies or defined their sites of origin. These maladies, different as they were perceived to be, could not be imagined throughout history without the crucially defining 'bum'. Both were failures, so to speak, in the rectum; or the rectum was the site of both afflictions even if it obviously was not the origin of these conditions. Sodomy is, of course, an old word designating what was once thought to be, in part, a medical condition; it is no longer used to refer to any meaningful syndrome. Its history is now almost entirely forgotten. For decades it has been politically incorrect to discuss the history of sodomy without reviling its former hangmen or exclaiming that they had always been persecutory, in church and state, court and seraglio.[4] No one sensible, and certainly no judicious cultural anthropologist or historian, has considered it (sodomy) even remotely proximate to the sexual orientations, amounting to life choices, brought about by such figures as, in Western Europe, the dandy (Georgian and Regency society), the Victorian and Edwardian homosexual (Havelock Ellis to EM Forster), the near closet-gay (Proust to WH Auden), the open gay (Cocteau to Genet), the liberationists (from Christopher Street to the Bastille), to the myriad queer lifestyles that have developed since Stonewall (1962) and AIDS (1980s). These lifestyles share many facets – the anatomical bum is not among them.

Nevertheless, for centuries the old sodomies – bestiality, inversion, pederasty, and perversion – were semiotically conceptualised as ailments adjudged to be

---

4 The exceptions have been largely academic – cultural historians and commentators who have formed a large block in the recent history of Western and non-Western homosexuality; see the many histories of sexuality written in the past few decades, especially those inspired by Michel Foucault.

every bit as deadly as cholera; 'semiotically' in the sense that their signs and symptoms were interpreted, read, compared and contrasted. However different the two were – in the original infecting agent, onset of the disease, pathways taken in the body, the time from infection to death, hence their chronicity – they were nevertheless mentalised as profoundly similar in their nether anatomical geography. The diseased male bum was the perceived site of both conditions. Indeed it was unimaginable to conjure either condition – cholera or sodomy – apart from the fundament. Cholera in which flowing rivers of filth were retained within the *corpora fabrica* was no cholera at all, as the requisite dehydration had not occurred; likewise, sodomy without penetration of the folds of the rectum was not sodomy but some minor offence hardly worth noticing in courts of law or medical surgeries.

The point is not that the two conditions – cholera and the old sodomy – were similar maladies in any empirical sense (clearly they were *not*, nor were they both maladies), but rather that they were *perceived* to share in this all-important common anatomical geography.[5] Stated otherwise, the mind internalised and visualised them as parallel universes so far as the body's predispositions were concerned. In the one (cholera) diseased fluids wreak the greatest destruction as they reach their delta: the filthy fundament, repository of accumulating faeces as filthy as Indian sub-continent rivers dragging in their currents the flotsam and jetsam of the ages. In the other (sodomy) an equally offending 'bum': a human organ whose hemispheres are parted, violated, penetrated, ripped apart, its folds torn and tattered, its tissues transformed from intact matter to desecrated meat in which the faeces stray and commingle with blood. An invading, almost steely-stiff male phallus is the offender in this imagined drama. So powerful is the visual fantasy that it took a veritable toll on human history, conceptualising these parallel universes – cholera and sodomy – as if co-existing, rather than as descriptions of actual physiological processes or real disease constellations. Mentalisations and fantasies, far more than realities, endowed medical conditions with their human vibrancy, as Susan Sontag, Michel Foucault, Sander Gilman, and – in particular for cholera – Francois Delaporte have all demonstrated.[6]

Human history should not have been infected with such distortion and fantasy, but it was. Even the briefest medical history makes the point in another, more empirical, key. The old *cholera morbus* had existed in Europe at least from the Middle Ages, as Dr Thomas Sydenham (1624–89) and his medical colleagues showed.[7] Rarely fatal, it was a loose disease condition amalgamating several types of diarrhoea and correlating them to geographical conditions of climate and,

5 This difference between empirical reality and popular mentalisation amounting to sheer fantasy could not be stronger. It has formed the basis of whole approaches to the public understanding of disease in cultural history, as in the work of Susan Sontag, Michel Foucault, Sander Gilman, Arthur Klineman, Roy Porter, Elaine Showalter, Barbara Duden, George Rousseau and many others. See also the important role of gendered male fantasy in cultural history: Theweleit (1992). For male fantasy and warm climates where diseases such as cholera flourished, see Aldrich (1993).

6 Delaporte (1986).

7 For Thomas Sydenham's writings on cholera, see Swan (1742) pp 133–55.

especially, heat. By the end of the eighteenth century, however, it had a new rival in *cholera Asiaticus*. Said to have arisen on the Indian sub-continent, it swept to the West from the 1780s and entrenched itself in the early nineteenth century. When Asiatic cholera first reached England in 1831, there was considerable argument amongst both physicians and the general public as to whether it was a distinctly new disease, or whether it was a merely a more severe variation of traditional English cholera or *cholera morbus*. No one could have predicted *cholera Asiaticus* in 1800; but even then, three decades before it arrived in Britain, for example, the public imagination connected filth and bowels, partly as the result of anxiety about new urban sprawl in Paris, Hamburg, London and elsewhere.

Cholera morbus was a bilious derangement arising from too great a secretion of bile, the bitter, brownish-yellow fluid secreted by the liver into the duodenum as an aid to digestion. It was attended with bilious diarrhoea, vomiting, stomach-ache and cramps, and it usually occurred in the late summer or early autumn – hence the appellation 'autumnal' cholera. Dysentery, meanwhile, is defined by the *Oxford English Dictionary* as 'A disease characterized by inflammation of the mucous membrane and glands of the large intestine, accompanied with griping pains, and mucous and bloody evacuations'. Contaminated food or water are the modern explanations for such disorders, which would have been exacerbated and transported in this period by poor hygiene and more plentiful airborne vectors – flies feeding off human, animal and organic waste in the streets and open sewers. Following a severe period of dysentery, *cholera morbus* and 'dysenteric fever' between 1669 and 1672, Sydenham explained that a succession of very hot and dry summers had meant that 'the blood and humors [...] arrived to a great adustion [sic] and sharpnesse' so that 'cholera morbus[,] gripeing in the bowells without stooles and dysenterys became very epidemicall'.[8] Heat, filth, faeces and waste combined in the fundament to produce the image of an epidemic that could wipe out human populations.

All such bowel disorders were generally attributed to two main sources: faults in the patient's diet or extremes in the weather, but new authorities in the Enlightenment were claiming that bodily regimen (hygienic cleanliness and evaporation of the body's fluids through dermal perspiration) and morality (elimination of body fluids through masturbation and sexual intercourse) played a role too. The most authoritative eighteenth century writer on bowel disorders was Sir John Pringle (1707–82), who became President of the Royal Society and physician to George III. Between Pringle's work and the appearance of *cholera Asiaticus* in Europe, theories on bowel disorders had changed relatively little. In *Observations on the Diseases of the Army* (1752), Pringle focused on the significant influence of air in causing dysenteries and fevers, and considered cleanliness an important preventative, but this was not for the hygienic reasons we would now understand. Perspiration was considered a necessary process for keeping the human body in equilibrium, which required the removal of excess matter, be it

8 Dewhurst (1966) p 123.

faeces, urine, menstrual blood or sweat. The elimination of fluid that occurs in masturbation and seminal ejaculation, he thought, was of another order and less salubrious. Elimination of fluid through the fundament was the most delicate operation of all. If any of these patterns was upset or irregular, or if the normal daily operation of the rectum was deflected or tinkered with, Pringle thought, debility followed. Thus, if the body could not eject unwanted matter through the skin as sweat, or faeces through the fundament, it would build up internally and cause damage to the bodily system: dysentery or *cholera morbus* represented the subsequent violent removal of an unnatural excess of bile or humours. (As such, some practitioners considered diarrhoea a positive rather than a negative physical symptom, illustrative of the body's attempt to heal itself, demonstrating how far from the popular (mis)conception the authoritative medical view was.) In Pringle's opinion, therefore, it was principally through the atmosphere, rather than contaminated diet, that diseases such as dysentery were transported. Filthy diet, in the end, was losing out to foul air, and he barely discusses the fundament or names it despite his awareness of its role in the elimination of waste.

Dysentery, moreover, had from time immemorial been rife in the military where sanitation and weather conditions were unpredictable. Diseases of the rectum flourished in the army and on the seas, as the military doctors of the pre-*cholera Asiaticus* world noticed. The trope of the inflammation of the bowels became a euphemism for a broad range of dysenteries, but as the new disease – the so-called 'Blue Cholera of India' – ravaged the West in the 1830s, the debates extended beyond contaminated diet and foul air to include foreign matter in the fundament (see Figure A). Thus, cholera was thought to attack those who were already *predisposed* by irritated bowels to be 'loaded with food and faeces', and who further exposed themselves by permitting contaminated matter to enter their lower bowel. Even one seemingly as morally uncontaminated as the English polymath and poet Samuel Taylor Coleridge (1772–1834) persuaded himself in 1832 – at the peak of the first wave of cholera hysteria in England – that he had contracted the illness this way.[9]

The two choleras were also distinguished in another way: their semantic profile. The doctors who pronounced on the old *cholera morbus* had never been certain of the degree implicated. They knew the rectum played a part but were unsure about degree and function. In the new *cholera Asiaticus* there was no doubt: if not the main villain, the bowel was nevertheless the site where infection and derangement occurred. Thus, WS Prior, an army officer who survived a clear case of Asiatic cholera in June 1832, blamed the increased mortality of the prevailing disease on filthy rectums.[10] However, bowel was a euphemism for rectum, itself a

9 Coleridge's explanation changed one crucial variable: being already *predisposed* by irritated bowels 'loaded with food and faeces', he believed that his exposure to a cold atmosphere had excited his nervous system and resulted in 'the spasms, the dejections, and the cold shivering' that gave him cholera. For a deep-layer discussion of Coleridge's gut and imagined cholera, see Rousseau and Haycock (2003).

10 Prior (1833).

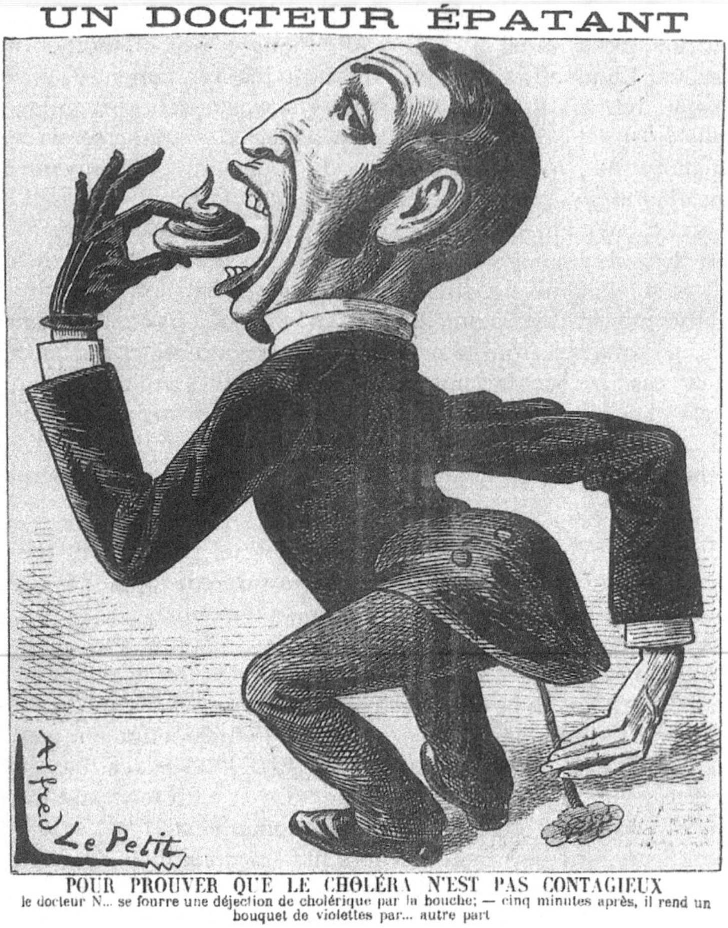
UN DOCTEUR ÉPATANT
Alfred Le Petit
POUR PROUVER QUE LE CHOLÉRA N'EST PAS CONTAGIEUX
le docteur N... se fourre une déjection de cholérique par la bouche; — cinq minutes après, il rend un bouquet de violettes par... autre part

Figure A: This caricature entitled 'Un docteur épatant' (an 'amazed doctor') and ironically claiming that 'cholera is not contagious', appeared in *Le Grelot* on 23 November 1884. This was after yet another outbreak of cholera terrorised the French public and just as Koch, in Germany, was discovering the germs responsible for its transmission. *Le Grelot* was a popular Paris magazine featuring cartoons of the diseased; hence its name taken from the bell sounding death to the afflicted. Here we see a doctor eating faeces and excreting a bouquet of violets. 'Doctor N' is allegedly a member of the anti-contagionist camp who believes that cholera is not spread through faeces. To his surprise, however, he excretes violets five minutes after consuming the faeces. The violets' blue hue reflects the then common belief that choleric victims themselves had a blue visage. Hence the common phrase 'La peur bleue' throughout the mid-nineteenth century indicative of the popular terror of contracting the disease. The cholera doctors were often confused by the patients' blue visage, for the patients' colouration was identical to those given arsenic, which also produced a blue effect on its victims. For further discussion of the caricature of cholera in this era, especially as 'La peur bleue', see Patrice Bourdelais and Jean-Yves Raulot, *Une peur bleue: histoire du choléra en France, 1832–1854*, 1987, Paris: Payot.

word describing an organ poorly understood in the early nineteenth century.[11] Set the chronological dials to c 1830 – when the new *cholera Asiaticus* entered Europe through Russia, spreading West to Germany, Britain and America – and rectum is still being used exclusively as a medical term, and is not yet in ordinary vocabulary. There the terms are consistently vulgar: in English 'backside', 'bum', 'ass' and other words that cannot be reproduced here, in French an even larger repertoire.[12] 'Fundament' had been a compromise: since the Renaissance it too was anatomical but had also appeared, if then only occasionally, in didactic and homiletic literature.

By the 1830s the rectum, or fundament, constituted the principal site of the tempestuous drama of the new disease yet – paradoxically – occurring in a precinct of the body that could barely be named except through euphemism and ellipsis. Had there not been another condition where infection occurred at the same site despite its inability to be named? The ancient and Renaissance doctors certainly thought so.[13] By 1600 the forensic doctors were sure that the most certain sign of sodomy could be read through the spoiled folds of the fundament. No other method of examination or interrogation was so reliable. Psychological and religious clues (what we would call disposition, personality and temperament) were indecisive. The convergence of sodomy and cholera – old and new, but especially in *cholera Asiaticus* as a result of its much greater emphasis on the role of the rectum – occurred in an anatomical zone, but the specific site could hardly be mentioned in polite society, certainly not its daily motions and evacuations, movements and derangements.

The pre-1830s (that is, pre-*cholera Asiaticus*) accounts of sodomy (of which there were many) resisted inclusion of the fundament for these linguistic rather than moral reasons. Arrests and court cases over two centuries (1630–1830) were unequivocal in the offending acts: the penalties for mere exposure and touching in

---

11 Another essay, longer than this one, is needed to trace this lexical history, especially uses – serious and comic – of the word 'bum'. Perhaps it is sufficient to note here how Freud interpreted the disgust giving rise to pressing need for ellipsis and euphemism: 'Where the anus is concerned it becomes still clearer that it is disgust which stamps that sexual aim as a perversion. I hope, however, I shall not be accused of partisanship when I assert that people who try to account for this disgust by saying that the organ in question serves the function of excretion and comes in contact with excretion – a thing which is disgusting in itself – are not much more to the point than hysterical girls who account for their disgust at the male genital by saying that it serves to void urine.' See Freud (1953) VII p 67.

12 Ditto the previous point; note concurrently the broad range of words then used for sodomites: *persilleuse, rivette, honteuse, travailleuse, tante* and others. Anthropologically considered, it would be profitable to extend the list to the fundament in non-Western languages, a task for which, however, I lack the philological competence.

13 This is made clear by the tradition in forensics from Aristotle and the pseudo-Aristotelian *Problemata* to the Renaissance commentaries of Avicenna and Dr Paolo Zacchias, the leading sixteenth century authority on the anatomically specific anuses of receptive sodomites, makes plain. For the Renaissance hermaphrodite's anatomical 'bum', see also Masten (1997) and Gilbert (2002). The Renaissance anus had also been, of course, the productive site for healthy evacuation, as evidenced in the then new successful cure for the fistula; see Arderne (1541). Nevertheless, the presiding view from the ancient world forward, in the Levant as well as the West, was that sodomites could not conduce their desire without this distinctive anal anatomy.

public places entirely differed from those for insertion and penetration of the anal folds. Even didactic works such as *Satan's Harvest Home* (1749), a manual explaining how to recognise sodomites in the streets, eschewed the word but covertly suggested that these profligates performed acts that cannot be named.[14] Such works dance around penetration of the fundament without ever naming it, culminating centuries later in the trope about 'the love that dare not speak its name'.[15] Another factor also commingled these two plagues – cholera and sodomy, as they were known down through the nineteenth century – in the popular psyche. This was their fierce degree of contagion.

Cholera Asiaticus was thought to be far more contagious than its predecessors by several quantum leaps. If, after 1830, it was the swiftest new killer, it was also the most contagious. Even the old *cholera morbus* was thought to be highly infectious. J-J Menuret, a Paris physician, thought it was so contagious that it could be spread in the air.[16] In his view, it was possible, as with SARS today, to catch the new cholera merely by breathing the air. Within a generation (1781–1831) the profile of cholera reached dazzling new heights of perceived contagion. Reading the medical history 1817–32 of *all* these choleras (they were far from being so neatly segregated then as they have since become), you see that what most distinguished old from new is contagion. The proof of contagion, however, lay in the speed with which the patient/victim dies. Early disease theory often arranged and even classified diseases according to their mortality and the swiftness of death they inflicted: consumption and gout being very slow if at all mortal, dysentery faster depending upon the type, post-1800 cholera the quickest of fatal illnesses and grower faster every day it then seemed. The new post-1830 theory of cholera rendered it the swiftest killer, if also the most contagious, among all nineteenth-century diseases all over the globe.

Where red-hot contagion lurks, barbarism does not lag far behind, so the argument went. In 1832 the march of barbarism assumed a triumph of tyranny: 'cholera would not be present among us had despotism not introduced it together with its ball and chain', Dr Prost emphatically proclaimed.[17] His medical colleague in Paris, Dr Metral, concurred, noting that: 'There is reason to think that if the peoples of the banks of the Ganges had the good fortune to live under free governments ... they would tame the plague that their river is vomiting forth to poison other parts of the earth. The arm of liberty would snuff out the impure monster at its source.'[18] Increasingly the new cholera – whatever its true taxonomy – stood for the primitive, as yet another French doctor proclaimed: 'the epidemics, some rare, some more frequent, that mow down human beings – those

14 Anonymous (1749).

15 Lord Alfred Douglas coined the phrase in his poem 'Two Loves', which was printed in the Chameleon in 1894.

16 *'Telle est la force de la corruption; tel est son pouvoir pour la production des maladies epidemiques'* ('This is the force of corruption: it is the power behind its production of epidemic maladies'): Menuret (1781) p 33.

17 Prost (1832) p 214.

18 Metral (1833) p v.

epidemics represent the triumph of ignorance.'[19] Yet another Parisian, J Guichard, chimed in that 'Scourges that seem to be reserved for races mired in ignorance' were the most severe.[20]

The year 1832 was thus a year of head-on confrontation between barbarism and civilisation, despotism and liberalism, ignorance and knowledge. This myth, the product of philosophical speculation pushed to extreme limit, played a vital role in the sign system accompanying the new global menace: not only did it justify colonisation by linking the new cholera to the alleged political and cultural inferiority of oriental nations, it also proved, to the delight of some Europeans, that the poverty of those nations stemmed from the temperament of their people. This was precisely the point Dr Berard, another Paris physician, had been asserting ever since the new cholera struck Paris, namely that 'a convincing explanation of [the] epidemic was therefore readily available: most contagious diseases – the great scourges of the human race – originated among and were spread by barbarous peoples'.[21] Here he echoed Dr Metral, already cited, in the view that 'This disease was particularly bent on destroying nations sunk in barbarism'.[22] By 'barbarous peoples' all these physicians alluded (if not as elliptically as in their rhetoric of the fundament) to subjugated and impoverished nations of the East, especially those around Bengal. Berard was explicit: 'India first and foremost.'[23]

Cholera was thus divine retribution among the vast realm of the primitive, filthy and sexually promiscuous. But it was not limited to easterners and Orientals. The imperiled Western fundament in the 1830s – even civilised French and English 'bums' – was proof that the new pollution of immorality was wrecking advanced civilisations. Campaigns for cleanliness, as well as the policing of prostitution in cities now swelling to unimaginable populations, soared. Semiotically speaking, smell was thought to be the sign of contagion. All faecal matter retains an odour that is often received as repugnant, but this odour is not necessarily that of putrefaction. Excretion in the fundament was the clue to pathology: the healthy rectum smelled but of another order than the diseased, especially the cholerically infected. J Morin, yet another Paris doctor, went so far as to make explicit these subtle discriminations among foul ordures, yet he could invoke the word rectum only once in the charged passage about *'Parvenues au rectum'*.[24]

All this while sexology marched ahead – it had been developing as something of a science of sex from the mid-eighteenth century. One of its prime tenets was the notion of a third sex: an intermediate gender between male and female

---

19 Lauvergne (1836) p 216.

20 Guichard (1832) p 36.

21 Berard (1826) p 107; see pp 102–07 for the rhetoric of his polemic against primitive nations who spread miasma and the pollution of the new disease.

22 Metral (1833) p 5.

23 Berard (1826) pp 103–04.

24 Morin (1835) pp 94–95. Morin uses the word 'anus' once.

partaking of the characteristics of both and inherently flawed by being weaker than either. Lamarck and other pre-Darwinian degenerationists influenced its development and by c 1830s – when the cholera epidemic was taking its toll in Europe – the sodomitical type or 'third sex' was theorised as especially vulnerable to disease and, more specifically, endowed with an inherently defective rectum. After 1859, the third male sex (whether called androgyne, urning, Uranian or any number of other names) was said to be evolving as an increasingly defective body, its main flaw delimited to the rectum. Vulnerability was medicalised as pathology in which the folds (membranes within the rectum) are distressingly weak and thereby particularly capable of absorbing foreign matter, germs and bacteria, especially of the type carried by the new cholera. Few authors in France did more to popularise these notions than Joseph Morel de Rubempré, who set himself up in Paris as a specialist in syphilis and brought out multiple editions of *La médecine de Vénus sans le médecin* (*The Medicine of Venus Without the Doctor*), each edition fuller than the previous one, all tinged in semi-medical titillation.[25]

It is not, however, Morel's *médecine de Venus* which captures the homology of cholera and sodomy, but a work of his from 1842.[26] No other work, in any language, is more germane to the theme of this essay than this one. Here, in his 'pornology or new history of debauchery and prostitution [...] in France', he provides in great detail histories of ancient and modern sodomy, accounts of notable debauchees from Socrates to Sade, methods of spotting mignons, sodomites and hermaphrodites, descriptions of all sorts of diseased fundaments and – most crucially for the point – confirmation that the barbaric sin of cholera and sodomy are commensurate by being both localised in the same anatomical region:[27]

---

25 There is no reliable biography of Joseph Morel de Rubempré (1812–86), who is not to be confused with other Morels of his generation. Study of this Morel's life and works would well repay the effort: physician, romancier, pornographer, popular commentator, he holds an important place in the history of Western sexology because he antedates the German sexologists by at least a generation.

26 See also Morel de Rubempré (1842).

27 The reader must approach this typical passage of Morel with care, for he is a masterful rhetorician. His language is charged and coded; see, for example, the use of 'involuntary'. He has just invoked it, a paragraph earlier, of the male prostitute's touch: 'This contact, initially seemingly involuntary, is the masculine prostitute's skilful way of approaching you [...] he comes closer and [...] it will not be long before you see the [...] audacious carnal touching: this is the hideous provocation of that miserable prostituted human creature [...] this strange sodomitical creature also has, like the sluts, his home, his places of triumph, his house of call [...]' In the passage cited at the top of p 147, however, it is rectal discharge which is 'involuntary'. Repetition of the word provides an encoded moral narrative: from first bodily temptation to ultimate bodily consequence. Morel routinely uses morality as a mask; here his lurid account of anatomical signs is genuine. He was one of the few Paris doctors to articulate his disgust at the symptoms, unlike the nineteenth-century dysentery specialists who glanced that way but were silent. Morel, however, also creates a bathetic effect, compiling the terror of history's worst scourges and completing the crescendo's crest in the miserable creature's eroded anus vomiting 'greenish discharges'. Here he additionally mocks hysterical readers of his treatise who react to sodomy even more viscerally than plague. His final disclaimer caps the folly: just having described in nuanced and lurid French the greatest grossnesses of his subject, he claims he can 'no longer speak French'.

> Sodomy should be seen in terms of hygiene and medicine. This fatal propensity, this deplorable practice is liable to reproduce the same terrible effects of lesbianism among women, and moreover, that cruel rectal discharge (from the anus), those ulcerations of the anus, those cankers in the same place, the fistulas and other unfortunate accidents, which together all too often give birth to a triple evacuation of blood, pus and fecal matter, constitute one of the most hideous complicated diseases of humanity. I have seen cholera, I have seen typhus, I have seen the plague, the most hideous scabs and lepers; but nothing seemed to me more miserable than a miserable creature whose anus is eroded by numerous phagedenic [that is, caused by the cholera bacteria] ulcers, whose rectum, source of the most fetid greenish discharges, and through which escape *involuntarily* [my emphasis], and often at all moments of the day, those substances which one can only dispose of in the latrines at certain times of day. I close the subject, for I no longer know how to speak French when it comes to describing things like this.[28]

'I no longer know how to speak French.' Given that Morel makes this disclaimer *after* the event, after he has described in lurid French the most intimate grossness of his subject, we are reinforced in the impression that he has been double dealing – no less so than the refined voices of his age decrying *cholera Asiaticus* as a barbaric disease. And why is the male prostitute's rectal discharge involuntary? The doctor cannot help himself from being touched by his patients, any more than he (the prostitute) can prevent the discharge. Morel's intentions in this work are ambiguous. In any case, this is not the place to dwell on his treatise except to notice how it combines cholera and sodomy in the specific geographical site of the 'bum'. He was one of the few doctors openly to avow disgust for the symptoms themselves – other cholera specialists hardly even suggest that it might be unpleasant. Morel constructs the terror of the world's most sublime scourges by claiming that what is even more miserable than they are is a wretched creature's eroded choleric anus.[29]

The road from Morel and his fellow sexologists of the 1840s and 1850s – especially Dr Ambroise Tardieu (1818–1879) of *Herculine Barbin* fame[30] – to the evolving 'intermediate sexes' of Edward Carpenter, and Havelock Ellis, is not tortured. It passed through the edifices constructed by Charles Darwin in his 1859 *Origin of Species*, Karl Maria Benkert's neologism of the 1860s about an evolving homosexual type, the degeneration theories of the 1860s and 1870s, culminating in the German sexology of the 1880s and Krafft-Ebbing's *Psychopathia Sexualis* (1884) – all pronouncing in one way or another on the invert's anatomical differences. Dr Tardieu almost represents the culmination and convergence of these theories. He rose quickly to the top of his profession without any of the doubts that lingered for Morel. A leading doctor in French prisons, he soon became the chief forensic exponent in France and a pioneer in its developing sexology. He provided the first description of the battered child syndrome, now known as the '*Tardieu Syndrome*'.

---

28 Morel de Rubempré (1842) pp 44–45.

29 Note his repeated uses of 'miserable' for these creatures of the bum: whom exactly among his readers does he address?

30 Foucault drew his portrait of Herculine's hermaphroditical fundament from Dr Tardieu's treatise.

He pronounced on all sorts of sexual irregularities and abnormalities – no wonder Foucault was so engrossed in his works, especially his '*Étude médico-légale sur les attentats aux moeurs*', of which *De la pédérastie* is the third part). He was therefore doubly an authority in this area, and known to be working on his *Question médico-légale de l'identité* (1874). He trained, among other medical students, Antoine Proust, father of Marcel Proust, the great novelist. More germane, perhaps, for our purposes, he pronounced at length on *both* sodomy and cholera: no doubt lingers about his views on either.

Tardieu believed that the anus is the most vulnerable region of the hermaphrodite's, or evolving new sex's, anatomy as well as the pederast's. Hence, when examining a typical pederast:

> ... the anus presents the most characteristic traces of sodomite violence. Apart from the deep infundibulum [funnel shape] that the anal region forms, the sphincter is completely loose, and the orifice is dilated to the point where it no longer contains fecal matter, and the simple opening of the edge of the anus gives rise to the emission of abundant gases.[31]

Tardieu joined the two again in a 'Treatise on epidemic cholera; being lectures delivered under the authority of the faculty of medicine of Paris'.[32] Despite his inability to name the rectum in the presence of his medical students to whom these lectures are delivered, he leaves them in no doubt through euphemism that the rectum is the chief site of cholera. Constitutional and moral influences were conjoined and loomed large in his theory, the individuals most susceptible to the new cholera being those already 'exhausted by antecedent diseases'. Tardieu's resort to polite euphemism did not alter significantly over the next century. It is little wonder then that the nonagenarian EM Forster, when commenting on his novel *Maurice* in great old age, pointed to homosexuality's chief sign in the semiotic of the bum. Forster, the informed novelist of *A Passage to India* (1924), was well-read in Indian sub-continent cholera, as well as post-Carpenterian theories about homosexuality. It required no great imaginative leap to combine medical plague and sexual stigma. Indeed, Forster could have taken the step without becoming versed in the new medicine or sexology of his maturity. Proof lies in his 1962 postscript to *Maurice*. Construed carefully it forms a cultural explanation of the genesis of the old, pre-Darwinian sodomy which had segued into the new homosexuality of his Edwardian adulthood, but Forster, like his predecessors, could never bring himself to name the anatomical spot.

Bibliography

Anonymous, *Satan's Harvest Home*, 1749, London: np.

Aldrich, Robert, *The Seduction of the Mediterranean: Writing, Art and Homosexual Fantasy*, 1993, London: Routledge.

Arderne, John, *Treatise on Fistula in Ano*, 1541: np.

---

31 Tardieu (1858) vol 9, part 3, '*De la pederastie et de la sodomie*', pp 146–224.

32 It originally formed part of his *Manuel de Pathologie Medicale* (1848). The 1849 English translation was by Samuel Lee Bigelow, MD, Boston, MA: Ticknor, Reed and Fields.

Berard, Frédéric, *Discours sur les ameliorations progressives de la santé publique*, 1826, Paris: np.

Coleridge, Samuel Taylor, *The Complete Poems*, 1997, London: Penguin.

Delaporte, François, *Disease and Civilization: The Cholera in Paris, 1832*, translated by Goldhammer, Arthur, 1986, Cambridge, MA, and London: MIT Press.

Dewhurst, Kenneth (ed), *Dr Thomas Sydenham (1624–1689): His Life and Original Writings*, 1966, London: Wellcome Historical Medical Library.

Forster, EM, *Maurice*, 1971, London: Edward Arnold.

Freud, Sigmund, 'Three essays on sexuality, and other works', in Strachey, James, (ed), *Standard Edition of the Complete Psychological Works of Sigmund Freud*, vol 7, 1953, London: Hogarth Press.

Gilbert, Ruth, *Early Modern Hermaphrodites*, 2002, London: Palgrave.

Gilman, Sander, *Difference and Pathology: Stereotypes of Sexuality, Race and Madness*, 1985, Ithaca, NY: Cornell University Press.

Guichard, J, *Relation statistique et pathologique du choléra morbus dans le quartier des invalides*, 1832, Paris: np.

Lauvergne, H, *Choléra-morbus de Provence*, 1836, Toulon: np.

Masten, Jeffrey, 'Is the fundament a grave?' in Hillman, D and Mazzio, C (eds), *The Body in Parts: Fantasies of Corporeality in the Early Modern World*, 1997, London: Routledge, pp 129–46.

Menuret, J-J, *Essai sur l'action de l'air dans les maladies contagieuses*, 1781, Paris: np.

Metral, *Description naturelle, morale et politique du choléra-morbus a Paris*, 1833, Paris: np.

Morel de Rubempré, J, *Traité des dégénérescences physiques intellectuelles et morales de l'espèce humaine*, 1842, Paris: Baillière.

Morel de Rubempré, J, *La pornologie ou histoire nouvelle universelle et complète de la débauche et de la prostitution et autres dépravations dans tous les pays du monde, notamment en France particulièrement dans Paris depuis les temps les plus anciens jusqu'à nos jours, et moyens infaillibles de remédier à ces fléaux et de diminuer le nombre des prostituées sans employer la rigueur*, 1857, Paris: Terry.

Morin, J, *Manuel théorique et pratique d'hygiène*, 1835, Paris: np.

Pringle, John, *Observations on the Diseases in the Army*, 1752, London: A Millar.

Prior, WS, *A Treatise on the Mistreatment of Cholera Morbus (1832)*, third edition, 1833, London: np.

Prost, A, *Traité du choléra-morbus considéré sous les rapports physiologiques, anatomico-pathologiques, thérapeutiques et hygièniques*, 1832, Paris: np.

Rousseau, George S, *Perilous Enlightenment: Pre- and Post-modern Discourses – Sexual, Historical*, 1991, Manchester: Manchester University Press.

Rousseau, George S and Haycock, David, 'Coleridge's choleras: cholera morbus, asiaticus cholera, and dysentery in early nineteenth-century England' (2003) 30 *Bulletin of the History of Medicine* 298–331.

Swan, John (ed), *The Entire Works of Dr Thomas Sydenham, Newly Made English from the Originals*, 1742, London.

Tardieu, AA, *Manuel de pathologie médicale*, 1848, Paris: np.

Tardieu, AA, *Treatise on Epidemic Cholera*, 1849, Paris: np.

Tardieu, AA, *Question médico-légale de l'identité*, 1874, Paris: np.

Tardieu, AA, *'Etude médico-légale sur les attentats aux moeurs'* in *Annales d'hygiène publique et de médecine légale*, second series, vol 9, 1858, Paris: np.

Theweleit, Klaus, *Male Fantasies, Vol 2: Male Bodies: Psychoanalyzing the White Terror*, translated by Conway, Stephen *et al*, 1992, Minneapolis, MN: University of Minnesota Press.

CHAPTER 10

BEHOLD THE (SICK) MAN

Michael Worton

The title of this chapter is, of course, a modification of the celebrated Biblical phrase, 'Behold the man' or *Ecce Homo.* This phrase marks a key moment in the public life of Jesus Christ and, as will be seen later, has come to be much used as the title of exhibitions representing the male body (as well as of Nietzsche's celebrated autobiographico-philosophical work of 1888, which is tellingly subtitled 'How one becomes what one is'). In this chapter, I take this culturally resonant phrase as a starting-point for the examination of some photographic representations of illness in men which seem to me to interrogate in interesting ways the nature both of masculinity and of mortality.

The Biblical context of *Ecce Homo* is that, in the hours leading up to his crucifixion, Jesus was taken through a series of quasi-legal proceedings that flaunted any sense of justice. At one point, Pilate, the Roman governor, ordered that he be whipped; after this, the soldiers mocked him by placing a crown of plaited thorns on his head, clothing him in a purple robe and pretending to worship him as a king. Pilate then ordered that Jesus be led out and displayed to the jeering crowd:

> Then Pilate therefore took Jesus, and scourged him,
> And the soldiers platted a crown of thorns, and put it on his head, and they put on him a purple robe. And said, 'Hail, King of the Jews!' And they smote him with their hands.
> Pilate therefore went forth again, and saith unto them, 'Behold, I bring him forth to you, that ye may know that I find no fault in him'.
> Then came Jesus forth, wearing the crown of thorns, and the purple robe. And Pilate saith unto them, *'Behold the man!'*
>
> Gospel according to St John 19:5

This is the moment of the *Ecce homo*. The words *Behold the man* are those of Pontius Pilate, who brings Jesus out before the crowd in order to disculpate himself and to state publicly that he can 'find no fault in him'. As governor of Jerusalem, Pilate is bound by tradition to release one prisoner at the time of the feast; he offers the crowd the liberation of Jesus, but the crowd of Jews vociferously choose Barrabas, a convicted robber, demanding that Jesus be crucified. Pilate then, in a symbolic gesture which has as much cultural weight as his words of presentation, washes his hands before the crowd, saying 'I am innocent of the blood of this just person' (Matthew 27:24). The 'Ecce Homo!' is thus a powerful expression of belief in the *innocence* of a victim who is destined to be a scapegoat (and, in Jesus' case, the archetypal scapegoat as ultimate saviour).

It is important to note that the phrase 'Behold the man' is found in an Old Testament prophecy that heralds the coming of Israel's Messiah:

> Thus speaketh the Lord of hosts, saying, 'Behold the man whose name is Branch': and he shall grow up out of his place; and he shall build the temple of Jehovah; even he shall build the temple of Jehovah; and he shall bear the glory, and shall sit and rule upon his throne; and he shall be a priest upon his throne; and the counsel of peace shall be between them both.
>
> Zechariah 6:12–13

The theological relationship between the Old and New Testaments is that what is foretold in the Old is realised in the New. The repetition of the 'Ecce Homo' phrase thus 'proves' theologically that Jesus is indeed the Messiah, the saviour of Israel and the deliverer of the Jewish nation, and he becomes the saviour through passing through mockery, unjust accusations, crucifixion, death and finally resurrection.

However, for my purposes, what is particularly significant about the episode and especially about Pilate's phrase is the dimension of display, of exhibition whereby Jesus – as God made *Man* – becomes an object of monstrosity,[1] a freak to be publicly displayed and mocked. In the history of Western art, the theme of *Ecce Homo* is rare before the Renaissance, but thereafter it becomes one of the most powerful of Christian images. The most famous early painter of this theme is Hieronymus Bosch, whose best-known version is perhaps the 1485–90 one now in the Philadelphia Museum of Art, which portrays a bestial, baying crowd presided over by a distant, impervious Pilate who refuses even to open his eyes and watch. The *Ecce Homo* subject as such comes in two distinct versions in art. The first of these is a full *narrative account*, in which Christ is shown wearing the emblems of kingship with which the mocking soldiers have invested him – the crown of thorns, the purple cloak and often a reed sceptre. In this tradition, the *Ecce Homo* painting is more than a historical or Biblical work: it serves as a reminder that the judgment of one's contemporaries and peers is often flawed, blind and riven with self-interest. In my view, the painting which best and most powerfully represents this tradition is Bosch's version of 1490, now in the Städelsches Kunstinstitut in Frankfurt, where Jesus is portrayed as intensely human, as he stands stooping, dejected and humiliated, before the hostile crowd (Figure 1). Jesus as the Son of Man stands for all humanity, but in this image he is very much a male figure, as opposed to an otherworldly one, as in many other depictions of this scene (including Bosch's earlier version). The humiliation and shame that he undergoes are thus assaults on his masculinity as well as on his claims to divinity.

The other major tradition is very different and centres on Jesus himself, with the jeering crowd or other spectators virtually absent, figuring in the paintings only as a frame for the image of Christ wearing a crown of thorns; indeed, often the painting presents only the head of Christ who accepts his suffering and looks forward to his crucifixion and death. In such images, the painting is intended as a

1 Here I would emphasise the etymological fact that 'monster' and 'monstrous' come from the Latin 'monstrare', to show. In other words, a monster is not inherently ugly or frightening or whatever, but derives its 'monstrosity' from the fact of being an object of display; its identity is not innate but is determined by the gaze and the presuppositions (and prejudices) of the crowd.

devotional image, which, as an aid to meditation, can facilitate recognition both of the place of suffering in the world and of the possibility of (deferred) transcendence. One of the most moving examples of this type of *Ecce Homo* is Correggio's beautiful work of 1525–30 in the National Gallery in London (Figure 2), where Christ gazes over and beyond the imploring look of his mother into the future that awaits him. While his head is most definitely male, his torso, his arms and especially his hands are very feminine, thereby making of him an androgynous figure who symbolises all humanity, both men and women, in their thirst and hope of transcendence.

More recently, the phrase 'Ecce Homo' has been used as the title of a variety of exhibitions. Three examples will serve to give a flavour of how widely this phrase is now used. The first is that of the Swedish artist Elisabeth Ohlson (1961–), whose exhibition of 1998–99 was inspired by Biblical themes and by the work of Michelangelo, Caravaggio and Doré and consisted of 12 photographs of the figure of Jesus in the company of modern-day homosexual men and women, thereby provoking public debates about the nature of Christianity, the body, sexuality and sexual orientation.[2] A second example is that of the Lebanese-American painter, Chawky Frenn, who in 2001 exhibited under this title a series of paintings which he describes as 'dream cabinets' and which were inspired by altar pieces and museum dioramas as well as by his memories of confrontations with death and mortality in war-torn Lebanon. These works explore the relationships between death, desire, memory and longing, the *Homo* here being mankind in general, although usually figured as male.[3] A third and very different exhibition under this rubric was the 1997 collective exhibition by 24 sculptors on the theme of 'What is the nature of Mankind now?'.[4] The central project of this *Ecce Homo* exhibition was to interrogate whether humanity has changed over the past century or millennium, especially in the light of major changes in healthcare, in the role of the media, commercialisation, globalisation, etc.

These examples show how differently the title of *Ecce Homo* can be used in the art world, but my purpose here is not to chart the compulsively fascinating history of this theme in Western art. Rather, I want to take the Biblical statement and the artistic genre that has resulted from it as my starting point, since there is a cultural force and a cross-cultural resonance in the *Ecce Homo* which, in terms of the representation of suffering, are more complex and perhaps, in today's largely

---

2 When shown in Uppsala Cathedral, the exhibition caused great controversy and opposition within the church and led to the Pope cancelling an audience with the Swedish Archbishop, K-G Hammar, who had invited Ohlson to show her works in Uppsala Cathedral. The exhibition toured Sweden, the rest of Scandinavia and several other countries in Europe, but the European Parliament in Strasbourg eventually banned it. For details of the exhibition, together with all the images, see www.eccehomo.nu/eng/indexeng.html (accessed 4 February 2004).

3 The exhibition was shown in a variety of venues in the USA in 2000–01, beginning in the Johnson Centre and Fine Art Galleries, George Mason University, Fairfax, Virginia, where Frenn is Assistant Professor of Painting.

4 This exhibition organised by the Art Foundation Hazart was held in the sculpture garden and gallery of De Hazelaar Sculptures near Amsterdam, June to September 1997.

secular cultural psycho-politics, more important than those generated by representations of the Crucifixion – which is a specifically Christian event. I intend therefore to consider four images by different photographers, each of which engages – astonishingly, provocatively and, above all, movingly – with the problematics of representing and seeing illness. The illnesses involved are smallpox, AIDS and varicose veins, but the common illness that they all both engage with and make present is the more insidious but truly mortal disease of *intolerance*.

I would argue that the artistic representation of suffering in the West almost invariably has a religious, not to say a theological, dimension: we cannot forget the suffering of Jesus, even if we are non-believers or followers of another faith than Christianity. However, alongside the Christian tradition (which dominates Western art even today), there is another tradition, one which stems from Ancient Greece but which serves to reinforce the Christian message about the place and function of suffering. Since Aristotle associated art with catharsis, the aesthetic has been held to have a moral function. Indeed, from Aeschylus onwards, Western culture has privileged the notion of *pathei mathein* ('suffering alone teaches'), thereby making of illness an ethical and epistemological phenomenon and ensuring that the *aesthetics* of illness and even the *representation* of illness remain largely unexplored areas.

Susan Sontag has convincingly argued in different places that the metaphorising of cancer as a judgment on the individual is complicit with modern secular ideas of selfhood and that the metaphorising of AIDS in pre-modern terms as a 'plague' enables collective judgments to be passed on communities and even whole societies.[5] Illness can thus be used as a social weapon, being a potential tool of and for societal and inter-societal manipulation and even oppression. One function of the artist of disease is therefore to combat such usage of human suffering by alerting spectators to the fact that ultimately disease will always escape coding, be this coding medical, social, moral or theological. Epidemiology teaches us much about how diseases function, spread and determine social behaviours, but we must remember that everyone suffers in his or her very own way and that almost every individual ill person fails to conform in detail to the scientific pattern established for the disease.

I have become fascinated by the way in which photographers, as opposed to other artists such as painters, sculptors, or even writers, can represent illness and suffering in ways which are particularly interesting, exciting and challenging. The four I have chosen to consider here (Ajamu, Rotimi Fani-Kayode, Duane Michals and Joel-Peter Witkin) are very different, although their works were all created within a period of seven years (1985–92). What binds them together is the fact that each of them is highly culturally aware and engenders in the spectator a process of speculation about meaning and meaningfulness. This process often begins with aesthetic pleasure (and sometimes with enjoyment of the humour in the images), but it can also be one which combines a certain anxiety with creativity, as these

5 See Sontag (1979) and Sontag (1989).

works draw their spectators first into a recognition of their presuppositions and prejudices and then away from these and into fresh thinking and seeing.

Photography and mortality

The patron saint of photography is St Veronica, the woman of Jerusalem who felt compassion for Jesus as he painfully carried his cross to Calvary and wiped his sweating face with a cloth – on which was left an image of his features.[6] This was therefore the first 'photograph' in history! Veronica's name can be anagrammatised into *vera icon*, thereby permitting photographers the delightful fantasy that their art fuses transcendental truth (*vera*) and concrete reality (*icon*) in their images. I would highlight in passing that the metaphors of Veronica's veil and the Shroud of Turin are used almost interchangeably by many theorists of photography, thereby unconsciously equating the mark of mortality and death with the proof of existence.[7] According to Susan Sontag:

> Photography is an elegiac art, a twilight art. [...] All photographs are memento mori. To take a photograph is to participate in another person's (or thing's) mortality, vulnerability, mutability.[8]

In a more personal, whilst equally theoretical vein, Roland Barthes reveals in *Camera Lucida* that, when being photographed, he suffered from a sensation of inauthenticity and experienced a micro-version of death – which he defined as 'parenthesis'.[9] Almost all modern theories of photography are, in fact, grounded in anxiety – about time, about loss – and conceptualise the semantic and representational functioning of photographs as analogous to the work of mourning. Perhaps the most beautifully considered definition of a photograph is offered by Mary Price: 'a picture of that which is about to become a memory, a capturing of what, in the present which is about to become the past, is to be remembered.'[10] Photography is therefore (about) loss. However, it also provides a sense of 'having been there' and thereby contributes to the diminution of solitude.

Although it may in one sense be true that one always suffers alone, there is also always a need to fracture or transcend that solitude, to attempt to do something with the suffering, to make it matter. Our (Western) culture has instilled in us the belief that suffering can open up an ethical dimension within the sufferer, in the sense that an individual's pain – which surely has no point in itself – can nonetheless take on a charge of meaning if it becomes the occasion for the empathetic, even suffering response of a reader or spectator. Furthermore, while

---

6 Although there is no reliable evidence for this event, a cloth which is claimed to be 'Veronica's Veil' is held in St Peter's in Rome.

7 See, for instance, Guibert (1981) pp 93 and 127.

8 Sontag (2002) p 15

9 Barthes (1982) p 14.

10 Price (1994) p 163.

pain is a fundamentally solitary experience, it is also deeply social; indeed, in many ways it is a socially constructed and *relative* phenomenon. Consequently, although we feel totally alone and separated from our culture and society when experiencing acute pain, it is impossible to write about or visually represent our suffering in a wholly individualistic way, since both the pain and our experience of it are shaped by that very culture from which we feel cut off.

Jean-Paul Clébert, the biographer of Alphonse Daudet, the nineteenth-century French writer who died after suffering severely in the tertiary stage of syphilis, has suggested that 'When one discovers that one is ill, one finds the words to say it'.[11] This is, I would suggest, quite simply not true. When we contract a disease, we often set about learning the specialised vocabulary of that disease, but in the reality of our experience of pain, the only words we have to describe our pains are those that are socially determined – and these are usually dead metaphors, such as a stabbing pain, a dull ache, a feeling of being drained, etc.

To experience pain does not consist in being wholly centred on one's physical suffering; rather, it is an experience between selfishness and engagement with others. As Alphonse Daudet himself puts it in his account of his own suffering:

> Unless you want to behave like an abominable egotist, you have to avoid giving expression to your pain so as not to upset those around you. [...] Our pain is always new to us, but becomes quite familiar to those around us. It soon wears out its welcome, even for those who love us the most. Compassion loses its edge. [...] the only real way to be ill is to be by yourself.[12]

Furthermore, suffering through being ill has more than a physical and a social dimension: it also has an ontological dimension, even if most of us do not conceive or articulate of it in those terms: as David Morris argues, 'Pain in effect spends its existence moving in-between the extremes of absolute meaninglessness and full meaning'.[13] This is an important insight – and it helps us to understand just how difficult it is to represent suffering, since the very experience of pain is itself so extraordinarily torn, dichotomous, inexplicable.

Visual artists working on the representation of illness and suffering necessarily work within a social and cultural tradition; they recognise that their works are necessarily the product of a tradition. My four chosen photographers are all working within the tradition of the representation of the male, which includes as a major dimension the heritage of *Ecce Homo*. The challenge they set themselves is to create works that will use the familiarity of social codes of representation to make us think again about the individual(s) attacked by the disease – whether these individuals be those represented (as in Witkin's *John Herring*) or those evoked and invoked (as in Fani-Kayode's *Sonponnoi*). Furthermore, the interrogations that they mobilise will focus to a great extent on the sick and decaying body as an object that needs to be *seen* and not occulted or made invisible as if it were something of which to be ashamed.

---

11 Clébert (1988) p 194 (my translation).

12 Daudet (2002) pp 76–78.

13 Morris (1991) p 35.

Historically, men, unlike women, have not needed to explore their own body image, because their relation with the world is not mediated by the body in the way that women's social place and role have been constructed by their biological functions. Indeed, in order for men to preserve the hegemony of male power, it has been essential to keep the body at a safe distance, even if it cannot be rendered completely invisible. The body is always there, but rarely accorded (by men) its place as a fundamental structuring principle.[14] Indeed, in order to retain their power, men have collectively refused to interrogate their bodies, which have thereby become unhealthily protected from public (and often private) scrutiny. Illness changes all that and makes the body urgently present, albeit in a state of deterioration and decay.

As soon as the social structure is shaken, as it has been through such different phenomena as the creative challenges of feminism and the ravages of AIDS (for long perceived – in the West – as a gay male plague), traditional certainties about masculinity begin to dissolve and the male body becomes the site of interrogation rather than of affirmation and confidence, and this means that masculinity needs to be increasingly recognised as a personal narrative or representation. However, this personalising of the body is no privatisation, no appropriation or imposition of power through secrecy and willed invisibility. It is a staging of difference, a play of and with representation that entails a repositioning of the question(s) of gender outside the traditional binary oppositions of male/female and heterosexual/homosexual.

So what can photography bring to representation that is unique and why is it special? To a large extent its distinctiveness is due to its realism, which paradoxically makes it a problematic and troubling medium. This is because, as we know from literary theory, realism is about communicating an *effect* of the real rather than presenting or imitating the real itself: in other words, mimesis is a performance rather than a representation. And if 'photography's realism creates a confusion about the real',[15] this is particularly true of photographs of illness which, whether they are of an individual or a group, make present and therefore give a certain ontological status to their subjects, thereby making icons of things that should remain images. This ontological confusion is responsible for the ambivalent status of photography, in both aesthetic and socio-political terms, for the photograph seems to issue directly from the physical world, yet it is also (and it is perceived anxiously as) an intervention into – and a manipulation of – the world of empirical experience.

---

14 Barthes (1977) p 175, argues that 'the body is irreducible difference, and [...] is also at the same time the principle of all structuration'.

15 Sontag (2002) p 110.

Photographic perspectives on illness

Rotimi Fani-Kayode[16] was influenced by the work of Robert Mapplethorpe in his quest to create images which fused desire, ritual and the black body – beautiful images which were made to be gazed upon and savoured. However, he was also greatly influenced by his Yoruba heritage. Fani-Kayode's family were forced to leave Nigeria in 1966 as political refugees, so his experience of life was always as an outsider, neither wholly Nigerian nor wholly English; furthermore, he was (a) an artist, (b) gay, and, towards the end of his life (c) a Person With AIDS (PWA). He thus suffered a sense of exclusion and marginalisation from his culture, which nonetheless he sought to incorporate into his work, both as images and in terms of his creative thought-processes.

His family had the title of Akire or 'Keepers of the Shrine of Ifa', Ifa being the oracle divinity in the Yoruba religion and second only to the all-powerful god Olorun with respect to wisdom and foreknowledge. This heritage suggested to him the practice of seeking to emulate the 'technique of ecstasy' through which the Yoruba priests became possessed and communicated with the gods: Fani-Kayode's aim was to communicate with the unconscious mind and also to fuse Yoruba and Western, often Christian traditions and iconographies, in order first to seduce his spectators aesthetically and thereafter to oblige them to think. This is clearly seen in his work, *Sonponnoi* (Figure 3).

In the Yoruba religion, beneath Olorun there are several hundred *orisha* or minor gods, one of the most powerful being Sonponnoi, the god of smallpox, who is dreaded because he is a manifestation of the wrath of Olorun, and punishes offenders with smallpox. He became particularly important in the smallpox plagues that were transmitted by various inter-tribal wars – indeed, he became so feared that some Yoruba were too frightened even to pronounce his name. Also, Sonponnoi was not to be worshipped in towns, and all sacrifices and offerings to him had to be taken to the country. Indeed, as a result of threatening the other divinities with smallpox, he was forbidden to associate with them and became an outcast, living in uninhabited parts of Yorubaland. The divinity himself was therefore in a sense marginalised, ostracised, even when he was at his most powerful. Furthermore, smallpox was considered a disgrace, because of the unsightly nature of the disease, and its victims were ostracised, just as lepers were in the Middle Ages (Figure 4 and Figure 5).

Significantly for Fani-Kayode's work, Sonponnoi's shrines were painted with a design of spots: these spots have been transposed by the artist to the headless and therefore anonymous, marginalised body in the photograph.

---

16 Fani-Kayode was born in Nigeria in 1955 and died in London in 1989. A photographer who studied first economics and then fine art in the USA, he was a founding member and the first chairperson of Autograph, the Association of Black Photographers. His photographic world focuses on the body as a means of exploring the relationship between erotic fantasy and ancestral spiritual values.

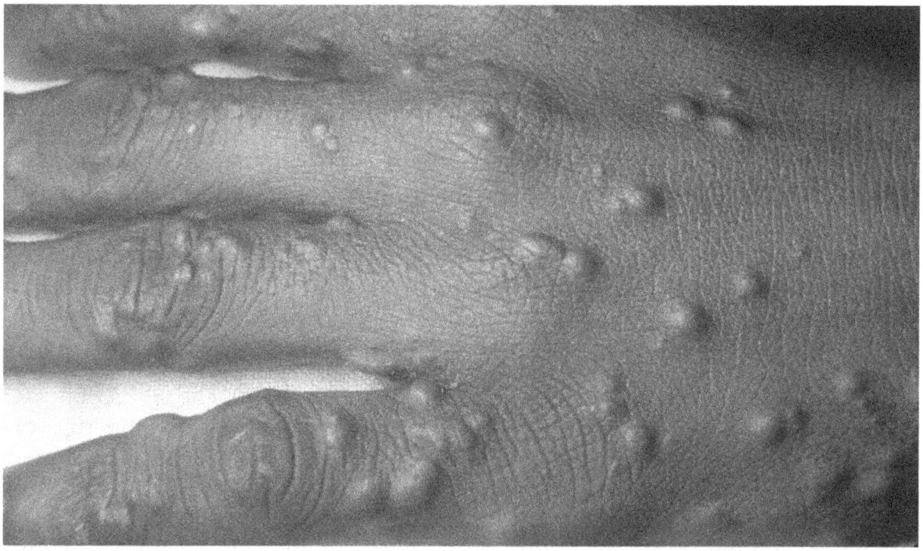

Figure 4: *Smallpox on the Hand* © The Wellcome Trust Picture Library, London.

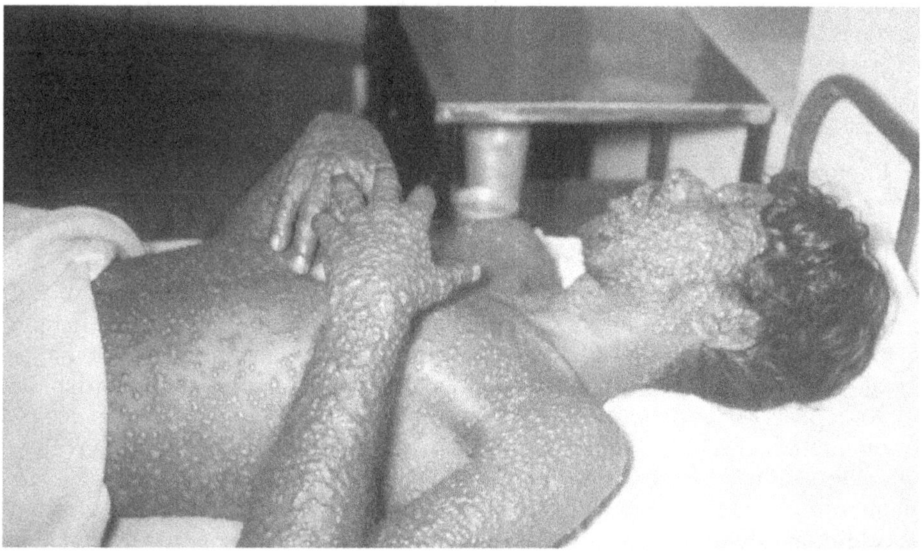

Figure 5: *Smallpox on the Torso* © The Wellcome Trust Picture Library, London.

In 1980, the World Health Organisation officially declared smallpox eradicated from the globe. However, the spectre of smallpox remains very powerful in Africa. The priests of Sonponnoi may have lost their power as the cult vanished as a practice, due to the fact that the British Government forbade his worship. Nonetheless, the force of the cultural memory of Sonponnoi remains very strong. Fani-Kayode's transposition of the spots from the shrine to the seated body with its ritual necklaces obliges those familiar with Yoruba beliefs to rethink the meaning of those spots, which both represent the pustules of smallpox and evoke tribal markings. Furthermore, the figure is holding in his groin – like a phallus – a burning triple candle which evokes both the force of sexuality that continues even in sickness and the trinitarian Christian faith that replaced the Yoruba religion, whilst also bringing through its missionaries relief from diseases like smallpox.

We look at Fani-Kayode's work and marvel at its sensuality and seduction; we also realise that we do not fully understand it, whether we are Nigerian or European. This is no piece of exotic, tribalist art reworked for a Western audience. Nor is it a piece of Western art gesturing nostalgically or gratefully to a lost (colonial or other) past. It is neither Yoruba nor European. It is both beyond and within the different traditions that made it possible. This is the key point about why Fani-Kayode's works are important and powerful: they are not to be decoded and then forgotten; they are to remain in our minds and memories as images that we know to be meaningful because they speak of something deep, of something beyond individual cultures, of something that is calling to us.

Sonponnoi provokes in the spectator musings around the nature of illness and its place in society, and about marginality and exclusion as well as about how one can (and must?) belong to more than one culture – if not wholly to any single one. Thus, art, by reflecting on itself and by referring to its multiple origins, can make us as spectators actively enter the present, excavate our (individual and collective) past and seek new ways into the future.

Photographs normally represent only what people or things looked like at the moment that the photograph is being made. However, we must remember that what is captured is, in a sense, invisible, since the photograph snatches a millisecond of existence out of the flow of time. The human brain processes the mobile information it receives (mobile because the eye scans the static image) and fashions this information into a visual memory. This image-memory is a fiction, an invention, what I have elsewhere called an 'interpretation-collage which makes sense, rather than a replica of a fragment of reality'.[17] In other words, the photograph is an *analogon* of reality. However, this does not mean that it is a representation of reality. Rather, it exists in a relationship of analogy with reality, whereby neither identity nor total and exact reproduction is posited. The photograph is, as Barthes puts it, an 'emanation of *past reality*';[18] I would propose an additional definition: it operates – and is – a translation of reality, and this translation is semantically (and even visually) mobile, as the spectator-reader

17 Worton (1995) p 737.
18 Barthes (1982) p 88.

speculates on the presence and absence of meaning. Furthermore, the image also compels the viewer to go on looking at it. Whether this process of spectating is therapeutic or not is perhaps ultimately not the main point; what matters is that the viewer looks and looks and looks, and finally sees the body as both alien and similar.

Joel-Peter Witkin adopts a very different approach to portray illness, choosing in *John Herring, PWA, Posed as Flora with Lover and Mother* (Figure 6), to present a real individual John Herring who proclaims his masculinity (through his moustache) in the very instant that he is posing as Flora, the goddess of fertility.[19] The persona he is assuming is in direct opposition to his status as a PWA, for Flora, as well as being the goddess of flowers, was the goddess of fertility, abundance, nature and motherhood. This tension is manifested in the contrast between the lavish watered silk eighteenth-century dress and the various pieces of improvisation such as the crumpled tissue paper base on which he is standing, the crude masks on the faces of his lover and his mother, the hastily thrown-on curtain material that passes for antique tunics for his naked lover and his mother whose polka-dot dress is visible beneath, etc. The photograph is explicitly a staging, with John Herring absolutely centre stage in front of a painted backdrop, dominating the image. The photograph evokes eighteenth-century formal portraiture in order simultaneously to exploit and to challenge its signifying processes and to demand that the spectator examine every detail in a quest for its meaning. The first, most forceful, tension is of course that between a moustachioed aging hippie posing as a female goddess and dressed in an elaborate gown. However, one quickly notices that the whole portrait is made up of a series of imaginative, but hasty, improvisations. Allusions to eighteenth-century formal portraiture abound, but the spectator does not need to be informed or aware of any precise references; rather s/he enjoys the sheer fun of this image, whilst also recognising that it abounds in tensions and contradictions. When one has done a tour, as it were, of the image's inventiveness, one turns back to its central point: the face of John Herring, who gazes out calmly at the spectators. What is compelling in the context of the time in which this picture was made is that a man suffering from AIDS offers himself with poise and composure as a 'monster' to be looked at. Through dressing up as Flora, he deliberately draws attention to himself and makes the spectators look at him and interrogate him. He offers himself as very consciously visible, as a presence that cannot be avoided, thereby making of AIDS something to be confronted, but not to be feared. Also, as the title makes explicit, he is not alone: in his living with AIDS as in his posing as Flora, he is accompanied by both his lover and his mother. He is part of a supportive community. In other words, this PWA reveals through the photograph that he is not to be excluded, marginalised or made invisible, as many people at that time would have wished. John Herring may not be an important historical

---

19 Joel-Peter Witkin (1939–) is one of the most influential of contemporary American photographers. He works with uncomfortable subject matter and models, sometimes taking as his models individuals who are already physically disadvantaged or 'freakish', as he puts it, and then rendering them even more outlandish. Fascinated by form and artistic history as much as by the grotesque, he produces images that haunt the spectator.

figure, but through the photograph he ensures that his condition and that of all other AIDS sufferers is considered, thought about and *seen*. John Herring, PWA, has a life-threatening disease; he can also invent; above all, he can also have fun being inscribed into an aesthetic and tradition which both values and creatively undermines cultural history and tradition.

If the Witkin photograph achieves its impact through the presentation of public exposure and provocation, albeit through the means of theatricality and dressing-up, a very different approach is used by Duane Michals in his *The Dream of Flowers* (Figure 7).[20] This work consists of an apparently sleeping man whose head becomes progressively covered with flowers, to the point at which it is almost completely obscured. The first of the four images also has a quality of Narcissus to it, in that the man is like a head on a reflective surface, and this dimension of reflection gives a *specular* quality to the image and encourages the reader into speculation around it. The series of images has a gentle, melancholic feel as, from image to image, the head is gradually submerged under the flowers, with the hair disappearing under a veil created by sprays of delicate blossoms. This work has, on the one hand, evocations of the 'Flower Power' culture of San Francisco in the 1960s; it also evokes the *Ophelia* (1851–52) of the pre-Raphaelite painter John Edward Millais (1792–1881), which represents Ophelia covered in flowers and floating down the river after her suicide. These cultural evocations take on greater significance when one notices that there is a letter written in a shaky hand beneath each image. The word is not complete until the last image, when the head has virtually completely vanished under flowers which can now be read as a form of funeral wreath, for the four-letter word is AIDS. The references to the Flower Power of San Francisco (where AIDS was first diagnosed in the USA) and to Millais's Ophelia-imagery of flowers symbolising death draw the reader into a meditation on the ultimate outcome of AIDS, but Michals's work is in no way seeking to aestheticise or sanitise AIDS through his beautiful images; rather, he draws the spectator into a reflection on the *interactions* of life, death, beauty, and ephemerality.

Fani-Kayode deals with a deadly epidemic (smallpox) that ravaged the world for centuries and Witkin and Michals deal with AIDS, one of the most devastating of today's global health problems. On the other hand, Ajamu[21] chooses a much less serious medical condition, varicose veins, as the focus for one of his explorations of black male sexuality. As often in his work, he uses humour as a

---

20 Duane Michals (1932–) is one of the USA's foremost art photographers. He began his artistic career as a water-colourist. However, in 1956, on a trip to the Soviet Union, he borrowed a friend's camera to take snapshots, and realised when he saw the resulting pictures that he had found his true vocation. In 1966, he started to experiment with what was to become one of his trademark elements: the addition of handwritten texts to his photographs.

21 Ajamu (1963–) is a British photographer who defines himself as 'black and queer' and whose work is grounded in a culture of *otherness* from which he explores issues of race, sexuality and physical difference. Taking as his starting point mainstream notions of the 'normal' body (the stereotype), Ajamu seeks to represent and revalue so-called freaks and freakishness on the basis that the terminology of the freak can be seen as a metaphor for those who are dislocated, estranged and alienated from, and marginalised within, contemporary culture.

way of 'hooking' the viewer and ensuring that s/he looks more closely at and thinks more carefully about his images. *Silver Heels* (Figure 8) makes the viewer initially smile at the sight of muscled but varicose-veined male legs crammed into a pair of women's shoes. Traditional male masculinity is interrogated here, but questions are raised also about femininity and the tyranny of fashion – and about the *visibility* of varicose veins, which are so often hidden beneath support stockings.

Although not life-threatening, varicose veins are extremely common: in the UK, for instance, approximately 20% of the adult population suffers from this venous disease. The condition increases with age, with more than half the population over the age of 65 suffering from it; it is also more common in women than in men at all ages, with 70–80% of pregnant women developing the condition during the first trimester. Furthermore, it is much more prevalent in Westernised and industrialised countries than in developing countries, due to the Western diet with its high fat content, low fibre content and overabundance of refined sugar. In other words, varicose veins are mainly associated with Western pregnant or elderly women. The photograph is witty; it is also provocative. By presenting a black man's legs with the condition (and with his feet in a pair of ladies evening shoes and placed at an angle that is very much a feminine pose), Ajamu challenges several stereotypes at once, demanding that we rethink our presuppositions about masculinity, sexual orientation, blackness, body-building and musculation, women's fashion – and also varicose veins. Programmed by the title, we first of all look at the shoes, then realise that the legs in them are a man's, and finally note that these firm legs are seamed by prominent zigzagging varicose veins. It is at this point that we realise that a significant assault is being launched on all our processes of presupposing and pre-judging as well as on medical diagnostic practices: the anonymous black man *should not* have varicose veins, since he does not fit the profile (a pregnant or elderly Western woman), and yet the proof is there, literally before our eyes. So just as assumptions about black men are contested, so also are presuppositions about who gets what disease and why. Ajamu's photography makes us smile; it also makes us review our ways of seeing and judging the world through the prism of prejudice.[22]

These four photographers all work repeatedly and in different modes with the male body, but I would argue that their photographs dealing with illness are particularly important because they are works of committed and thought-through witnessing. Each of them is playful in one sense or another; each also visually articulates an awareness and a *knowledge* of the complex personal, social and cultural ramifications of being ill. There is a certain elegiac quality in the Witkin and the Michals images, but there is also defiance (in the Witkin) as well as beauty and hope of transcendence through the medium of cultural memory (in the Michals). Fani-Kayode reminds us of how both the divine and the Other may

22 In the context of the gender blurring that Ajamu operates here and elsewhere, it is worth noting that, in a recent interview, he states that his main role models are his mother and his grandmother. See Ajamu (2004) p 23.

illuminate the dark fear of dying, and Ajamu uses the display of a partial presence (the black man's legs) to bring into our conscious musings old Western women as well as young black men. These photographs challenge; they also *help*. As Ross Chambers states in *Facing It*, his beautiful and thoughtful book on AIDS diaries:

> The reason witnessing mitigates the pain it cannot cure seems to lie in the fact that an act of witnessing, contrary to the circumstances of trauma themselves, implies a certain belief in there being a future. [...] the act of witness can never be immediate or direct, but must always be oblique and deferred with respect to its object.[23]

To face a representation of AIDS or smallpox, be it a textual one or a visual one, is to confront more than intimations of mortality, it is to stare the reality of dying in the face. Or is it? What happens, rather, is that one sees something else than what is being represented. An artwork representing illness is radically different from a medical illustration. This is so for two reasons: first, because the creator of the artwork has modified the reality s/he sees, senses or intuits; and secondly, because the spectator-reader approaches the artwork differently, *expecting* a deviation from reality.

The spectator's response will be varied: empathetic, repulsed, charmed, intrigued, etc, and much will depend on the cultural position from which and within which the spectator is viewing the images. Inevitably, however, whatever one's position, to gaze on images of illness can be tantamount to intrusion, as well as being a supportive act of witness. In the four works I have considered (as in many others), we find a radical new conception of the *Ecce Homo*. Here it is man/men as mortal who is/are being presented for mockery. Their specificity, specialness and marginality are foregrounded, yet each of them plays the role of scapegoat and thereby stands for Everyman. Thus, each of these works fulfils (and develops) the dual purposes of the *Ecce Homo* genre, both facilitating meditation and reminding us through their implicit narratives to beware the judgment of our 'fellow men'. And to conclude, I would ask you actively to remember and to *see* the title of this chapter. At the risk of sounding overly Barthesian, everything is in the parenthesis. Sickness is certainly present in these images, but it is in a complex relationship to the 'monstrous men' on display: they are men first, rather than being sick first – although perhaps the sickness is a defining quality of their mortality and their manhood. To see them is to wonder – to wonder at them and to wonder about them. It is also to wonder and to speculate on the meaning and purpose of life. Suffering may not always purify, but the *sight* of it transformed into artworks can certainly change our minds, our hearts – and our prejudices.

Bibliography

Ajamu, 'In the family' (2004) 80 F:S (Winter).
Barthes, Roland, *Roland Barthes*, translated by Howard, Richard, London: Macmillan, 1977. (Originally published as *Roland Barthes*, 1975, Paris: Seuil.)
Barthes, Roland, *Camera Lucida: Reflections on Photography*, translated by Howard,

23 Chambers (1998) p viii.

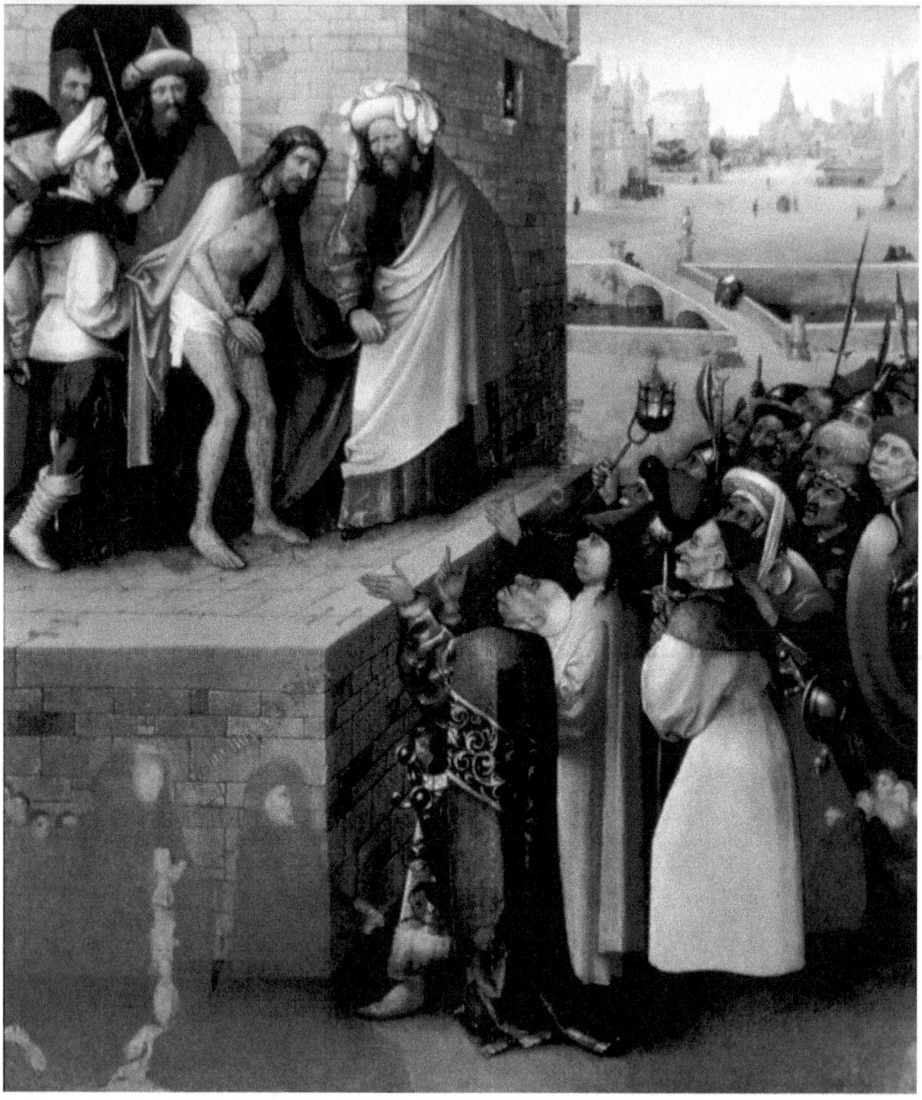

Figure 1: *Ecce Homo*, 1490, Hieronymous Bosch © Städelsches Kunstinstitut und Städlisches Galleria, Frankfurt am Main.

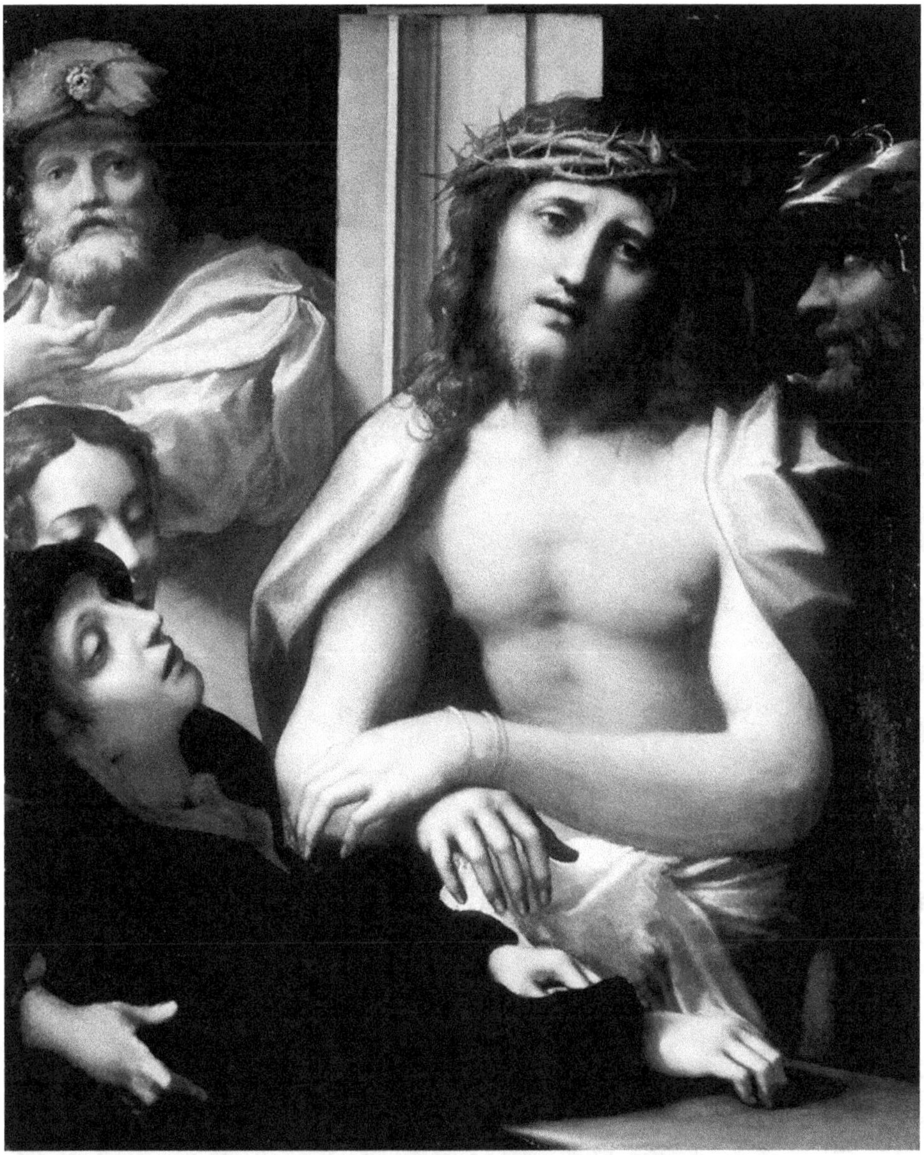

Figure 2: *Christ Presented to the People (Ecce Homo)*, c 1525–30, Antonio Allegri Correggio © The National Gallery, London.

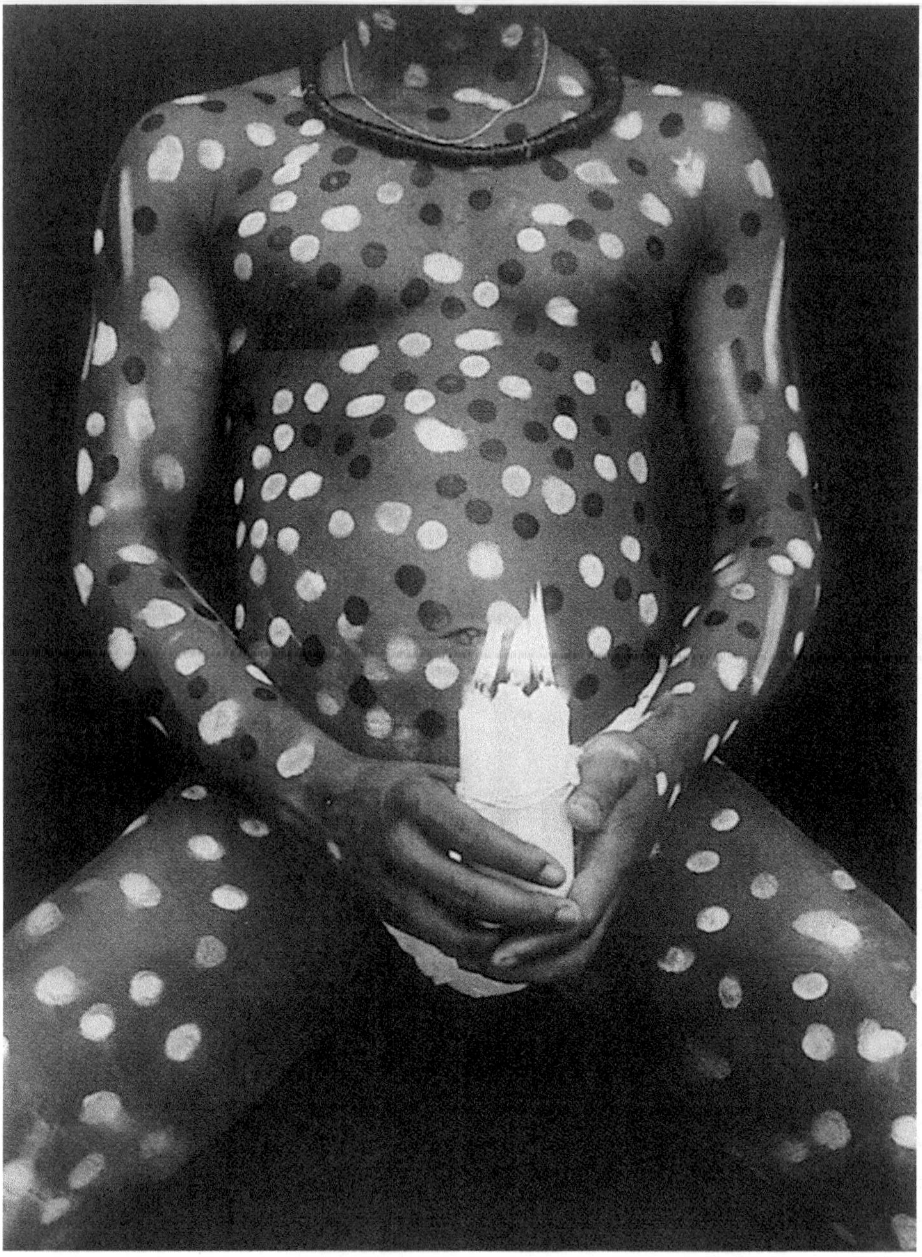

Figure 3: *Sonponnoi*, 1987, Rotimi Fani-Kayode © The Estate of the Artist. Courtesy of Autograph ABP Ltd.

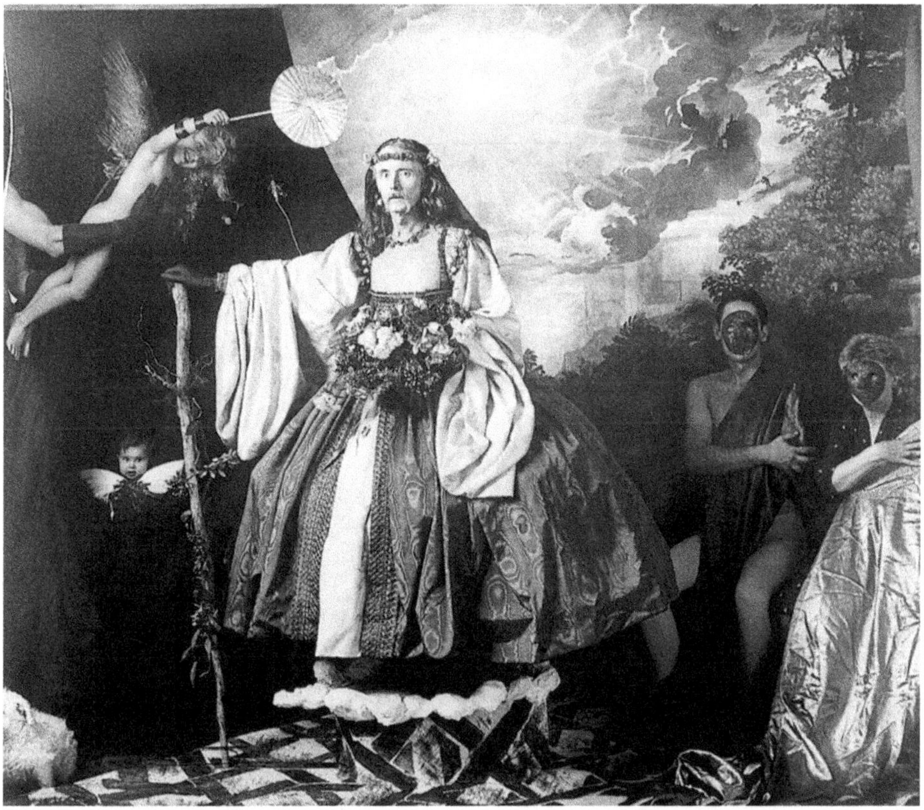

Figure 6: *John Herring, PWA, Posed as Flora with Lover and Mother*, 1982, Joel-Peter Witkin © The Artist. Courtesy of the Fraenkel Gallery, San Francisco.

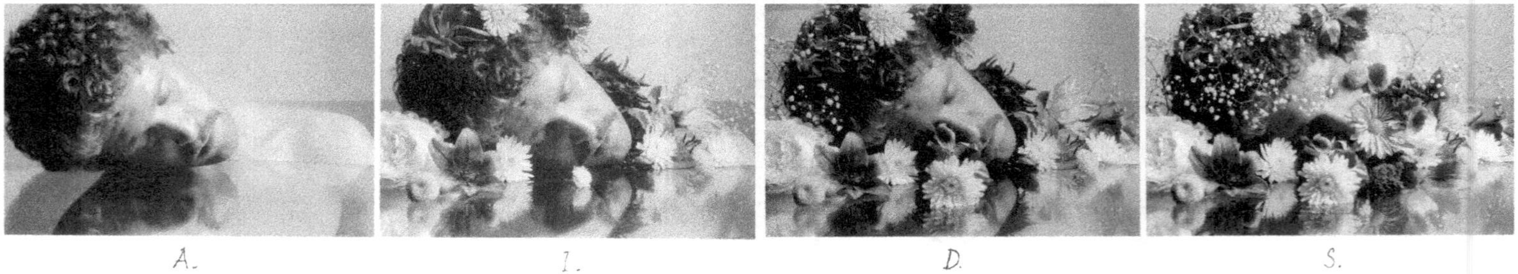

Figure 7: *The Dream of Flowers*, 1985, Duane Michals © The Artist. Courtesy of the Pace/MacGill Art Gallery, New York.

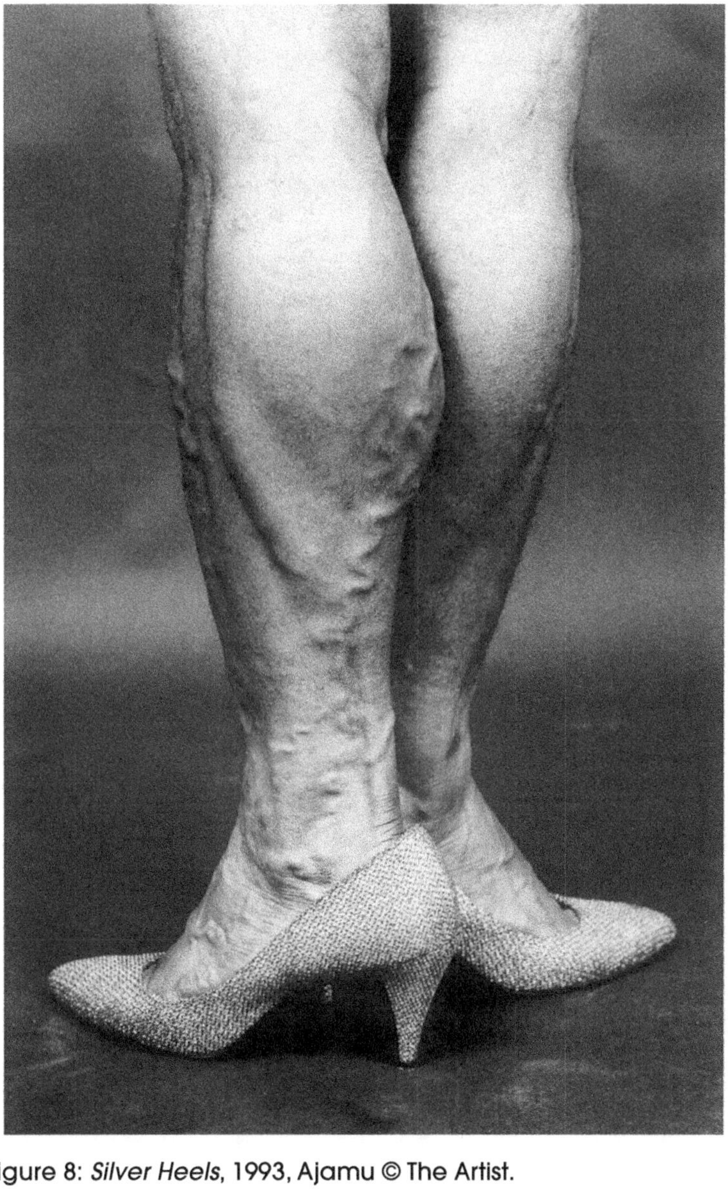

Figure 8: *Silver Heels*, 1993, Ajamu © The Artist.

Richard, 1982, London: Vintage. (Originally published as *La chambre claire: note sur la photographie*, 1980, Paris: Gallimard.)

Chambers, Ross, *Facing It: AIDS Diaries and the Death of the Author*, 1998, Ann Arbor, MI: University of Michigan Press.

Clébert, Jean-Paul, *Une famille bien française: Les Daudet: 1840–1940*, 1988, Paris: Presses de la Renaissance.

Daudet, Alphonse, *In the Land of Pain*, translated by Barnes, Julian, 2002, London: Jonathan Cape. (Originally published as *La Doulou (La Douleur): 1887–1895* et *Le Trésor d'Arlatan: 1897, Œuvres complètes illustrées*, vol 17 of *l'Édition Ne Varietur*, Paris: Librairie de France, 1930.)

Guibert, Hervé, *L'image fantôme*, 1981, Paris: Les Editions de Minuit.

Morris, David B, *The Culture of Pain*, 1991, Berkeley, CA, Los Angeles, CA, Oxford: University of California Press.

Price, Mary, *The Photograph: A Strange Confined Space*, 1994, Stanford, California: Stanford University Press.

Sontag, Susan, *Illness as Metaphor*, 1979, London: Penguin.

Sontag, Susan, *AIDS and its Metaphors*, 1989, London: Penguin.

Sontag, Susan, *On Photography*, 2002, London: Penguin.

Worton, Michael, 'Thinking through photography, remembering to love the past', in Streiff-Moretti, Monique *et al* (eds), *Il senso del nonsenso: scritti in memoria di Lynn Salkin Sbiroli*, 1995, Naples: Edizioni Scientifiche Italiane, pp 733–53.

PART III
LEARNING FROM SICKNESS AND HEALTH

CHAPTER 11

INFECTIOUS SOCIAL CHANGE: TUBERCULOSIS AND EXILE AMONG TIBETAN REFUGEES IN DHARAMSALA

Audrey Prost

This chapter offers an ethnographic exploration of the relationship between tuberculosis, gender and social change, based upon research conducted during a year of fieldwork in the Tibetan exile community of Dharamsala (Himachal Pradesh), India, between 2000 and 2001. The first part of the chapter is an overview of the incidence of tuberculosis in the Tibetan refugee community, while the second part offers a case study focusing on the treatment of one female tuberculosis sufferer in Dharamsala. Through this case study I propose that the epidemiology of tuberculosis, as presented in part one, is echoed and transformed by the social meanings given to it by the community. Social change linked to exile is discussed and critiqued through the 'medicalisation' of social groups effecting change: thus, newcomer refugees who have come to India post-1980 come to be seen as 'contagious', and young 'modern' women to be perceived as a 'risk group'.

Tuberculosis centre stage

Tuberculosis has been reported as the biggest health threat to the Tibetan refugee communities of India. This heterogeneous population of approximately 110,000 Tibetans, divided in 37 communities, includes first, second and third generation refugees,[1] as well as Tibetans who fled the Tibetan Autonomous Region in the 1980s and are generally referred to as 'newcomers' (*gsar 'byor ba*). The original Tibet-born refugees now comprise 35% of the exile population. According to the Central Tibetan Administration in Dharamsala, some 35,000 cases of tuberculosis have been reported in the exile community since 1959.[2] The burden of tuberculosis was described by a leading Tibetan allopathic doctor in Dharamsala as a 'humanitarian crisis', thereby underscoring the urgency and gravity of the situation. Indeed, tuberculosis mobilises the entire spectrum of healthcare

---

1 While the first group of Tibetan refugees that arrived in India in the aftermath of the 1959 exodus were granted refugee status by the Government of India, their children and Tibetans that left the Tibetan Autonomous Region after 1980 were no longer accorded this status. However, since Tibetans refer to themselves as refugees (*btsan byor ba*), I have confounded the legal distinction that demarcate the first, second and third generations by referring to all as refugees.

2 Information given by the Department of Health, Central Tibetan Administration.

practitioners and ritual specialists in Dharamsala: doctors from the institute of traditional medicine (*Men-Tsee-Khang*) know how to recognise the pulmonary form of the disease; local Tibetan and foreign allopathic doctors screen and care for patients in the local hospital; oracles (*mo pa*)[3] deal advice on the best course of therapeutic action in both traditional and allopathic systems; neighbours act as health workers in the Direct Observation Treatment Short course (DOTS) adopted by the hospital; lamas deliver protective threads (*srung dus*) to guard against misfortune and perform funerary rites for the deceased. The diagnosis and therapeutic management of tuberculosis therefore involves a wide range of social agents. Consequently, *ti bi na tsha* (the illness of TB) is constructed out of the symbolic meanings mapped onto the disease by each of these intervening groups.

Quantitative studies of TB incidence among Tibetan exiles indicate notable variations in infection rates between regions, age and occupational groups, but no qualitative study to date has sought to correlate how popular perceptions of TB affect the spread and treatment of disease in the community. The sufferer's experience of TB must, moreover, be understood in the context of the physical and mental hardship caused by displacement. The obvious socio-economic constraints linked to the Tibetan refugees' status have confirmed the prevalent perception of tuberculosis as a disease of poverty and inequality. Refugees also often describe the suffering of exile as an 'embodied' maladjustment to their surroundings, and TB as a further exacerbation of this dis-ease: exiles are often heard complaining that, in India, the weather is too hot, foods rot too quickly, germs and disease abound. Older tuberculosis sufferers born in Tibet lament that there are more diseases in India than in the homeland. Tibet's mountainous, wind-swept expanses are often contrasted to the crowded Indian settlements where dust and pollution can make one sick. The change of environment occasioned by exile itself is thus seen as a source of ill health.

At the time of my fieldwork, a play about the local hospital was put on by local performers in an annual drama competition organised by the Tibetan Institute of Performing Arts (TIPA). The final act of this highly anticipated theatre show depicted the local hospital where TB patients were quarantined. On the stage, two beds face the audience. In the first, an emaciated young Tibetan boy is breathing the characteristic wheezing of tuberculosis, occasionally coughing out bloodstained sputum. In the second bed, a rotund diabetic Tibetan elder grumbles over the measly portions of hospital food given to him, attempting to bribe relatives to bring him sweets and *chang* alcohol. The tuberculosis patient tells the audience and his ailing roommate the story of his escape from Tibet. Why risk one's life crossing the border, he says, just to find oneself in a crowded camp in India with no employment prospect, away from one's family, and afflicted with disease? 'Why carry on?', he asks the audience. 'Rather die', he adds, with youthful bravado. Acting up this last comment, he hides the tuberculosis medication under his pillow without taking it. The nurses go about their rounds and fail to notice that he has stopped taking the pills, or that he is regularly sneaking out to the balcony to smoke the cigarettes provided to him by his

3 A *mo pa* is a ritual specialist or oracle who is empowered to perform *mo* (dice divination).

diabetic roommate. The duo devise a final strategy to fool the hospital personnel: the diabetic patient smuggles in cigarettes through his visiting wife and daughter, which the tuberculosis patient exchanges for his share of food and sweets. In this emotion-laden scene, the two Tibetan refugees, a newcomer and an earlier settler, bond despite the social differences that had previously kept them apart, but their trickery is soon exposed as the nurse discovers the pills hidden under the tuberculosis patient's pillow. It is already too late: in a dramatic flourish, the young TB patient rises from his bed, his face-mask tainted in blood from expectoration, and collapses on stage. Meanwhile, the diabetic elder, who has been feasting on rich foods and Tibetan butter tea gives in to a great convulsion and falls dead into the arms of his weeping wife and daughter. In the audience, the commotion and laughter caused by the two men's performance descends into an uneasy silence. On stage comes the doctor, and gives the following pronouncement: 'Because we are Tibetans, we are kind to each other, we help each other. But if we do not listen to the doctors, if we do not listen to the nurses, we are putting each other in danger. If we all get sick here, if our children die here, how will we go back to Tibet? If you want to truly help each other, be vigilant to disease.'

Although the play was clearly being utilised as a vehicle for health education, a dramatised and moralised depiction of reality, the characters of the young tuberculosis sufferer and the elder diabetic did exist in Dharamsala. One would meet these patients, or rather their real-life models; they were often described as emblematic of the connection between health and the social disorientation characteristic of the changing exile community. In the following section I will give a brief introduction to the demographics of TB among Tibetan exiles before offering two case studies of female TB sufferers and the social meaning of illness in the community.

The distribution of tuberculosis in the exile community

TB incidence is highest in the more densely populated Tibetan settlements. It is prevalent among Tibetan seasonal workers such as sweater-sellers, and also among the unemployed across all settlements. This clearly links TB incidence to environmental and mobility factors: Tibetan sweater-sellers spend 3–4 months of the year in impoverished and densely crowded Indian cities where exposure to the TB bacillus is likely (for example, Ludhiana, Delhi), or travelling from one city to another selling hosiery. Once infected, they may have difficulty adhering to a prescribed drug regimen while pursuing their trading activities. Age-wise, TB incidence peaks among the 15–29 age-group and among the elderly (over 65).[4] A survey conducted by the Tibetan Department of Health also revealed that the number of years spent in the refugee settlements was linearly associated with the risk of TB: the longer people stayed in a given settlement, the higher the risk of contracting the disease, which has particular significance in the case of monks and

4 In Bhatia *et al* (2002) p 1.

nuns who spend long periods of time in religious institutions and are at great risk of catching TB. Conditions for an epidemic spread of TB are present in the Tibetan exile settlement: many impoverished newcomer refugees spend months in crowded, enclosed housing where they are at risk of prolonged exposure to the TB bacillus.[5] The exiles' immune response to the disease is often weakened by other medical problems, poor nutrition and low morale. The problem is further complicated by the presence of multi-drug resistant (MDR) TB.

The Tibetan Department of Health's survey was a pioneering effort to gather data on health conditions in the Tibetan exile community, but it revealed some disturbing statistical curios. The first was a striking absence: about 30% of TB cases reported gave no record of sputum examination, which was recorded as 'unknown'. Secondly, an average 20% of cases had no known outcome, meaning that the doctors did not know what had happened to the patients after the initial diagnosis. Many patients seemed to escape the net of medical surveillance. The researchers attributed this to the precariousness of the medical equipment in the hospital and to patchy administration. They did not question, however, whether the 'disappearance' of 20% of TB patients might have been caused by social obstacles to treatment compliance, and possibly to the presence of a social stigma attached to the disease. In order to explore these possibilities, I now turn to an investigation of popular perceptions of TB and persons affected by TB in the Tibetan exile community.

As illustrated by the theatre vignette presented at the onset of this chapter, the narratives provided by the actors offer an explanatory model of their illnesses, in the construction of which the individual's personal interpretation of events comes to play a crucial role. In the play, the young man afflicted by tuberculosis made explicit references to the traumatic incidents that led to his flight in exile, and also to the hardships he suffered there. TB was often described to me as a disease of exile, not only because Tibetans often contract it upon arrival in India, but because it is specifically associated with the predicaments of exile lifestyles: poor lodgings, economic deprivation and contact with the alien, socially and epidemiologically 'contagious' Indian population. As anthropologist and psychiatrist Kleinman famously argued, 'meaning of a social kind is stamped into bodily processes and experiences'.[6] Among Tibetan refugees, popular discourse about tuberculosis has become focused on a few, discrete segments of the population, and associated with specific social ills, linked to gender roles and social change.

Popular perceptions of the disease started to materialise as one asked Tibetan doctors and patients why many adolescents were falling ill with TB. Adolescent boys' TB was perceived as linked to the harsh conditions of exile educational facilities and generally identified with the 'suffering of exile'. Girls' TB, however, had a different symbolic aetiology. A significant number of exiles said that being slim, dieting, was a 'new disease' that girls had contracted in India. One of my

---

5 www.tibet.ca/en/wtnarchive/1995/4/10-3_1.html (accessed 11 February 2004).

6 Kleinman (1988) p 10.

older woman friends pointed out girls on the marketplace who displayed the characteristic brown spots of malnutrition on their cheeks (*sha rdags*, or marks on the flesh). She frowned disapprovingly, and said that they should eat and not be so concerned with their attractiveness. The innocence of older female settlers who had been brought up in Tibet was contrasted to the attitude of the India-raised new generation to which the young 'dieting' women belonged. One woman, who had arrived in India at the age of 16, told me how she would find and collect condoms in her college precinct and use them as hair bands, oblivious to the hilarity which this triggered among her more savvy classmates. Young exile girls' quest for attractiveness and sexual freedom was morally reprehensible. When young women starved themselves to look good, this made them more susceptible to catch rampant diseases such as tuberculosis, which thrived on weakened immune systems. The association between tuberculosis and changing lifestyles was made explicit in older women's concern with perceived changes in girls' morals and the community's more general identification of TB as a 'disease of exile'.[7]

Girls and older women: the construction of TB 'risk groups'

The following section presents two contrasting case studies highlighting differences in the social construction of tuberculosis among two exile 'risk groups', namely girls and older women.

Eighteen-year-old Dolma, one of the patients who came to the hospital regularly to get her TB medicine, explained to me how her family had immediately assumed she had tuberculosis when she started coughing heavily and losing weight. The symptoms of TB are clearly known in the community, including by traditional Tibetan doctors, who co-operate with the allopathic hospital in the screening of patients. Dolma was worried by her parents' constant reference to TB, especially since one of her sisters had already suffered from the disease. She had a boyfriend, Tsultrim, who was studying in the nearby faculty of Chandigarh. Soon after they had met, however, he left Dharamsala to continue his studies, enjoining her to take good care of her health and study hard to complete her studies. Dolma's family often remonstrated with her for neglecting her school work, even though she had had repeated health problems, including chest and stomach pains that warranted frequent visits to the local biomedical hospital. When we talked about these symptoms, Dolma told me she was afraid of having developed breast cancer, which she had read about in Indian women's magazines. A few weeks later, however, her parents, alarmed by her worsening symptoms, decided to send her to the TB clinic. She appeared more and more gaunt and, when her birthday came, refused to eat the foods she would normally enjoy, getting angry when her sisters and mother teased her for acting lovelorn when she should have been getting better and concentrating on getting back to school. Her

7 Prost (2003).

preoccupation with Tsultrim, they said, had caused all sorts of trouble, making both her mind and body weak.

Dolma's sputum test proved positive, denoting an exposure to the TB bacillus. She then received a long-awaited letter from Tsultrim, who recommended her to go and see a *mo pa*, a lama who would perform divination with dice (*phyag mo*). Although Dolma's parents were sceptical about this, Tsultrim thought that the oracle would be able to ascertain the diagnosis. Exiles are aware of the number of contagious youths that walk around without masks, seeking to escape quarantine at home or in the hospital. They are also aware that the hospital laboratory sputum tests are done quickly and in poor laboratory facilities, and that the diagnosis can sometimes be flawed. In this atmosphere of diagnostic uncertainty, the culturally appropriate scheme, which involved going to the oracle, was an actual mode of practical clarification which complemented rather than contradicted the biomedical approach. Tsultrim did not only recommend a *mo* because he thought the oracle would be able to offer a culturally sensitive explanation of the illness, by linking it to ideas of karma or spirit intervention for instance, but also because he would be able to ascertain the biomedical diagnosis. Because the biomedical hospital staff is held in high regard, the diagnosis is rarely questioned in the context of the clinical encounter. Doubts and questions as to primary and proximal causes of the disease are directed toward members of the family with experience in dealing with TB, or, as in this case, to oracles.

Three months later, though, Dolma had developed a serious case of TB. While her sister had stayed in hospital during her own illness episode, Dolma had followed Tsultrim to New Delhi, where she was supposedly undergoing treatment. I offered to go and visit her, but her relatives said that it was no use: she was not staying in hospital but resting in her boyfriend's apartment. She looked very thin, they explained sadly, and did not want to go out of the flat. According to her sister, Dolma had left town to be with her boyfriend, but also not to be seen around town suffering from the illness. She had many close friends in Dharamsala, all of whom wrote to her and sent presents, wishing her a prompt recovery, but among her relatives and elderly women, however, she was seen as having taken unnecessary risks and deliberately endangered her life.

This story suggests a stigmatisation of young Tibetans' TB and its identification with a lifestyle disease linked to changing morals and increasing disorientation among the younger generation of refugees. Dolma's story was by no means exceptional, as was explained to me by the nurses and doctors in the biomedical hospital. They claimed that most patients saw the DOTS as an opportunity to take the treatment into their own hands, and affirmed that perhaps as many as half of the patients consulted an oracle at some point after the diagnosis. Concern with the changing mores of young female adolescents was reflected in the stigmatisation of girl's TB as a disease of exile modernity, embodying a growing preoccupation with bodily appearance and defiance of the older generation's advice. This was in turn linked to the emancipation of young women in exile and their increased access to education and employment, which was perceived as a sharp transition from the older female refugees' lifestyles.

In Dharamsala's medical circles, doctors and nurses often referred to the higher rates of compliance of Tibetan patients, in comparison to those of local Indian TB sufferers.[8] They argued that the Tibetans' better record of compliance was due to the impact of health workers and the implementation of the DOTS programme. The community's involvement in patient support, in reporting and monitoring the progress of TB sufferers as part of DOTS, was seen as the Tibetans' key asset in fighting the disease. Over a hundred community health workers, both men and women, have been trained in Dharamsala's allopathic hospital and the community health program is the second largest expenditure of the exile Department of Health, after the TB Control Project itself. Women play a key role in the community support for TB patients, not only as health workers, but also as supportive neighbours and colleagues.

One may also speculate that the participation of older women as community health workers in TB prevention may have contributed to a further stigmatisation of young girls' TB as older refugees tend to view the rapidly changing lifestyles of exile youth rather negatively.

A few months after Dolma's initial sputum test, TB struck again in a family close to me. Ani Tseyang, a 62-year-old woman, had fallen ill after an outbreak of the disease in her nunnery. She had a middle-aged son and relatives living in other settlements. Tseyang had decided to become a nun after the death of her husband. Her son's wife had left Dharamsala for Canada, from where she sent money home to the family. Tseyang recalled the circumstances in which she first experienced TB:

> I didn't feel good at all. And I had breathing pains. I started to cough continuously, no blood, just coughing. Sometimes it was so much I wanted to throw up, but I couldn't. One of the nuns in my nunnery, my friend, had just been sick with TB. I had helped her go down to the hospital, prepared [made ready] her medicine, and sometimes brought her food when she was down [in the hospital]. I had a mask when I helped her but sometimes I took it off, when I made food, when I talked, or when I recited *ma ni*.[9]

During the winter, Tseyang left the nunnery and moved in with Norbu, her son, in the upper settlement of McLeod. Up in his two rooms located in a quiet part of town, she seemed to recuperate as her son cooked and cleaned for her. Norbu told me that he was certain she had TB, and that he even put an ear to try and detect the wheezing sound or the 'crackle' that the doctors looked out for with they examined patients in the clinic.

Tseyang continues: 'Norbu took me to the hospital for the first time. I wanted to have a *mo* to find out if I would die soon. I am old, so I thought: it is time.' Norbu said his mother had nevertheless been patient and courageous with the disease, and that she had intensified her religious practice in preparation for her passing away once the diagnosis had been ascertained. From our talks, I gathered

---

8 According to Wares *et al* (2000) p 35, there is a higher default rate for smear-positive pulmonary cases (47.3% for Indians and 10.7% for Tibetans), and a lower cure rate for Indians (43.2% versus 80.1% for Tibetans).

9 Recitations of the mantra of the deity Avalokiteshvara (Tib Chenrezig) *'om mani padme hum'*.

that she thought the disease was not necessarily fatal, but that she believed she was too old to survive it. Her apprehension grew when she learnt how long the treatment would last. Norbu nevertheless insisted on taking her to the Tibetan TB specialist who regularly checked her X-rays and delivered the prescriptions. By that time, Tseyang could not walk down the road safely on her own, and had become weaker through the effect of the medicine, which was giving her tremendous leg pains.

I accompanied her during one of her weekly visits, along with her son and a neighbour. After the staff had taken the chest X-ray, Norbu, Tseyang and I waited outside the TB consultant's office for her appointment. One elder toothless nun came to greet Tseyang, inquired about her health, than started on a litany about her own pains. The medicine had made her old she said: her teeth had fallen out and she could no longer eat the food given to her. She insisted on giving Tseyang some bananas she said she would not be able to eat. After that episode, Tseyang was increasingly reluctant to go down to the hospital, and, although she did not openly oppose the trips, she wore her protective mask and folded her robes over her head so that she would not be recognised.

Soon after, however, Tseyang and Norbu found an ally in one of their neighbours, a non-practising nurse who had offered to give Tseyang her daily injections so that she would not have to stay in the hospital or constantly travel up and down the hill to receive her medication. At home she would lie on the bed, rest and recite *ma ni*. Her young neighbour's children would often come and visit, and the two neighbours would regularly bring cooked food and help with the house laundry. Surrounded by friends and family, Tseyang now seemed to be headed for a speedy recovery. Rinchen, Tseyang's neighbour who was moonlighting as a nurse, shared some thoughts on TB while ceremoniously preparing the injections in her flat:

> These TB patients sit the whole day by themselves, just thinking about their illness, being sad … They cannot get better that way! And they don't eat tasty food, good quality food, only dal, rice, potato, *tingmo* [Tibetan bread]. TB patients, they should get a high protein diet. I know, I trained in a hospital, as a nurse […] They need a really special diet, TB patients: vegetables and meat, and lots of protein, because this TB disease is very powerful, and if you don't take food and medicine, your body gets weak and you can die. Their mind is also weak, so they need to see people, and they need to talk. This is very important. If there is a lot of TB, you have to give lots of talks. Do they give lots of talks? Nurses or social workers, every week there should be talks, on what to do, how we can prevent it. […] These people really need help. Sometimes I see nurses who are really not good. They go and see the patient, they do [she makes the gesture of slamming medicine down on the table]. No, when we were training we learned, we should stand near the patient's bedside until he takes the medicine, and we should talk, we should encourage them, and say 'you should be happy that you are here in hospital now, we are here to take care of you and you are going to get well with this medicine'. Sometimes these nurses just say, 'here is medicine, take, eat, *eat*!' […][10] The patient might throw away the medicine, or hide it under the bed […].

10 This parodies Tibetan expressions of hospitality, when a host forces food onto a guest using the same injunction.

I prompted Rinchen to talk about Norbu's mother, asking if her condition had improved:

> Yes, but she's very weak, all the time. Of course, she's taking medicine. Until she's better she has to. That's why people get sick, young ones, boys, girls, they take medicine for a while, then they feel better so they don't care. And then they go out till late, they go to parties, dancing, without eating well. OK, if you go to a party, fine, then sleep. Many young get ill. My opinion is, it is because they don't sleep in time, they don't eat in time, they don't have a proper diet. They think 'Oh, I'm getting fat, I can't be fashionable, I should not get fatter'.

These two narratives show how differently TB is perceived between the two statistical 'risk groups', that is, adolescents and older refugees. For adolescent girls, the disease has become associated with poor self-discipline along with an increasing concern with bodily appearance and affluent lifestyles. It is thus linked to the perceived dangers of social mobility and emancipation. For young boys, however, it was more often described as a result of the physical and psychological hardships of exile, and the risky behaviour to which unemployed, idle young men were led to, generally out of desperation. The case of the elderly nun presented another side of this illness, one in which her life-experience, ideas about moral retribution, her individual relationship with aging and the aging Tibetan community came into play. TB is commonly depicted as a lifestyle disease, more specifically an exile disease related to modernity and social change. This is further illustrated by the fact that practitioners of traditional Tibetan medicine argue that prevalent medical problems such as AIDS, TB and hypertension are recent disorders which have arisen due to the moral degeneration of modern society, a process inscribed in the cosmology of both Buddhism and Hinduism.

Medical anthropologists have argued that chronic illness is the privileged ground for cultural constructions of disease, where local aetiologies, prevalent beliefs about health and well-being, and individual life-experiences are expressed through illness narratives[11] I contend that infectious diseases such as TB, because they affect vulnerable groups like adolescents and the elderly, catalyse interest around the topic of social change, and give rise to powerful discourses about the responsibility of sufferers in effecting change and shaping the well-being of the community at large. Adolescents and elders are often the central protagonists of conversations about social change, as debates offset the virtues of older settlers with the changing lifestyles of exile youths. By the same token, narratives and discussions relating to TB often encompass concerns with social change and the specific issues confronted by the two 'risk groups'.

Conclusion

The perception of infectious diseases such as tuberculosis is deeply influenced by what one might call the 'medicalisation of social change' in popular culture (for example, the stigmatisation of skinny, fashion-conscious girls). The community

---

11 Kleinman (1988), Kleinmann (1995), Lock and Scheper-Hughes *et al* (1987), Hahn (1995).

generates discourses about illness through the informal categorisation of 'risk groups', thereby underscoring the perceived social causes of the disease. Thus, concern both with the growing emancipation of women and with the disorientation of young people has been mapped onto the high incidence of TB among young adolescent girls. I would contend that Tibetan exile discourses about TB focus on adolescents and elderly sufferers in part because the vulnerability of these two groups has come to embody the vulnerable state of exile society at a time of profound social change, when the original generation of refugees is disappearing and giving way to new generations of exile, half of them born in India and the other in Tibet. The exile community is apprehensively chronicling the growing cultural chasm between the younger India-born generation of exiles, newcomers and older settlers. In this context, popular perceptions of tuberculosis have become stamped with social meanings that shape the disease's aetiology and therapeutic resolutions on the basis of the perceived flaws and qualities of the 'risk groups' concerned.

Bibliography

Bhatia, Shushum, Tsegyal, Dnanyi and Rowley, Derrick 'A social and demographic study of Tibetan refugees in India' (2002) 34:3 *Social Science and Medicine* 411–22.

Connor, Linda and Samuel, Geoffrey, *Healing Powers and Modernity: Traditional Medicine, Shamanism, and Science in Asian Societies*, 2001, London: Bergin & Garvey.

Hahn, R, *Sickness and Healing: An Anthropological Perspective*, 1995, New Haven, CT: Yale University Press.

Inhorn, Moucia and Brown, Peter, *The Anthropology of Infectious Disease: International Health Perspectives*, 1997, Amsterdam: Gordon & Breach.

Justice, Judith, 'Can socio-cultural information improve health planning? A case study of Nepal's assistant nurse-midwife' (1984) 19:3 *Social Science and Medicine* 193–98.

Kleinman, Arthur, *The Illness Narratives: Suffering, Healing, and the Human Condition*, 1988, New York: Basic Books.

Kleinman, Arthur, *Writing at the Margin: Discourse Between Anthropology and Medicine*, 1995, Berkeley, CA: University of California Press.

Lock, Margaret and Scheper-Hughes, Nancy, 'The mindful body' (1987) 1:1 *The Medical Anthropology Quarterly* 6–41.

Prost, A, 'Exile, social change and medicine among Tibetans in Dharamsala' (2003) unpublished PhD thesis, University of London.

Wares, DF, Sadutshang, TD, Beecjomg, NJ and Davies, PDO, 'Control of tuberculosis amongst the Tibetan refugee community in Northern India' (2000) 47:1 *Indian Journal of Tuberculosis* 35–41.

CHAPTER 12

ANGRY WOMEN AND THE EVOLUTION OF CHINESE MEDICINE[1]

Shigehisa Kuriyama

The voices of souls long dead echo in your speech, but you scarcely hear them. By habit, you suppose the words emerging from your mouth to be uniquely yours, direct expressions of what *you* think and feel, here and now. You do not listen.

Stop to lend an ear, though, and you soon discover that much of your language is in fact strangely opaque – that often, you have little notion of why you say what you say. As if waking into a dream, you begin to hear yourself mindlessly intoning phrases inherited from an unknown past, like a puppet mouthing sounds for some ghostly ventriloquist. Chinese speakers today no longer know why they speak of 'a great rush of liver-fire' (*dadong ganhuo*) to describe someone who is enraged. They may be vaguely aware that the expression comes from traditional medicine, but for most, *ganhuo*, liver-fire, is simply a set formula – a synonym for fury, nothing more.

It wasn't always so. There was once a time when *ganhuo* named not an arcane abstraction, but a vivid, intimate feeling. Indeed, it is the force of that original feeling, its persisting inertia, which makes people continue to speak of raging liver-fire, still now, when they no longer comprehend its sense.

The voices of souls long dead echo in talk of fire raging in the liver. My question is, what do these voices relate? The answer, I shall urge, speaks to how issues of gender have powerfully shaped the development of Chinese medicine in hitherto unsuspected ways.

Modern narratives of traditional Chinese medicine accent a vision of human life conceived as a microcosmic reflection of a grand macrocosmic order. The same dynamic of the *wuxing*, or five phases, whose interactions of mutual birth and suppression framed the rhythm of the seasons, the structure of space, the shifts of winds and weather, also governed change in individual lives. People's inner organs and outward behavior, their facial colour, their feelings, even their tastes in food, were uniformly governed by correspondences that mapped these organs and actions, colours, feelings, and tastes onto the cosmic grid of the five phases:

---

1 Grateful acknowledgment is due to the Chiang Ching-kuo Foundation, which supported the research for this chapter, and to Dr Li Jianmin, from whose help and advice I have benefited in countless ways.

Five Phases:	Wood	Fire	Earth	Metal	Water
Five Feelings:	Anger	Joy	Worry	Sadness	Fear
Five Viscera:	Liver	Heart	Spleen	Lungs	Kidneys
Five Directions:	East	South	Centre	West	North
Five Seasons:	Spring	Summer	*Tuyong*[2]	Autumn	Winter
Five Colours:	Green	Red	Yellow	White	Black
Five Tastes:	Sour	Bitter	Sweet	Spicy	Salty

Charts of this sort thus anchor nearly every synopsis of Chinese medical theory and, in the past, much of this scheme would have been common knowledge, even among laymen. All would have known fire as one of the five phases, and the liver as one of the five viscera; and insofar as one remembered how the correspondences between the five viscera and the five feelings made the liver responsible for anger, invoking the liver in evoking rage would have seemed natural enough.

For those curious about the particular meaning of liver-fire, however, this chart offers no help. The correspondences between the five viscera and five phases, you can see, pair the liver not with fire, but with wood. Fire is represented by the heart. Liver-fire, in other words, had no place – and hence has no meaning – in the scheme of five-phase interactions.

And yet its importance in the Chinese medical tradition is certain. Browse through the patient case histories in an eighteenth-century collection such as Wei's *Xu mingyi leian* (1770/1979), for example, and we constantly find doctors invoking liver-fire to solve the mystery of sickness. One patient is embarrassed by incontinence, another is racked by coughing, the limbs of another are locked stiff in tension, and still another complains of fatigue and lack of appetite. These afflictions and the sufferings of scores of other patients manifesting scores of other symptoms are all, remarkably, traced back to fire in the liver.

We have to do, in other words, with a diagnosis that appears prominently in history, but which current accounts of Chinese medicine do not prepare us to interpret. Something basic, plainly, is missing from our accounts. The logic supporting the discourse of liver-fire must lie elsewhere, outside the framework of the microcosm-macrocosm resonances on which we habitually concentrate. Chinese doctors must have drawn inspiration from other, hitherto neglected sources. It is these other sources that led them to dwell on fire raging in the liver, and it is to these sources that we now must hearken.

We inhabit a world increasingly isolated from fire. Gradually, but inexorably, electric lighting, heaters, and stoves have displaced candles, campfires and the hearth, so that our encounters with fire now tend to be limited and occasional – the striking of a match, the dull glow of a cigarette, the burning of autumn leaves, conflagrations glimpsed on television. As our lives have drifted ever further from the patient, daily tending of flames, we have become steadily deaf to the overtones once heard in talk of fire.

2 Intercalary period devised to bridge the gap between the four seasons and five phases.

What is fire? Deep thinkers in the past have contemplated brightly burning flames, and often imagined themselves peering into the very ground of existence. At once so intensely present and yet so intensively changing, fire seemed to embody the ultimate secret of being and change. Heraclitus famously spoke of the world as 'an ever-living fire' (*pyr aeizōon*),[3] and the Stoics declared all things – from the stars in the distant heavens, down to the inner intimacy of the soul – to be composed of a fiery breath.

In China, the sixteenth-century philosopher Fang Yizhi glimpsed the ceaseless, inexhaustible activity of fire behind the birth, and activity, and transformation of all things. 'The operation of the universe is governed by fire,' he declared, 'and the human body too is governed by fire.'[4] This means that: 'We are born through fire, and die through fire; sickness originates in fire, but the cultivation of life too depends on the same fire.'[5] All distinctions and oppositions – the universe and the body, the yin and the yang, birth and death, health and sickness – thus merged, finally, in fire. For Fang, fire was the purest essence of the yang principle, but this yang was not a relative yang, not the traditional yang complemented by an opposing yin, but rather an absolute yang that unified both the yang and the yin. It underlay contraction as well as expansion, descent as well as ascent, the painful slowness of old age as well as the rash impetuousness of youth. It was a transcendent principle that comprehended all dichotomies.

Reviewing the history of the imagination of fire, Gaston Bachelard concludes, in a similar vein, that:

> Fire is a privileged phenomenon which can explain everything.
>
> If all that changes slowly is explained by life, all that changes quickly is explained by fire. Fire is a sort of super-life (*Le feu est l'ultra-vivant*). Fire is intimate and universal. It lives in our heart. It lives in the heavens ... Among all phenomena, it is really the sole that can so clearly accept contrary judgments: it is good and it is evil. It shines in Paradise. It burns in Hell. It is gentleness and torture. It is hearth and apocalypse.[6]

Fire, then, is absolute animation. Fire, then, is the transcendent union of contraries. Such are the guiding intuitions. Fang Yizhi's vision hints, further, at how they might be translated into a theory of medicine: fire is the source of all birth, growth, and vital vigour, he explains, but it is also and at the same time the origin of sickness and death, the source of a fatal fragility.

---

3 Heraclitus, Fragment 30: 'The world is an ever-living fire, parts of which are always extinguished to form the two other main world-masses, sea and earth.' (Kirk and Raven (1964) p 199.)

4 Fang (1978) p 14.

5 Fang (1978) p 15.

6 Bachelard (1949) p 23.

I cannot retrace for you all of the history of fire in China,[7] but it is essential that you at least know this: the rise of fire as a central theme in Chinese thinking about the body was a distinctly post-classical development.[8] Fire was already important, it is true, in various aspects of ancient medicine – in the pathology of summer heat, for example, and in the therapy of moxibustion, but the explicit insistence on fire as a pivot of all life and sickness developed only from around the thirteenth century onwards. Liver-fire, for example, the diagnosis that figures so ubiquitously in Ming (1368–1644) and Qing (1644–1911) case histories, does not appear anywhere in the *Huangdi neijing*, the foundational classic of Chinese medicine, nor does it appear in any other treatises of the ancient medical canon. The vision of a fiery body expressed a new direction in the Chinese imagination. It represented, indeed, the most significant change in Chinese medicine since the completion of a theoretical canon back in the third century.

At the core of this change was the sense of the duality that I have described – the intuition of fire as at once a vital necessity and a wild menace. The influential physician Zhu Danxi (1281–1358) thus imagined fire as the restless motor behind all activity in the world, all animation in the body. Without fire there was no life, yet, at the same time, fire for Zhu represented one of the greatest threats to life. All too often, all too readily, fire, being fire, could flare up in reckless agitation (*wangdong*) and scorch and consume a person's vital resources.[9] Such uncontrolled blazes accounted for much of human sickness. If intuitions of dynamic, universal flux provided the general backdrop for the discourse of fire, it was above all this sense of fire's volatility, its potential to wreak havoc, that made fire a compelling concern.

Proponents of the pathology of scorching inner fires would not fail to cite the authority of the *Huangdi neijing*, which already distinguished between a 'subtle fire' (*shaohuo*) nurturing the *qi* or vitality in the body, and a harmful 'blazing fire' (*zhuanghuo*) which disperses this *qi*.[10] In fact, the distinction had little visible impact on ancient medicine. In the *Neijing*, it is no sooner mentioned than dropped, and none of the other ancient treatises offer any elaboration. The notion of blazing fire became resonant only much later, in post-Song dynasty (960–1279) medicine, when it was interpreted as anticipating the theory of reckless fires.

Why did reckless fires come to loom large in Chinese reflection on human beings and their vulnerabilities? How should we understand the rise of the discourse of fire in Chinese medicine?

The general answer almost certainly must be sought in the close identification of reckless fire with fiery feelings. When Zhu Danxi and doctors after him spoke of the pathology of uncontrolled inner blazes, they invariably tied it to desire and

---

7 One review of fire in medicine that is more useful than most is Chapter 3, '*Er huo yu hengdong*': Xu (1997) pp 71–92.

8 Li (2001), has pointed out, however, that the imagination of fire played a vital if implicit role in the formation of the crucial ancient concept of *qi*, or vital breath.

9 Zhu (1993) pp 38–39.

10 *Suwen* (1987) p 19.

the volatility of the passions. 'Human feelings and desires,' Zhang Jiebin explained, 'frequently move recklessly, and once they are set in motion, they incite fire, and as this fire gains strength it damages the vital resources.'[11] Scorching flames did not flare up without cause, by chance. If fire sustained all vital motion, it was *emotion* that stoked this fire into a destructive blaze. The history of the imagination of fire in China is thus inseparable from the history of the passions. The new discourse of reckless fires mirrored a special emphasis on unruly feelings.

However, this answer by itself is clearly not enough. Doctors in antiquity, we know, were already keenly aware of how emotional disorder could disorder the body. To elucidate the particular motivations behind the new theory of fire, we need to look closer at how this theory was actually deployed in practice, and scrutinise the specific character of the feelings to which it was applied.

And here we return to the phrase with which we began, namely, the rush of liver-fire. In the scheme of the five phases, as we saw earlier, each of the five viscera governed a particular passion. The heart was thus responsible for joy, the liver for anger, the spleen for worry, the lungs for sadness, the kidneys for fear. In principle, the pathology fire could afflict any of these. There was theoretically no reason why the unruly blaze of emotion should not scorch the lungs or kidneys, say, just as readily as the spleen or liver.

The case histories in Ming and Qing medicine, however, testify to a distinct bias in practice: the preponderance of actual diagnoses of fire disorder concentrate on the liver; that is, on the organ at the root of anger. It isn't by coincidence, then, that Chinese to this day speak glibly of liver-fire, while an expression like 'lung-fire' is entirely unknown. Even 400 years ago, the latter was merely an abstract possibility, almost never diagnosed. The former, by contrast, was the implicit model inspiring the very notion of reckless fire, the paradigm case. If the pathology of reckless fire highlighted the great power of feelings over life, the stress on fire in the liver expressed, above all, a stress on anger.

What should we make of this bias? Chinese writings since antiquity offered a variety of lists, summing up the basic responses by which human beings engage the world. Confucian commentators typically referred to the *qiqing*, or seven feelings identified in the *Book of Rites*, namely, joy, anger, sorrow, fear, attraction, aversion and desire.[12] Chinese Buddhists, too, spoke of 'the seven feelings' (*qiqing*) as a formula, but on their list (*xi, nu, ai, le, ai, wu, yu*) fear was replaced by pleasure (*le*). There was likewise a medical discourse of 'the seven feelings' stemming from the *Neijing* but, in this case, the seven were joy, anger, worry, longing, sadness, fear and shock (*xi, nu, you, si, bei, ju, jing*). Then there were shorter lists of six feelings, five feelings, or four, which drop and shuffle elements from the lists of seven and, on occasion, add a new entry, such as resentment (*yuan*). If we sift through these inventories, however, we arrive at a notable fact:

11 Zhang (1980) p 42.
12 Kong (1990) p 430.

there are two – and only two – feelings that appear in them all. These two, moreover, are sometimes explicitly invoked by themselves, as a metonymic pair summarising the entire range of passions. They are *xi* and *nu*, joy and anger – the delight of things unfolding exactly as one would wish, and the frustration of actions and events confounding one's desires.

Anger, as the representative of negative feelings, the name of joy's opposite, had, in other words, long claimed a privileged place in Chinese conceptions of the passions. This is doubtless one factor that contributed to the pre-eminence of liver-fire, but a second look at the case history literature also points to other, more specific factors at work. We have already observed that diagnoses of fire disorder placed overwhelming emphasis on liver-fire. Further study reveals another telling trend, and that is that the great majority of patients diagnosed as victims of liver-fire were women.

It is in gynaecological treatises, in fact, that we first find doctors regularly blaming sickness on fire in the liver. If the discourse of fire as a metaphysical principle was supported by broad intuitions of a restless, dynamic universe, the perception of fire as a daily, intimate danger was nurtured especially in the context of diagnosing the afflictions of women.

To interpret this connection, we must appreciate that the very notion of *fuke*, of a medical branch specialising in women's diseases, only began, like the imagination of the fiery body, to take form in the Song dynasty.[13] We must appreciate, further, that the creation of this specialty was closely bound to concern with the emotions. Why create a separate branch for women's disorders, after all? The authors of the *Neijing* and other ancient texts saw no need. The essential elements of the body, blood and vital breath, and the basic forces that harmed or nurtured them – factors such as wind and cold, light and day, repletion and depletion, food and drink – were shared by men and women alike.

Proponents of the new specialty, while conceding this essential commonality, argued that two considerations still set women's disorders apart. The first were, of course, the uniquely female ailments related to menstruation, pregnancy and childbirth; the second was the greater sway of emotion in the lives of women. It was especially the latter, specialists urged, that so often made female afflictions so difficult to treat. Gynaecological treatises would often retrieve the judgment of the Tang dynasty doctor Sun Simiao on this point:

> The longing and desires of women are more intense than those of their husbands, and they are more stimulated to become ill. Add to this that in women envy and dislike, compassion and love, grief and sorrow, attachments and aversions are especially stubborn and deep-seated. They cannot themselves control these emotions; and from this the roots of their illnesses are deep, and their cure is difficult.[14]

---

13 On the development of Chinese gynecology, see the excellent study by Charlotte Furth (1999).

14 Sun (1955) p 16. (The translation is from Furth (1999) pp 71–72.)

In general, then, the close ties that subsequently formed between the pathology of fire and the disorders of women can be seen as the confluence of two intuitions: on the one hand, the reckless fires that scorched the body were fires of emotion; on the other hand, women were imagined to be especially susceptible to the empire of the passions. Chen Yan, however, the renowned Song dynasty doctor who compiled the first major compendium of prescriptions for women, specified more exactly: female disorders require separate discussion because the congested anger (*yunu*) of women is double that of men.[15] The problem, in other words, was not just emotion in general, but anger in particular, and not just any anger, but especially *yunu*, congested anger.

We come here to the final clue: time and again, in the case histories, the anger of the women suffering from liver-fire is further qualified as 'congested'. This phrase 'congested anger' is foreign to English, but the contexts of its use indicate that the feelings it names are not unfamiliar. We have to do with resentments that are chronic and recurring, longstanding frustrations allowed – or forced – to accumulate, often over the course of years. Congested anger is thus supported and elaborated by a congery of revealing qualifiers: the woman is 'quiet', 'reserved'; the feelings are 'habitual' (*su*) and 'long' (*jiu*), 'repressed' (*yi*) and 'oppressed' (*men*). Here is a patient who says that she has long ago come to hate her husband; here is another, childless, whose husband is eager to welcome a concubine.[16] The doctors in the case histories never propose social solutions to such situations, nor do they ever seek to alter the patients' feelings directly; instead, they prescribe assorted remedies designed to 'clear' the fire in the liver – as if congested anger were like a suffocating, turbid miasma, clouding and poisoning the soul.

This theme of congestion is suggestive. The imagination of the fiery body, I have said, marked the most significant new direction in Chinese medicine since the formation of the classical canon in antiquity, and I have argued that new direction was entwined with a particularly keen sense of how emotions can stir disorder. However, it would be wrong bluntly to cast this development in terms of a shift from a neglect of, to an emphasis on, the passions, for the passions figured importantly in ancient medicine too. What we discern, rather, is a modulation of accent, an emphasis on a new *quality* of feeling.

The *leitmotif* of the imagination of the body in classical Chinese medicine was not congestion but emptiness – not the frustration of desire, but rather submission to desire. The ancient discourse on regimen is suffused with the obsessive fear of depletion.[17] If people could only remain calm, and free of passion, and retain the vital essences fully within, the *Neijing* explains, they would be impervious to disease; fierce winds and bitter cold and all the other noxious dangers of the world simply would have no room to enter, but as it is, such detached calm is exceptional, and sickness and premature senescence prevail. Men routinely – and

15 Xue (1990) *juan* 2 p 1.

16 See, for instance, Xue (1990) *juan* 1 p 24.

17 On depletion in Chinese medicine, see Chapters 5 and 6 of Kuriyama (1999).

quite literally – lose themselves to desire, recklessly allowing their very life to flow out of them, in drunken orgies.[18] The implicit guiding model undergirding this fear of depletion was the male loss of semen in intercourse, for semen was the precious, all-too-limited seed of life, the very essence of vitality. Its careless expenditure inevitably aged a man, and made him vulnerable to sickness; its exhaustion meant death. Which of course is why the art of the bedchamber was integral to the cultivation of the body in ancient China, and why this art centred around techniques of seminal retention. Which is why, too, the market for *buyao*, drugs that compensate for depletion remain in great demand up to the present day.

Anxieties about the drain of vital energies, then, run through the entire history of Chinese medicine, but the rise of the discourse of fire speaks to how these anxieties were complemented in Ming times by a new consciousness of congestion – how, in one sense, anxieties about male dissolution were supplemented – though not supplanted – by keen attention to female frustrations. The voices that echo in the talk, today, of liver-fire are not least those of mostly anonymous women whose anger had been long forgotten.

18 Suwen (1987) pp 7–8.

Chinese Glossary

a. Terms and names

buyao 補藥

Chen Yan 陳言

dadong ganhuo 大動肝火

Fang Yizhi 方以智

fuke 婦科

ganhuo 肝火

jiu 久

juan 卷

le 樂

men 悶

nu 怒

qi 氣

qiqing 七情

shaohuo 少火

Sun Simiao 孫思邈

su 素

wangdong 妄動

wuxing 五行

xi 喜

xi, nu, ai, le, ai, wu, yu 喜怒哀樂愛惡欲

xi, nu, you, si, bei, ju, jing 喜怒憂思悲懼驚

yì 抑

*yuan*怨

yunu 鬱怒

*zhuanghuo*壯火

Zhang Jiebin 張介賓

Zhu Danxi朱丹溪

b. Texts

Fang Yizhì, *Wulun xiashi* 方以智 「物理小識」

Huangdi neijing zhangju suoyin「黄帝内經章句索引」

Jiaozhu furen liangfang daquan「校注婦人良方大全」

'Chanbao fanglun' 產寶方論

'Yueshui buduan fanglun' 月水不斷方論

Kong Yingda, *Liji*, 'Li yun' 孔穎達「 禮記」禮運

Li Jianmin, 'Huo zhi wei yao: *Bencao gangmu*▪ *Huobu* kaozheng' 李建民

火之爲藥—「本草綱目・火部」考證

Suwen 「素問」

'Yinyang yinxiang dalun' 陰陽應象大論

'Shanggu tianzhen lunbian' 上古天真論篇

Sun Simiao, *Beiji qianjin yaofang* 孫思邈, 「備急千金藥方」

Xu mingyi leian 「續名醫類案」

Xu Yiming, *Xingli yu Qi-Huang* 徐儀明「性理與歧黃」

Xue Lizhai, *Jiaozhu furen liangfang* 'Yueshui buduan fanglun'

薛立齋「校注婦人良方」月水不斷方論

Zhang Jiebin, *Jingyue quanshu*, 'Junhuo xianghuo lun'

張介賓,「景岳全書」君火相火論.

Zhongguo yixue dacheng「中國醫學大成」

Zhu Danxi, *Gezhi yulun*, 'Xianghuo lun' 朱丹溪「格致余論」相火論

Bibliography

—— *Huangdi neijing zhangju suoyin*, 1987, Taipei: Qiye shuju.
Bachelard, Gaston, *La psychanalyse du feu*, 1949, Paris: Editions Gallimard.
Fang, Yizhi, *Wuli xiaoshi*, 1978, Taipei: Taiwan Shangwu yinshuguan.
Furth, Charlotte, *A Flourishing Yin: Gender in China's Medical History 960–1665*, 1999, Berkeley, CA: University of California Press.
Kirk, Geoffrey S and Raven, John E, *The Pre-Socratic Philosophers: Critical History with a Selection of Texts*, 1964, Cambridge: Cambridge University Press.
Kong, Yingda, *Liji*, vol 1, 1990, Shanghai: Shanghai guji chubanshe.
Kuriyama, Shigehisa, *The Expressiveness of the Body and the Divergence of Greek and Chinese Medicine*, 1999, New York: Zone Books.
Li, Jianmin, *Huo zhi wei yao 'Bencao gangmu Huobu' kaozheng*, 2001: a paper presented at a workshop on the History of Material Culture, Institute of History and Philology, Academia Sinica, Taiwan.
Sun, Simiao, *Beiji qianjin yaofang*, 1955, Beijing: Renmin weisheng chubanshe.
Suwen, 'Shanggu tianzhen lunbian', in *Huangdi neijing zhangju suoyin*, 1987.
Wei, Zhixiu, *Xu mingyi leian*, 1979, Taipei: Hongye Shuju.
Xu, Yiming, *Xingli yu Qi-Huang*, 1997, Beijing: Zhongguo shehui kexue chubanshe.
Xue, Lizhai, 'Jiaozhu furen liangfang', in *Zhongguo yixue dacheng: 29*, 1990, Shanghai: Shanghai kexue jishu chubanshe.
Zhang, Jiebin, *Jingyue quanshu*, 1980, Taipei: Tailian guofeng chubanshe.
Zhu, Danxi, *Danxi yiji*, 1993, Beijing: Renmin weisheng chubanshe.

CHAPTER 13

READING GENDER IN ANCIENT EGYPTIAN HEALING PAPYRI

Stephen Quirke

I am Isis.

These words mark the start of several formulae recited by ancient Egyptian healers, and assert a direct identification of the healer with Isis, goddess of healing.[1] This is especially remarkable, because nearly all healers recorded in ancient Egyptian writing are men: a recent list of 150 individuals with the title *sunu* 'physician' includes only one woman.[2] Evidently, ancient Egyptian healing, as recorded in writing, presents a challenge to modern Western medical reading: first, in its very different manipulation of gender, and then, more broadly, to Western definitions of medicine and science, originally as a male terrain, against magic and religion, perhaps a female territory. Such categorisations fail our evidence. I take that challenge to be the justification for the comparative approach in this instance. Interdisciplinarity should contest its own claims: should an archaeological orientalism be represented in the volume?

In the case of Egypt, the interface between the world of writing and the world of healing can first be directly observed in manuscripts after 2000 BC. The contents of the principal published manuscripts of the second millennium BC indicate that the activities and knowledge of the healer fell into three categories, each category summarised in one Egyptian word:

shesau 'diagnosis' and 'prognosis' or more broadly 'treatment';

pekheret 'prescription' – the materials available for use, and their combinations and applications;

re 'formula' – the words to be recited to resocialise the patient from the exile of ill health into the world of the healthy, or to keep the individual in good health.

In most modern Western reception, this written tradition has been dissected into medical ('scientific') and magical ('religious') halves. However, in ancient Egyptian practice, the three activities complement one another; healing involved recognition and action (*shesau*), materials (*pekheret*), and the power of words (*re*).

---

1 For two examples from many sources, see Borghouts (1978) No 90, p 59 and No 91, p 62.

2 Nunn (1996) pp 211–14.

In general, manuscripts keep these three categories separate, but conceptually, in combination, they form a single field of healing, for which again there is an Egyptian term *meket hau*, 'protection of the body'. Titles to manuscripts specify that they were for use by any healer – they do not create three separate professions in healing. In inscription and manuscript sources, healers have distinct titles according to the broad type of ailment they treat, the most common titles associated with healing being:

> *sunu* treating external injuries, so loosely translatable as 'physician' – this is the title that has most appealed to modern Western doctors as an ancient Egyptian ancestor, and there is a higher level for this group at great courts, the *wer sunu* 'chief physician';
>
> *kherep Serqet* 'conjurer of Serqet' (water-scorpion goddess) treating the effects of scorpion bite and snake bite;[3]
>
> *wab Sekhmet* 'pure-priest of Sekhmet' (the fury in the ancient Egyptian pantheon, goddess of plague) treating ailments for which there is no identifiable source, with an emphasis on contagious disease and plague;[4]
>
> *sau* 'protector' perhaps a broad term for healer, but rarer than the previous three.

Again, the modern Western reception has violated the ancient categories in its pursuit and construction of an ancestral medical profession on Western terms. The translations 'conjurer' and 'priest' have warded off most modern medical commentators, and yet the written record indicates that these were involved in the struggle for good health as much as the 'physician'.

The earliest surviving book (in Egypt, a papyrus scroll) that deals with the treatment of women at, or rather just before, birth, dates to about 1800 BC.[5] The manuscript is preserved in the Petrie Museum of Egyptian Archaeology in London.[6] It was among a great haul of papyri retrieved by Flinders Petrie in 1889 during his 'rescue archaeology' excavation of a large town site at Lahun, roughly 100 km south of modern Cairo; Petrie called the site Kahun, and so the papyrus has entered histories of medicine, as well as Egyptology, under such Western medical terms as the Kahun Medical Papyrus or the Kahun Gynaecological Papyrus. Being wary of medical superscription, I prefer to refer to it by its current inventory number UC 32057, though number too can scarcely be neutral. The fragments of the papyrus came from the largest group of manuscript fragments found at the town, a group numbered 'Lot VI' in the publication, and comprising mainly letters and accounts from a rich household. The exact findspot of 'Lot VI' is not recorded, though excavation records perhaps suggest a palatial house at the centre of the town.[7] Placing this in social context, there were 11 such palatial houses in the area excavated, and about 250 smaller dwellings, all on an

---

3 Känel (1984).

4 Känel (1984).

5 Griffith (1898) pp 5–11; bibliography, discussion and translation in Bardinet (1995) pp 221–29 and 437–43.

6 Located at University College London, Gower Street, London, WC1E 0AH.

7 Gallorini (1998) pp 48–49.

orthogonal plan.[8] This sets UC 32057, and probably though not explicitly the women to be treated according to it, in an urbanised elite class. Class in a pre-industrial society may be a blunt category, but the politicising vocabulary of second-wave feminism still seems to me necessary; on these terms, ancient Egypt might be described as a male-dominated society in which those who write form a minority of the population asserting control over resources – writing belonged to the few. However, two qualifications modify this view, that also comes from the modern Western world:

> there is no monolithic literacy, but rather a spectrum of literacies and illiteracies that have yet to be charted and assessed in their operation in and over time;[9]
>
> patriarchy is barely an appropriate term in a society where men and women die young – the mythic prototype for sovereign power is not Osiris the father, but Horus the son, making ancient Egypt a prototypical filiarchy, where the young adult male has power.

In the reconstructed form attained by Griffith, UC 32057 is the best preserved of eight manuscripts identifiable as writings for health among the thousands of papyrus fragments from across the site at Lahun. Four of the manuscripts are in hieroglyphs, the most sacred script:

> the only surviving veterinary papyrus in the ancient Egyptian language (UC 32036);
>
> a small fragment with reference to serpents (UC 32117E);
>
> diminutive fragments probably from two separate manuscripts (UC 32106B and 32118A).

The remainder are in the more cursive script, known in Egyptology as hieratic, but at earlier periods not reserved for priestly purposes:

> UC 32057;
>
> three items from series of incantations for good health with instructions for use (UC 32091A, 32116A and 32271B).

In addition to these eight, there is one manuscript, from the same discarded set of papyri as UC 32057, for which the classification has been debated among Egyptologists, because its contents switched genre across time. This is a fragment of narrative, preserving part of an episode involving Horus, god of order, and Seth, god of disruption (UC 32158).[10] Six centuries later, the same episode appears in a longer narrative of the contendings of Horus and Seth, perhaps to be recited at a festival celebrating kingship (known from a single beautifully preserved manuscript, Papyrus Chester Beatty I).[11] It seems also to have been used as an

8 Kemp (1989) pp 149–57.
9 Cerquiglini (1989) p 35.
10 Griffith (1898), Lot VI 2.
11 See Broze (1996) and Verhoeven (1996).

incantation to be recited for good health, and so falls within the third ancient Egyptian category of writings for good health specified above.[12] By contrast, the version written down at Lahun, about 1800 BC, was written not to heal, but to entertain, to be read – it is a 'literary' fragment. I deduce this from the formal features: both layout and the related handwriting style are radically different from the eight contemporary healing manuscripts from Lahun. In the absence of any evidence that the papyrus was used by a healer in its time, I should strictly exclude it from this presentation. However, its contents touch on themes central to this volume, and this justifies a summary of the episode here.

The god Seth, the disruptive trickster of the tale, greets his nephew Horus with the phrase 'how beautiful are your buttocks' – Horus tells Seth that he is too big and painful for him, and after the act he goes to tell his mother Isis, goddess of healing. She advises him to put his fingers between his buttocks and catch the semen. The Lahun fragment breaks off at this point of the episode; the later longer version omits the repetition of the encounter, but presents the consequences. In the latter version of the tale, Isis puts the semen of Seth on his favourite food, the milky Cos lettuce, so that when Seth boasts to the court of the gods that his semen is in Horus, it emerges from his own forehead, because he has eaten it – instead of humiliating Horus, Seth has humiliated himself, and Isis has tricked the trickster.

In dialogue with ancient writing, a modern reader may forget how much he or she reads into the episode; this may be a primary risk for any writing, but it is tangibly acute for ancient writing. For example, assessment of this episode depends on the opinion the reader or hearer has about sodomy; within the episode as preserved from Lahun, Isis herself expresses no emotional reaction to the account of Horus being penetrated by Seth, producing only the strategy for stopping Seth from using this event to humiliate Horus in public. Similarly, the active partner seems free to declare his act in public, if he intends to humiliate the passive partner. The act itself is not being judged in the way that a London reader might have judged it in the year of the discovery of the papyri, 1889, or in 1898, when Griffith published his translation, discretely in Latin in order to protect the less learned from its contents. Most importantly for the early twenty-first-century reader today, in this tale foregrounding gender roles and homosexual acts, the age of the participants is not stated. Such missing information creates a double dilemma: the modern reader may not recognise the lack of crucial information, and/or may fill in any gaps whether more or less unconsciously. The reading becomes colonially constitutive rather than dialogic; only the anchor of the physical manuscript source itself preserves a chance of a dialogue.

The Lahun manuscript for the treatment of women

The largest surviving 'health manuscript' from Lahun is the papyrus scroll UC 32057, imperfectly preserved. It presents three 'pages' of 29, 30 and 28 lines respectively, written in a small cursive hand, in black and red as is usual for the

12 Westendorf (1987).

time. Thirty-four red (rubric) headings introduce treatments for the ailments of women and the sexing of the unborn child. The 17 on the first two pages have the heading *shesau*, the 17 on the third page are more miscellaneous, and less well-preserved, with headings such as 'determining the child to be born', 'determining a woman who will conceive as against one who will not (conceive)'. The second case illustrates the way in which the compiler arranged the material:

> Examination of a woman who is ill from her womb wandering
> You should say of it 'what do you smell?'
> If she tells you 'I smell roasting'
> You should say of it 'it is wrappings [?] of the womb'
> You should treat it by fumigating her with whatever she smells as roast.

Taking the contents as performative as well as communicative, the cast of characters may be defined as four roles, each of which constitutes a 'body', a spatio-temporal physical sphere open to gender negotiation:

authority – the unnamed source of the words;

healer – the person receiving the words and acting on them;

patient one – identified throughout as 'a/the woman' (note that at this period the Egyptian language has no definite or indefinite article);

patient two – child to be born, not present in all manuscripts.

My translation of the 34 passages of the papyrus has been online on the UCL website Digital Egypt for Universities (www.digitalegypt.ucl.ac.uk) since summer 2002, the occasion for an interdisciplinary seminar at UCL. Historians of medicine and Egyptologists, teachers and learners, men and women, participated at this to address the principal question whether a single translation can deliver content to more than one discipline in Higher Education in this country. Although the original intention was more the interaction with the disciplines of medicine and the history of medicine, the most challenging exchanges came from observations by Alison Roberts, whose research focused on ancient Egyptian goddesses.[13] Her comments forced us to appreciate the extent to which a healing manuscript bears or does not bear gender already inscribed at the moment of and by the process of writing, as distinct from the modern and equally gendering reinscription of content in translation into different but still written media of print and computer screen. Three issues in particular may be addressed in a modern reading of this papyrus:

healer-patient relations as expressed in masculine and feminine pronouns;

the effect of specialised vocabulary and verb forms for healer-patient relations;

the effects of introducing writing as a medium in healing (or in training for healing).

13 Roberts (1995).

By distinguishing in the second person singular between male and female, as modern Arabic does, the ancient Egyptian language appears to assign specific gender to healer (masculine pronoun) and patient (feminine pronoun). Roberts in particular raised the question of how a language with masculine and feminine pronouns would express neuter and common gender – those being the two genders specified in other languages: for example, in modern Danish. If an ancient writer intended 'he or she', that might well have been written with the masculine pronoun; in reading, the common gender is bound to be converted unthinkingly into male by a modern reader with specifically gendered expectations both of medicine and of an ancient society constructed in the mind as patriarchal.

The same point applies to the specialised verbal forms used in this and other healing manuscripts, on the model 'you should say … then you should do'; a reader presuming male domination is likely to read the healer-patient relations in these treatments of women as man controlling woman by imposing order. It remains possible that such control did exist, and was imposed through writing, taking us to the third point, the impact of writing in healing. Nevertheless, on the page, the words leave the gender open, with a variety of possible gendered readings:

- a man directs a man in the treatment of a woman;
- a woman directs a man in the treatment of a woman;
- a man directs a man or woman in the treatment of a woman;
- a woman directs a man or woman in the treatment of a woman.

Beyond the identity of the patient as 'woman', the modern reader is not given explicit information on the class, age, gender, or ethnicity, in other words on any of four primary variables in the social construction of identity, yet the modern reader may have decided all the answers to those questions automatically.

The precise manner of reading itself constitutes the greatest block to understanding, whenever readers overlook the complexity and variety of reading acts. This risk seems particularly acute with historical sources. The physical singularity of an ancient document can easily blind us to the plurality of individuals implied by the existence of the document – writer or writers, readers ancient and modern. Even, or especially, in the age of mechanical reproduction, an original manuscript may seem more the starting point of a straight line from past to present, rather than a node in an intersubjective web. The mystifying impact of unique status is compounded by the rarity of medium. The ancient script and its material support encourage us to privilege a technical expert in decipherment; that expert performs an apparently unidirectional transmission from written word to modern medium of communication, most often a printed book. No one else, it seems, can engage with ancient writing in the same authorised manner, and all others in modernity must resign themselves to accept the message issued by the expert as *prophetes* 'the one who speaks on behalf of (the source)'. These conditions leave little prospect of human engagement with the sources. The resulting reader may be recognised when Hirschkop summarises the way that

Pavel Medvedev criticised Formalists, in these terms: 'the subject facing the text is reduced to the status of a quasi behaviourist creature, reacting to meaningful contents as if they were merely signals.'[14] Not only has the humanity of the ancient writing disappeared, but the linear model of reading degrades its modern subject too by casting that subject as something less than historical, less than human. In practice, verbal communication never appears so one-dimensional, and reading too cannot be reduced to a simple line between writing and reader. As a particular form of speech act, access to the written word always generates multi-dimensional engagements between subjects. Even the unique written source becomes multiple from the moment that it is translated into sound by an act of reading, introducing new readers and hearers and ways of being read.

The claims of direct linearity remain seductive for anyone confronted with an inscription or manuscript in an ancient script. UC 32057 offers a particular challenge: it is written in a cursive version of the hieroglyphic script, and this requires additional training – creating a tiny minority within the already tiny minority of Egyptologists. Nevertheless, the claims of the privileged 'direct reader' can be put to the test urged by Said in *Orientalism* and, perhaps more, in his response to some Western critics.[15] The orientalist philologists profess more direct access to an ancient script and content, but their claim only holds within the limited frame of philological research. These experts may be able to offer a translation, a grammatical explanation, a certain style of commentary, and sometimes a point in space and time (if not an account of the historical background: philologists rarely display much awareness of the material cultures that produced the writing). However, philology cannot communicate content beyond the terrain sanctioned by the philological discipline: as soon as the words are out, they call for a far vaster cast of experts and readers. Moreover, by privileging their own technical expertise, and reducing other modern readers to passive recipients of whatever philology elects to convey, philologists expose the implicit political agenda of their supposedly apolitical craft. As Said argued, whatever their individual intentions, orientalists as a group have served not so much humanity as imperialism.[16] Not surprisingly, then, their direct route to the sources turns out to be the most prejudicial of all. From an understanding of language as intersubjective, the role of philologists can be brought back into the host of possible engagements with ancient writing. In his observations on heteroglossia, the internal differentiation of natural languages, Bakhtin wrote that 'all words taste of a profession, a genre, a movement, a party, a particular work, a particular person, a generation, an age group, a day and hour'.[17] That approach can be applied both to the modern reader, including the philologist, and to the ancient writing, always allowing for the transformative potential of the medium in creating specific communicative space. Intersubjectivity may offer the means to fight prejudice in reading ancient content, but the prejudices run so deep that, if

14 Hirschkop (1999) p 164.

15 Said (1995) pp 341–47.

16 Said (1995) p 342: 'I do say that the *guild* of Orientalists has a specific history of complicity with imperial power.'

17 In 'Discourse in the novel', Holquist (1981) p 293, discussed in Hirschkop (1999) p 19.

they are to be overcome, a strong new setting for reading must be found.

Any reader requires some social empowerment to read; reading is not a linear dialogue between writing and reader, but a multi-dimensional engagement. Whereas the ancient written source tends to be considered single, readers ancient and modern may be more clearly multiple at any time. The unique source itself is multiple from the moment of dialogue, as soon as it is translated into sound by the act of reading, introducing new readers and hearers and ways of being read. The most direct reading would theoretically be in the original cursive script, requiring particular training; the claims of this absolute linearity should be put to the test urged by Said in *Orientalism*.[18] By their customary arrogance, the direct routes may be the most prejudicial. Two of the possible routes out of prejudice are mentioned here.

The first is the ethnographic parallel, always alluring; this needs to be made explicitly different to the ancient Egyptian setting, especially when it is as sympathetic as the contemporary Egyptian village. The ethnographic parallel deludes most when it is read as a resurrection of the lost past, and when it therefore functions primarily as a prop to nostalgia. However, if instead the parallel setting is itself read with sensitivity, that other human social context may offer a broadening of experiential horizons. In this more sympathetic engagement, with fuller acknowledgment of the distinctive complexities of each human interaction, the 'ethnographic parallel' can do much to remove the assumptions that distort the view of a modern observer. In the case of UC 32057, a Western reader needs to be aware of the gulf between Western healing and other approaches, and descriptions of social anthropological fieldwork in a contemporary Egyptian village can help to provide such awareness.[19] They may take the modern Western reader out of the anaesthetised museum into the dirt and blood of a room where birth killed mother and child in a high proportion of cases – still in the early twentieth century, childbirth was the main killer in Egyptian life.

Audio renderings are my second option, more for rhetorical power perhaps, rather than an assertion of authentic performance. Hearing reading is an activity that can resurrect the past, by making the hearer aware of the plurality of voices and of readings, and of the modernity of the readings and the views expressed by them. Hearing may be more responsive to regional differences, gender differences, individual as well as social differences. A freely experimental philology has as much to offer the understanding of ancient writing as experimental archaeology has brought to the study of past technologies. For the online translation, audio is available for select passages, with my reading of the Egyptian version, and reading by my colleague Colleen McKenna of my English translation. The experiment needs, of course, to be transferred from dictated hearing to template for reader/hearer participation: an awareness of the different effect of voices of man and woman can only be a start, towards a more 'public

---

18 Said (1995) pp 341–47.

19 For example, see Morsy (1982).

square', where passive learning is replaced by active and sensitive engagement. Orientalist philologies have scarcely begun to learn from the experience of other disciplines in both sciences and humanities, in contemporary art, and in other institutions aiming at social inclusion and a more democratic public life. They hold, rather too tightly, extraordinary ranges of human experience locked in the languages and scripts of past societies. Unlocking that material may finally justify their presence in more open fora such as this.

Bibliography

Bardinet, Thierry, *Les papyrus médicaux de l'Egypte pharaonique*, 1995, Paris: Fayard.

Borghouts, Joris, *Ancient Egyptian Magical Texts*, 1978, Leiden: Brill.

Broze, Michele, *Les aventures d'Horus et Seth dans le papyrus Chester Beatty I: mythe et roman en Egypte ancienne*, 1996, Louvain: Uitgeverij Peeters.

Cerquiglini, Bernard, *Eloge de la variante: histoire critique de la philologie*, 1989, Paris: Seuil.

Gallorini, Carla, 'A reconstruction of Petrie's excavation at the Middle Kingdom Settlement of Kahun', in Quirke, Stephen (ed), *Lahun Studies*, 1998, Reigate: SIA, pp 42–59.

Griffith, Francis LL, *The Petrie Papyri. Hieratic Papyri from Kahun and Gurob, Principally of the Middle Kingdom*, 1898, London: Quaritch.

Hirschkop, Ken, *Mikhail Bakhtin: An Aesthetic for Democracy*, 1999, Oxford and New York: Oxford University Press.

Holquist, Michael (ed), *The Dialogic Imagination: Four Essays by Mikhail Bakhtin*, 1981, Austin, TX: University of Texas Press.

Kemp, Barry, *Ancient Egypt: Anatomy of a Civilization*, 1989, London and New York: Routledge.

Känel, Frédérique von, *Les prêtres-ouâb de Sekhmet et les conjurateurs de Serket*, 1984, Paris: Presses Universitaires de France.

Morsy, Suheir, 'Childbirth in an Egyptian village', in Kay, Margarita (ed), *Anthropology of Human Birth*, 1981, Philadelphia: FA Davies, pp 147–74.

Nunn, John, *Ancient Egyptian Medicine*, 1996, London: British Museum Press.

Roberts, Alison, *Hathor Rising: the Serpent Power of Ancient Egypt*, 1995, Totnes: Northgate.

Said, Edward, *Orientalism: Western Conceptions of the Orient*, reprint with new afterword, 1995, London and New York: Routledge and Kegan Paul.

Verhoeven, Ursula, *'Ein historischer "Sitz im Leben" für die Erzählung von Horus und Seth des Papyrus Chester Beatty I'* in Schade-Busch, Mechthild (ed), *Wege öffnen: Festschrift für Rolf Gundlach zum 65 Geburtstag*, 1996, Wiesbaden: Harrassowitz, pp 347–63.

Westendorf, Wolfhart, *'Ein neuer fall der homosexuellen episode zwischen Horus und Seth?'* (1997) 97 *Göttinger Miszellen (Universität Göttingen: Ägyptologisches Seminar)* 71–77.

CHAPTER 14

RENÉ AND THE '*MAL DU SIÈCLE*': A LITERARY ROLE MODEL FOR THE NEGOTIATION OF PROBLEMATIC SEXUAL IDENTITY IN NINETEENTH-CENTURY EUROPE – THE CASES OF CUSTINE AND AMIEL[1]

Caroline Warman

This chapter presents the case studies of two francophone men: one a French nobleman born during the French Revolution, Astolphe de Custine, 1790–1856; and one a Swiss philosophy professor and a generation younger, Henri-Frédéric Amiel, 1821–81. For each, the central story of his life was how he related to his own fragile gender and sexuality – Custine was, it emerged, homosexual, whilst Amiel defined himself as lacking in all those attributes of strength, energy and productiveness which he himself defined as truly masculine. The histories of their gender-ing (because it was a process) oscillate suggestively between illness and text. That is to say, their stories are about illness, actual or perceived, self-diagnosed or socially-determined, and their response – both in terms of diagnosis and resolution – is profoundly textual. By this I mean that they construe their problems in terms of a general cultural malaise exemplified by a piece of high literature, to which they respond textually, re-identifying themselves in the light of it and thus dramatising and playing out the tension between gender, sexuality, health and society that they had to live with. They therefore leave the label of ill health behind, and write themselves towards well-being. Or do they?

The 'general cultural malaise' to which I am alluding was what was known in France as the '*mal du siècle*' – the sickness of the century.[2] The text which defined, exemplified or even *caused* it (as a fashionable trend) is Chateaubriand's *René*, first published in 1802 as part of his five-volume pro-Christian polemic, *Le génie du Christianisme* (The Genius of Christianity).[3] *René* is the story-with-a-moral of a dispossessed young nobleman, in a state of undefined yearning, awash with emotion yet devoid of purpose in life. His older sister decides to become a nun, and on the verge of taking her vows breaks out with an admission of her incestuous feelings for him. This is the catalyst of self-realisation for René who in despair departs for America where he makes a sort of half-life with the Natchez

---

1 I would like to express my gratitude to the Leverhulme Trust – it was as a Leverhulme Research Fellow at De Montfort University that I first worked on these topics. I would also like to thank George Rousseau, director of that Leverhulme project, who introduced me to Custine and Amiel and with whom I wrote articles on Custine (2001) and Amiel (2002).

2 For a survey of this topic, see Hoog (1954).

3 Chateaubriand (1966).

Indians, married but childless and living separately from his Natchez wife. He is known for his mysterious melancholy. There he learns of his sister's death, and finally reveals his story to the tribal elders, who, reprimanding him, tell him to 'temper [the] character which ha[d] already wreaked such havoc'.[4] He fails to stop yearning and being melancholy, and meets death soon after in a battle. Chateaubriand explicitly – if rather ambiguously – frames this tragic story of impossible love in a disapproving context. He is, he says, painting a portrait, undiluted by adventure, of the 'indistinctness of the passions' whereby a 'great misfortune is sent to punish René and shake up those young men who, surrendering themselves up to pointless dreaming, criminally evade their dues to society'.[5] The 'pointless dreaming' very clearly refers to René's forbidden obsession with his sister while the 'criminal evasion of society's dues' as clearly refers to his refusal to take an active patriarchal role in the tribe and to start a family. That is to say, the problem arises from unacceptable sexual desire, construed as anti-social, even as destructive of society.

There is, furthermore, a specifically literary aspect to the delusion, or *'mal'* – primarily meaning illness here but also the term for 'evil' – of this class of young men, and it is reading. The problem, says Chateaubriand in his framing remarks, is that these young men have read more than they have experienced and that their imaginative life has therefore overtaken their real life: 'the large number of examples to be seen, the multitude of books on the subject of man and his feelings, confer knowledge without experience [...]. One lives, heart bursting, in an empty world.'[6] To the twin themes of forbidden love and evasion of social duty is added here therefore the issue of reading about 'man and his feelings', that is to say reading about things which might not have been experienced and which are manifestly seen as tainting. Here Chateaubriand is extending the eighteenth-century debate about the corrupting effect of novels on women to a new group of vulnerable corruptible individuals.[7] Inappropriate knowledge and inadequate experience combine to create corrupted literate 'criminals' who 'evade their dues to society'. This is clearly a not particularly coded allusion to behaviours that did not conform to the patriarchal sexual mores of the time.[8]

---

4 Chateaubriand (1962) p 203. *'Modère seulement ce caractère qui t'a déjà fait tant de mal.'* (All translations are by Caroline Warman unless otherwise noted.)

5 Chateaubriand (1962) p 173. Extract from the 1805 preface to the first separate edition of René: *'Ce n'est pour ainsi dire, qu'une pensée; c'est la peinture du vague des passions, sans aucun mélange d'aventures, hors un grand malheur envoyé pour punir René, et pour effrayer les jeunes hommes qui, livrés à d'inutiles rêveries, se dérobent criminellement aux charges de la société.'*

6 Chateaubriand (1962) p 170. *'Le grand nombre d'exemples qu'on a sous les yeux, la multitude de livres qui traitent de l'homme et de ses sentiments, rendent habile, sans expérience. [...] On habite, avec un coeur plein, un monde vide.'*

7 For an excellent overview of this debate and especially of the views of the *philosophes* about it, see Trousson (1996).

8 The explicit mention, let alone discussion, of non-heterosexuality was extremely taboo in francophone society of the time: see Aron and Kempf (1979) pp 141–57.

It is difficult to give an adequate idea here of the extent to which Chateaubriand really was felt to have touched a cultural and emotional nerve: the noble melancholy of René was both identified with and in fact imitated, and also condemned in accordance with Chateaubriand's own dialectic. Suffice it to say that the extremely influential French literary critic Sainte-Beuve – who himself had been overwhelmed by *René* when he had first encountered it[9] – wrote in 1849 that 'René's sickness ... has been the sickness of our entire age'.[10] In short, we can say four things: that this illness/evil seems to be created and framed by textual engagement; that it was viewed in terms of a cultural phenomenon; that its symptoms were alienation, marginalisation and withdrawal from mainstream patriarchal productive society; and that at its core is sexuality, forbidden sexuality moreover. It thus simultaneously provides society with a coded way of naming – or euphemising – suspect sexuality, and also offers a possible identity or role model for those who might actually 'suffer' from such a malady.

Custine was one such. He came from an ancient and respected noble family – his grandfather was Adam de Custine, general of the armies of the North until 1790, and his father was also a soldier. Both were guillotined during the terror, when Astolphe was three years old, and his mother, Delphine, was imprisoned for six months during the same period. In the preceding year he had already lost his older brother, then six, to the smallpox vaccine that their mother had bravely yet trepidaciously given them. The decimation of the family – of its members, wealth and status (although these last two aspects were partially reconstituted under Napoleon) – was clearly traumatic. As an adolescent and young man, he was an extremely troubled character. In 1811, his mother wrote that 'Astolphe feels he is the most unhappy person in the world, and between you and me the particular cast of his spirit and character has condemned me to a life of ever-lasting tears'.[11] Custine himself informed his mother that his 'indisposition is an illness whose cause is much more serious than its effects: people are often in much worse pain without being as ill as I am'.[12] This statement seems almost wilfully obscure. In fact what happened to Custine in these formative years – his twenties – is that he repeatedly bumped his head extremely seriously – it occurred on his travels with his mother around Europe in 1811, 1813 and again in 1815 – at the Congress of Vienna – and each time he was bedridden for months.[13] Such was his

9 'I read René and shuddered ... what I saw in it was a perfect image of myself' (*J'ai lu René et j'ai frémi ... je m'y suis reconnu tout entier*), cited by Waller (1992) p 170.

10 As quoted by Hoog (1954) p 42.

11 '*Astolphe se trouve l'être au monde le plus malheureux, et par la tournure de son esprit et de son caractère, condamne ma vie à des larmes éternelles; mais que ceci soit entre nous*', 17 September 1811, Delphine de Sabran to her mother; quoted by Maugras and Croze-Lemercier (1912) pp 438–39.

12 '*Mon indisposition est une maladie grave par sa cause bien plus que par ses effets; on est souvent beaucoup plus souffrant sans être aussi malade que je le suis*', 27 January 1815, Astolphe to his mother: quoted by Maugras and Croze-Lemercier (1912) pp 483–84.

13 See Luppé (1957), Muhlstein (1996) and Tarn (1985).

susceptibility that he began to dream of a special helmet head-protector.[14] Farcical as this sounds, Custine himself always made the most extensive claims for his malady. In 1817, he wrote to a friend that 'I have suffered internally from incomprehensible ailments [...] I shall never be able to communicate the pain that has been hounding me since childhood.'[15] To an intimate young male friend (Edouard de la Grange) he writes repeatedly about his illness. At a crucial point in his self-revelation he talks in veiled terms about his head injuries:

> ... a series of [...] accidents, [...] repeated with a sort of fatality, [...] gave me an illness of the brain from which, for three years, I suffered morally and physically as much, I believe, as it was in me to bear. If I were able to tell the precise story of my soul during that terrible crisis, it would make a significant chapter in the book of human misery. Yet, however great the loss incurred in descending, against my will, into the very depths of my being, where the two natures meld and where physicality and morality no longer have any limits, I am still not sure whether I would prefer to have back the force of youth and life that I lost there at the price of the wisdom I gained.[16]

This curious passage is simultaneously vague in terms of specifics, sublime in its claims for misery and emphatic about the actual problem: again and again he refers to 'moral' *and* 'physical', to 'the two natures', to 'physicality and morality' unfettered by 'limits', to the fact that he suffered this 'against his will'. To be inferred is, I think, a reference to physical desire in mortal combat with the moral will. Neither appears to have won or lost: instead, we have the allusion to extreme suffering, and to the self-knowledge achieved, which seems to have been worth it. Custine had met Edouard de la Grange at a ball in 1818 and for a couple of years they corresponded very passionately, at least Custine did. Custine, at age 28, was about six years older than his friend, more experienced perhaps, and this letter is one of many that allude to impossible suffering, unspeakable feelings and intuitions of fundamental harmony. La Grange seems never to have responded in kind, yet Custine's hints cannot have passed unnoticed. In tandem with his many references to illness are his many references to *René*. Custine's mother, it should be said, had had a real-life love affair with Chateaubriand.[17] Custine tells La Grange

---

14 'I'd like to have a special head-protector made, a sort of reinforced wire hat, perhaps a cap of polished sheet metal, what do I know? If I were king, I'd get my entire privy council on the job!' (*J'ai envie de me faire un étui pour la tête, un bonnet double de fil de fer, un bourrelet de tôle vernie, que sais-je? Si j'étais roi, je convoquerais tout mon conseil pour imaginer un garde-tête!*), 27 January 1815, Custine: quoted by Luppé (1957) p 56.

15 '*J'ai souffert intérieurement de maux incompréhensibles [...] je ne pourrai jamais dire la douleur qui m'a poursuivi dès mon enfance*', 1817, Custine to Rahel de Varnhagen: quoted by Luppé (1957) p 67.

16 '*Ce sont des accidents pareils, mais renouvelés avec une espèce de fatalité, qui m'ont causé une maladie du cerveau, dont, pendant trois ans, j'ai souffert moralement et physiquement tout ce qu'il m'est donné, je crois, de supporter. Si je pouvais faire l'histoire exacte de mon âme pendant cette terrible crise, ce serait un chapitre important des misères humains. Quelque perte que j'ai faite en descendant malgré moi dans les profondeurs de mon être, où les deux natures se confondent, où le physique et le moral n'ont plus leurs limites, je ne sais si je voudrais retrouver la force de jeunesse et de vie que j'y ai perdue, au prix des lumières que j'y ai acquises*', 27 July 1818, Custine to the Marquis de la Grange: Custine (1925) pp 25–26.

17 See Luppé (1957), Maugras and Croze-Lemercier (1912), Muhlstein (1996) and Tarn (1985).

about the enduring impression *René* and its author made on him: 'I recognise in my anxious heart the echo of the sentiments and words of *René*, and I cannot go near its author without being afraid of what is analogous in myself to his innate sadness.'[18] I am René, says Custine, inviting his friend to transpose the interpretation. Many are the occasions on which he dramatises himself in the same romantic manner as René, talking of streams and torrents, abyss and chasm, incompleteness, love and yearning.[19] Custine makes it clear that René's veiled incestuous feelings convey an important message about his own. Incest, being socially taboo, becomes analogous to homosexuality.

La Grange evidently chose to be deaf to his meaning and in fact halted the correspondence altogether once scandalous evidence relating to Custine's homosexuality emerged in 1824, disgracing him, casting him out of polite society and forcibly relieving him of the necessity to communicate via mysterious codes and allusions. However, *René* was never left behind, and the extent to which Custine had internalised it as a role model is evident from a fragment from *Letters from Russia*, the book for which he was and remains best known: 'these reveries, I know, are no longer appropriate for someone of my age; M de Chateaubriand was too great a poet to paint us an ageing René. [...] yet my destiny [...] was to show you how a man born to die young grows old; a subject which is more sad than interesting, oh thankless task of all thankless tasks!'[20] In brief, Custine was an 'ill' person, ill essentially because of his impermissible sexuality, actually ill and ill according to his accounts of himself, but as he points out 'it is extremely stupid to think that the malady is always where it appears to be. Problems start and end in the mind'.[21] As we have seen, he uses the descriptions of his sufferings to do something other than communicate in a straightforward way his symptoms: he wants to talk about illness as code. In this context, illness is not what it seems, it is the mind talking – and specifically in his letters to the man he hopes to woo, Custine uses illness to allude politely to the unmentionable. By heavily emphasising the epic, even sublime, nature of his anguish, and by identifying himself as a René, he creates a non-sinful, unpornographic, unthreatening version of the sexual misfit which is also admirable, noble, even desirable. Illness is the code used by society to encrypt taboo desire – thus René is diagnosed with a mysterious malady – and it is illness again that Custine recodifies into text and intertext in order to communicate his essential nobility.

---

18 *'Malgré les efforts que j'ai faits pour me soustraire à son empire, malgré de longues absences, malgré ses propres conseils et le soin qu'il a pris lui-même d'effacer en moi les premières impressions qu'il y avait produites, et dont il craignait la vivacité, je reconnais, à chaque occasion, dans mon coeur inquiet, l'écho des sentiments et des paroles de René, et je ne puis me rapprocher de son auteur sans m'effrayer de tout ce que je trouve en moi d'analogue à sa tristesse innée'*, Custine, 19 October 1818: Luppé (1957) p 123.

19 See Luppé (1957) p 31.

20 *'Ces rêveries, je le sais, ne sont plus de mon âge; M de Chateaubriand était trop grand poète pour nous peindre un René vieillissant. [...] pourtant mon destin [...] était de vous montrer comment vieillit un homme né pour mourir jeune; sujet plus triste qu'intéressant, tâche ingrâte entre toutes les tâches!'*, Letter 21: Custine (1843) p 125.

21 *'C'est une grande bêtise, que de croire que la maladie soit toujours où elle parait. L'esprit commence les maux, et je crois que c'est lui aussi qui les finit'*, Custine to Rahel, 20 July 1817, Letter 35: Custine (1870) p 213.

Amiel shadows *René* in a less masterful and more hopeless way. Not rich or well-connected like Custine, Amiel miserably performed the functions of a philosophy professor in Geneva from 1849 until his death in 1881. What makes him remarkable is his exhaustive, hypochondriac diary, all 17,000 pages of it.[22]

Amiel's illness was chronic if undefined, his male gender vulnerable to the attacks he himself launched on it in his diary. Barren, sterile, onanistic, 'femmelette' in the evocative French term – perhaps womanlet, sub-woman in English – these are all insults he fires at himself.[23] His illness is a more advanced version of the *'mal du siècle'* (illness of the age) that Custine also suffered from but in the end overcame and turned to his advantage. Amiel also used it as a cultural identifier, also searched for intimacy, also located himself within its constituency.[24] When still a very young man – 24 years old – he announced that the notion that 'everything [was] to be found in books' was a delusion and expressed the fear that he had 'lost [his] life to [books]'.[25] In fact he was to live his life irrevocably textually, through the pages of his private diary, a genre of personal outpouring that *René*, again, had done much to launch.[26] He became stuck in the intimate confessional form. He had read too much, done too little, was unable to 'pay society's dues' and marry, remained awash with emotion that needed an outlet. I would stress that this is not my diagnosis but his own; at one point, for instance, he writes: 'What, really, am I doing here, quill in hand? I am day-dreaming, listening to the deepdown murmur of feelings and fears. Where does it lead? To the knowledge of one's misery. And that's not the way to get better. To ruminate over pain only exacerbates the weakness of the patient.'[27] Over the course of his 30-year daily dedication to the diary, it becomes his drug – 'my pharmacy' Amiel calls it, in 1850, and so it is, in more ways than one:[28] 'this diary is an outlet; it lets out my virility, which evaporates away in the sweat of ink. It has often dispensed me with the need for a friend or wife [...] it still delivers me from my active self. I have sometimes thought that producing these pages was a

---

22 Amiel (1976–94).

23 29 March 1858: Amiel (1979) vol 3, p 484.

24 See for example the following passage: 'Link with Pellegrin. We met more than a year ago at Rolle and are now friends. Intimate and confessional letters have already been exchanged; he made me read in his soul; I tried to do the same. The thing is concluded. A sensitive, delicate, religious soul, he is worth much more than me, but he loves me, and that makes us equal' (*Liaison avec Pellegrin. Nous nous sommes connus il y a plus d'un an à Rolle, maintenant nous sommes amis. Des lettres de confidence intime ont déjà été échangées; il m'a fait lire dans son âme; j'ai tâché d'y répondre. La chose est conclue. Âme sensible, délicate, religieuse, il vaut bien mieux que moi, mais il m'aime, et cela nous égalise*), December 1840: Amiel (1976) vol 1, p 185.

25 Amiel (1976) vol 1, pp 206–07.

26 Girard (1986), and Didier (1976). For a summary see Rousseau and Warman (2002) pp 238–39.

27 *'Au fond, que fais-je ici, plume à la main? je rève tout éveillé et j'écoute bruire en moi la tempête des impressions et des craintes. A quoi cela mène-t-il? A connaître ses misères. Ce n'est pas ainsi qu'on les guérit. Cette rumination de ses peines ne fait qu'augmenter la faiblesse du malade'*, Amiel, 18 July 1872: Amiel (1989) vol 9, pp 349–50.

28 A decade later, he writes *'[le journal intime] est ma pharmacie, et doit chercher à être mon miroir; non à m'amuser'*, Amiel 7 April 1850: Amiel (1976) vol 1, p 689.

replacement for life, a sort of onanism, a ruse of cowardly egotism, a way of escaping duty, of betraying society and Providence.' It is a malady which multiplies textually through cumulative self-diagnoses. For Amiel, the confessional role model, that noble, literate, mysterious, brooding young man, turns sour – in fact, it turns back on itself. The diary dramatises its preoccupation with narcissism, making great stockpiles of self-description which routinely crush their author with their accusation of non-performance. One such is the following: 'a private diary is the portrait of an individual given over to two sterile occupations, chasing after or savouring himself.' Amiel was not able to write himself out of illness: in his culturally-inherited perception, writing is not only an addiction from which he cannot free himself, but also the illness itself. He never combats the notion that self-reflexive writing, or more simply writing about feelings, was a morally corrupting force. Instead he derives his entire self-denigratory self-definition from his status as an (ill) writer. Reading and writing seem to have been pathologised – if reading is a symptom, writing is the full-blown disease, yet it seems to have been a disease that people wanted to infect themselves with. When, after Amiel's death, the diary was published – for which, it should be noted, Amiel had made extremely careful arrangements – it was hugely popular, quickly translated into English, German, Italian and Russian, running into five editions in four years. Tolstoy and Nietzsche are just the most important of the figures to have responded to it.[29] The diary whose topic was predominantly lack of health and sterility itself gave birth to a hundred diaries. Marie Bashkirtseff, Paul Claudel, André Gide and Paul Valéry all wrote diaries which were to some extent inspired or influenced by Amiel's.[30] It seems possible to advance also that the areas of private subjectivity that he explored and deplored were the ones most intensely focused on by psychoanalysis and literary modernism, both of which he foreshadows.

To conclude: my two case studies present two individuals of vulnerable sexuality or gender both subsumed within a particular literary and textual approach to identity and more specifically to ill identity, given then a particular name: the '*mal du siècle*', the illness of the age. So perhaps I could end by claiming that nineteenth-century francophone culture developed and dealt with issues of gender, sexuality and health through the medium of self-conscious literature such as *René* as well as through the parallel medicalising discourses that Foucault concentrates on in his *History of Sexuality*. When I say 'dealt with', I mean that society was able to disapprove, diagnose and offer cures all at once. This literature provided a platform to discuss – via the languages of euphemism and emotion – those tensions, giving access both to the 'doctors' of society (to be understood within the broadest sense) and to those who were diagnosed as sick. This sickness was internalised by its sufferers – via identification with René and his literary progeny – and its sufferers were then able to claim it as a special sort of identity. Thus, disapproval, diagnosis and 'perversion' or illness were all able to co-exist. This phenomenon is attested to by the fact that, although Custine and Amiel may

29 Merian-Genast (1931).

30 Stroev (1993).

have been socially marginalised in terms of the patriarchal structure of society, their works were widely read. This was also the case for the numerous 'René-poets and René-prosers', as the contemporary literary figure Maxime du Camp called them, throughout the century.[31] Perhaps we may feel therefore that what nineteenth-century francophone culture was doing – as well as condemning and repressing – was creating a literary space which allowed private subjectivity to flourish and which rehearsed the issues of gender, sexuality and health.

Whether it enabled subjects to write themselves towards well-being, as was posited at the beginning of this piece, is another question. In both cases touched on here, writing is a confessional and self-conscious process, as much about self-discovery as about revelation of the soul to others. Writing about the vulnerable self allows it to emerge into visibility, to gain an identity where none had existed, yet its virtuality quality – that is to say, the fact that this fledgling identity exists and looks at itself primarily in textual form, and more precisely in confessional writing – confines that existence to a sort of ghostliness. The writer may know and define his or her self, but that self-definition exists in a private and intimate space – a diary or a letter, for example. This self therefore is not public and does not have a recognised existence in the wider society where its specifically vulnerable quality, as defined by weakness and sensitivity on the one hand and non-patriarchal sexuality on the other, remains problematic. If it is forcibly made public, that self is invaded and imperilled, its private quality torn open. When left intact in the intimate sphere, it still leaves the individual vulnerable or compromised in society, as the written self has no public equivalent. So the problem remains that although new, hesitant identities were being developed in textual self-referential spaces, they were confined to them. Their private quality meant they could not create an equivalent public category to inhabit. This construction of the textual self as marginal and marginalised was perpetuated, of course, by the parameters within which it was conceptualised. Thus, as has been shown, the very activity of reading was construed as harmful to the youth who were supposedly tainted by impossible dreams and unreal experiences. Society allows the textual parallel world to exist, and yet condemns it both for its virtuality and for its all too real effects. Chateaubriand's *Le génie du Christianisme* is a case in point: he himself both creates and damns the vulnerable René. Custine and Amiel both suffered from and extended this sense of being confined to the textual self. The more they experimented in new definitions of the self, the greater the discrepancy between lived and conceptual self-reflecting selves grew, hence Custine's curious feeling, mentioned above, of being the living materialisation of a long-dead character in a book; hence also, in Amiel, the increasingly fevered relationship between convoluted and denigratory self-description on the one hand and attempts to stop writing and 'start living' on the other. So, if nineteenth-century confessional writing brings new marginal identities into textual life, it situates them in almost impossible tension to a normative society which denies them any real public equivalent, and this means, of course, that these fledgling identities never get to breathe with any ease: they are condemned to remain sick.

31 Camp (1991) p 29, cited by Call (1988) p 4.

Bibliography

Amiel, Henri-Frédéric, *Journal intime* (12 vols), edited by Gagnebin, Bernard and Monnier, Philippe, 1976–1994, Lausanne: L'Age d'Homme.

Aron, Jean-Paul and Kempf, Roger, 'Triumphs and tribulations of the homosexual discourse', in Stambolian, George and Marks, Elaine (eds), *Homosexualities and French Literature: Cultural Contexts/Critical Texts*, 1979, Ithaca, NY and London: Cornell University Press, pp 141–57.

Call, Michael J, *Back to the Garden: Chateaubriand, Senancour and Constant*, 1988, Saratoga, CA: Anma libri.

Camp, Maxime du, *Mémoires d'un suicidé*, 1991, Paris: Editions de Septembre.

Chateaubriand, François-René de, *Atala, René, le dernier Abencérage*, edited by Letessier, F, 1962, Paris: Garnier.

Chateaubriand, François-René de, *Le génie du Christianisme*, edited by Reboul, P, 1966, Paris: Garnier-Flammarion.

Custine, Astolphe Louis Léonor de, *La Russie en 1839*, 1843, Paris: Librairie d'Amyot.

Custine, Astolphe Louis Léonor de, *Lettres du Marquis A de Custine à Varnhagen d'Ense et Rahel Varnhagen d'Ense accompagnées de plusieurs lettres de la comtesse Delphine de Custine et de Rahel Varnhagen d'Ense*, 1870, Brussels: C Muquardt.

Custine, Astolphe Louis Léonor de, *Lettres inédites au Marquis de la Grange*, edited by de Luppé, Albert Marie Pierre, 1925, Paris: Les Presses Françaises.

Didier, Beatrice, *Le journal intime*, 1976, Paris: Presses Universitaires de France.

Foucault, Michel, *The History of Sexuality*, 1979, London: Allen Lane.

Girard, Alain, *Le journal intime*, 1986 (1963) Paris: Presses Universitaires de France.

Hoog, Arnand, 'Who invented the "*mal du siècle*"?' (1954) 13 *Yale French Studies* 42–51.

Luppé, Albert Marie Pierre de, *Astolphe de Custine*, 1957, Monaco: Editions du Rocher.

Maugras, Gaston and de Croze-Lemercier, Pierre, *Delphine de Sabran, Marquise de Custine*, 1912, Paris: Plon.

Merian-Genast, Ernst, 'HF Amiel im Spiegel der europäischen Kritik, 1881–1931' (1931) 21 *Die Neueren Sprachen*.

Muhlstein, Anka, *Astolphe de Custine (1790–1857): le dernier Marquis*, 1996, Paris: Grasset. (Translated by Waugh, Teresa as *A Taste for Freedom: The Life of Astolphe de Custine*, 1999, New York: Helen Marx.)

Rousseau, George and Warman, Caroline, 'Made from the stuff of saints: Chateaubriand's *René* and Custine's search for a homosexual identity' (2001) 7/1 *GLQ* 1–29.

Rousseau, George and Warman, Caroline, 'Writing as pathology, poison or cure: Henri-Frédéric Amiel's *Journal intime*' (2002) 33 *Studies in Gender and Sexuality* 229–62.

Stroev, Alexandre, '*Henri-Frédéric Amiel et la littérature de son temps*' (1993) 4 *Etudes de lettres* 71–84.

Tarn, Julien-Frédéric, *Le Marquis de Custine*, 1985, Paris: Fayard.

Trousson, Raymond, 'Préface' in Trousson, Raymond (ed), *Romans de femmes au XVIIIe siècle*, pp i–xxxiii, 1996, Paris: Laffont.

Waller, Margaret, 'Being René, buying Atala: alienated subjects and decorative objects in postrevolutionary France', in Melzer, Sarah and Rabine, Leslie (eds), *Rebel Daughters: Women and the French Revolution*, 1992, Oxford: Oxford University Press, pp 151–77.

CHAPTER 15

POETRY, PICTURES AND THE SEXUAL DEMOGRAPHICS OF HEALTH

Deborah Kirklin

What do we mean by health and well-being? How is medical culture constructed and in what ways? What do we – patients, carers and professionals – want from medicine, and are we realistic or justified in demanding it? How can we achieve a shared understanding of health and well-being, one that recognises both the unique experience of every individual who is ill and the commonality of what enables human beings to flourish?

These difficult questions may seem, at first sight, the domain of philosophers and politicians. It is, however, important to acknowledge the fundamental role that can and must be played by careful, informed and interdisciplinary analysis of both the politics and the representations of illness in answering these questions.

This understanding necessarily involves respect for each other's perspectives, values and goals. It also depends upon having both the willingness and the opportunity to learn about and appreciate the world, both physical and psychological, that the Other inhabits, and thereby to have better insight into what makes the Other who s/he is.[1]

The use of the arts and humanities in this context is ambitious and philosophical in nature, and the ideas offered in the next few pages are undoubtedly open to challenge. However, I would emphasise that the work of medical education described later in the chapter is grounded in the day-to-day realities of medical practice. A brief introduction is therefore provided, offering non-medical readers an overview of the clinical perspective on the impact of sex, gender and sexuality on health and health service provision.

At the practical level, the work described aims to help doctors meet the challenge of providing better healthcare for men and women. It explores how poetry and pictures can be used with medical students and established practitioners in order to enhance their appreciation of how their own sex and gender and those of their patients can influence the concept of equitable access to healthcare. The work described represents tentative, early steps within medical education and society to acknowledge the sexual demographics of health.

---

1 Kirklin (2003).

One of the basic tenets of medicine is, of course, that patients should be treated justly; that is to say, without favour or prejudice. For this to happen, there must be equitable access to healthcare service providers and to the provision of the most appropriate services for the specific needs of the patient. Some services, whilst clinically centred on the health needs of one sex (for example, obstetrics care for women or testicular cancer services for men), have important implications for the well-being of people of both sexes. Every pregnant woman bears some man's child; every man with testicular cancer is some mother's child. A balance in emphasis is required, one which recognises the needs of individuals in the wider context of their lives.

The term 'the sexual demographics of health', that I have coined, brings together in my view a number of important issues that, as a medical educator, I need to address. It encompasses not only the impact of the sex of patients on their health, but also the relevance of a patient's sex to the amount of scientific evidence there will be relating to their health status, about whom they are likely to see or choose to be seen by, when they are unwell, and the type of encounter that will be.

The delivery of healthcare should, of course, be guided by the healthcare needs of individuals and populations, with the chosen treatments underpinned by rigorous research into what is most effective. An important way in which researchers identify health needs is by interviewing representative samples of the population and asking them about the health problems they are experiencing. An appreciation of gender issues is key to both framing the questions that are asked and interpreting the results. In a Spanish medical paper published by Rohlfs *et al*,[2] which examines the importance of gender perspective in health interview surveys, the authors state:

> Gender is an analytical construct based on the societal organisation of the sexes that can be used to better understand the conditions and factors influencing women's and men's health *beginning* with the social roles that each culture assigns to people based on their sex.[3]

Rohlfs's paper makes clear that for health survey questionnaires to provide meaningful information about how gender affects health, there must be much deeper probing than merely asking whether the respondents are male or female. It is essential to ask about the individual's reproductive work, productive work, social class, social support, self-perceived health status, quality of life, mental health and chronic conditions. Furthermore, Rohlfs and his colleagues argue that a gender approach to gathering this data would be 'characterised by the analysis of the social relations between men and women, taking into account that sex is a determinant of social inequalities'.[4] Thus, even at the fundamental level of

2 Rohlfs *et al* (2000).

3 Rohlfs *et al* (2000), p 146. I am aware that it important to make a distinction between sex and gender, sex being the biological status of being either a man or a woman, whereas gender is a socio-cultural construct, which has implications for one's identity, role and function within the society within which one lives. In the rest of this chapter, however, I shall use the term 'gender', because this is the term still used in much discussion by healthcare professionals.

4 Rohlfs *et al* (2000), p 146.

identifying the particular health needs of individuals and the determinants of health status, an understanding of gender issues is essential.

Another key research-related phenomenon has to do with how medical researchers choose subjects for their research. Until relatively recently, women have largely been excluded as research subjects and, when they have been included, the data has traditionally not been analysed by sex. There are a number of reasons for this. The first is that researchers are reluctant to expose women to experimental risk during childbearing years, in case the mother's fertility and/or any future offspring are adversely affected. Secondly, there has also been a misconception that certain disorders, such as cardiovascular disease, do not affect women to the same extent as men. Thirdly, there is an economic imperative: for statistical reasons, if both men and women are used in research, one simply needs more research subjects in order to get an equivalent level of significance. Finally, there is often the assumption that women and men are affected by health problems in the same way and that research results obtained using men as research subjects can be used to guide the care of women.

Only recently have medical researchers begun to understand the pitfalls of these overly simplistic assumptions. At a Yale conference entitled 'Factoring in gender: women's health research', the question was asked: 'Why should we focus on women's health and sex specific differences?'[5] The need to understand disorders that are *unique* to women (such as ovarian cancer), that are more prevalent in women than in men (for example, osteoporosis), and conditions that affect women and men differently (such as drug addiction) was highlighted, whilst it was emphasised that the differences between the health of men and women are poorly understood and that more – and better conceived – research is needed.

Gender issues also have a bearing on the patient's choice of doctor, and consequently on the mix of patients that doctors see; these issues therefore have an impact on the 'comfort' level and confidence of doctors when caring for patients of different genders. Some patients, given a choice, will seek out or avoid a doctor of a particular sex. This can be for reasons of modesty or physical shyness – or alternatively because of perceptions about consulting styles or the tolerance and understanding of an individual doctor regarding particular types of problems that the patient wishes to discuss.

Women doctors are often assumed to be more comfortable with and more tolerant of the desire of patients to discuss emotional or psychological issues. Gay men and women have a tendency to seek out female practitioners, and I personally have had a number of patients of both sexes who feel more comfortable with how a female doctor interacts with them than with the way a male doctor responds. This is not to say that patients' assumptions will be proved correct in all cases. Some female doctors do not feel comfortable with talking about psychological concerns and are far from having a 'touchy feely' approach. Conversely, many male doctors provide excellent, respectful and empathetic care

---

5 http://info.med.yale.edu/womenshealth (accessed 29 June 2003).

for patients, irrespective of sex or sexual orientation. However, patients' perceptions are important, and we need both to respect their preferences and try to understand whether there is any foundation for their concerns.

Of course, many patients do not actively seek out a doctor based on sex. Either they 'take what they get' or other factors about that doctor (such as experience, expertise or local reputation) may be more important to a particular patient. In some cases, the patient simply has no choice, as when there is no other doctor in the neighbourhood. A key question is whether the sex of the doctor relative to that of the patient will have any impact on the care that the patient receives. One possible effect is related to the fact that patients tend to seek out doctors of the same sex; this means that doctors in training tend to see more patients of their own sex and proportionately fewer of those of the opposite sex.

In an interesting study, Paluska and D'Amico examined the 'comfort' of family practice doctors in training with regard to caring for patients of the opposite gender.[6] They found that 93% of female doctors felt they had seen enough female patients during their training but only 54% felt they had seen enough male patients. 76% of the male doctors felt they had seen enough male patients but only 31% felt they'd seen enough female patients. This perception of inadequate experience was reflected in how 'comfortable' they felt when it came to performing diagnostically important, but intimate, examinations. Male doctors were significantly more comfortable performing a prostate examination or checking for testicular problems than their female counterparts, who in turn were significantly more comfortable performing breast examinations than their male colleagues. So, in some ways, patient preference, based on differential skills of male and female doctors, is a self-fulfilling prophecy and leads to de-skilling of doctors.

These are just some of the elements that contribute to the sexual demographics of health. There are many complex and subtle issues that need to be addressed, and addressed on many levels. In this chapter, I shall now consider one area where literature and art can play a part, through the education and training of doctors.

The main purpose of medical education is necessarily to prepare doctors to deal with diseases – which are often more common in particular sex groups, ethnic groups, occupations or social classes. Doctors are trained to look for patterns, to formulate differential diagnoses, to follow a trail of clues left by each patient's life story, symptoms and signs. Whilst it makes sense to use the information contained in patterns to help in complex decision-making, this brings with it a challenge. A doctor must not only learn from the accumulated wisdom and evidence-base of medicine, s/he must also retain a real and vital appreciation of the uniqueness of the person in front of her/him.

Doctors, in common with other human beings, have a natural tendency to try, in their encounters with people, to make sense of the mass of data reaching them

6 Paluska and D'Amico (2000).

about each individual: they automatically want to classify them and thereby to explain and understand them, and ultimately to try to help them. Young, old, educated or not, male, female, black, white: these are useful pieces of information in healthcare, which do alert us – at least in general terms – to the sorts of lifestyles, behavioural tendencies or diseases that might be relevant to the individual patient.

However, it's the 'might' that is crucial here. The human tendency to put people in boxes may be an irritation when it happens in day-to-day encounters; it is potentially much more serious than that when the person doing the 'labelling' is a doctor or other healthcare professional. It may have profound implications for the healthcare choices given to a patient. One last example from medical research graphically illustrates this point.

A couple of years ago, Modell *et al* published longitudinal data from patients with thalassaemia.[7] Thalassaemia is a genetically inherited blood disorder. If the patient has one gene for thalassaemia it is a minor inconvenience. However, if s/he has two, this can lead to a severe disease associated with grave health problems and significant amounts of treatment. It is possible to screen couples at risk for this condition during early pregnancy and many couples will choose to terminate an affected pregnancy rather than proceeding with it. Thalassaemia disproportionately affects certain ethnic groups, including British Pakistani Muslims. Modell and other geneticists had been keeping a detailed register of all the patients tested for thalassaemia and all babies born affected by this disease. After about 20 years, they re-examined the history behind the birth of these babies in order to determine the extent to which each birth was the result of an active choice made by the parents. What they discovered was that a disproportionate number of births of babies born affected by the disease were to British Pakistani women.

One plausible explanation for this was that, for religious reasons, these women had refused both screening and termination of affected pregnancies. However, when the researchers looked back at the events leading up to these births, a persuasive alternative explanation emerged. The data showed that the number of women opting for termination after screening in the first three months of pregnancy was unaffected by ethnicity: just as many Muslim women chose to terminate their pregnancies as women of other religious or ethnic backgrounds. The big difference came when screening was offered after three months. At this later stage in pregnancy, the British Pakistani women were significantly less likely to choose termination. What was happening was that these women were much more likely not to be offered early screening than other women so that, by the time that they did have screening, it was too late for them to have real choice: everyone knew they were pregnant and therefore for many women in the British Pakistani Muslim community, termination simply was no longer an option. The authors conclude that an assumption, conscious or unconscious, seemed to be in play on the part of the doctors and midwives involved in offering screening. This false

7 Modell *et al* (2000).

assumption (that British Pakistani women would not opt for termination) had resulted in a failure to offer screening in the first place.

Gender and sexuality are just two of the many complex and interrelated factors affecting the interaction between patients and doctors. What follows is an example of how the arts and humanities can help to improve doctors' understanding and appreciation of these issues. The educational initiative described does not didactically teach students about theories or models of gender, nor does it aim to fill gaps in knowledge about different cultures, health beliefs or religious practices. Rather, its aim is to open minds to new possibilities in a non-threatening and inclusive way.

The teaching described takes place within the Women's Health course at the Royal Free and University College Medical School, London. Women's Health is a new of way of designating what is traditionally known as obstetrics and gynaecology – the name itself is a most welcome development. Interestingly, this new name also represents a challenge, in that there is a danger that the interests of the men who are the partners, fathers and sons of these women may be sidelined. The Women's Health course involves the students spending much of their time 'on the job', learning from contact with real patients being cared for in the hospital setting.

One session, lasting 90 minutes, is devoted to bereavement. A key aim of this session is to broaden the students' appreciation of exactly what constitutes a loss or bereavement in this context. By the end of this session, the students should understand that infertility, miscarriage, neonatal loss, the birth of a less than perfect baby, termination of pregnancy and the menopause are all types of loss. These are difficult, often distressing topics for these 20-year-old students. A number of approaches are used, including looking at a poem by Anne Sexton called 'The Abortion'.[8]

The practice of abortion evokes strong feelings within our society. The religious and cultural factors behind these strong feelings are reflected within medicine and medical practitioners. Whatever their personal feelings about abortion, doctors are required to provide good care to patients requesting terminations, and to ensure that the law relating to abortion is complied with. Students do receive both legal and ethical training, as well as professional guidance, to help them meet these dual responsibilities. However, an understanding of the ethical, legal and professional aspects of abortion only obliquely acknowledges the patient's experience of termination of pregnancy. For each women, and her partner, a termination is rarely a simple choice between good and bad, right and wrong.

For the students, reading Anne Sexton's poem aloud, one stanza at a time, carefully and clearly, with their colleagues listening, can shed new light on this complex human experience. They are invited to comment on what they feel about

8 Sexton (1961) pp 20–21.

the piece and to identify any passages or phrases they find particularly interesting or thought provoking. Importantly, they are not asked what they think about abortion: the focus is explicitly on their thoughts and responses to the poem itself. Although this is a fairly basic approach to textual analysis, for these students it is a radical one. Traditional medical training is essentially about acquiring knowledge and skills, and about developing appropriate attitudes, many of which are handed down from older colleagues as received wisdom. One of our students on another course a few years ago said that, after two weeks of working with literature, art, film, drama and creative writing, he felt like a student for the first time. When asked what he meant by this, he explained that it was the first time in almost four years of medical training that anyone had been interested in what he thought rather than in what he knew.[9]

This comment is, of course, partly an indictment of current medical education, but it also provides an insight into the potential role that literature could play. Reading a poem such as Sexton's 'The Abortion' and discussing the poem as text rather than debating abortion from a medical or ethical point of view may be the first opportunity that students have had to try to understand abortion as it affects an individual rather than as an abstract moral choice with which they engage in large part as a result of their background, religion and personal experiences. For many people, abstract moral choices are black and white, but the human experience rarely is: analysing a poem like this can help young students start to understand the complexity of human needs and to comprehend the concerns behind the choices that have to be made by the women they may meet in the consulting room.

Students also spend a couple of hours in a session that addresses more general issues in women's health. The session, developed and delivered by Dr Claire Elliott, focuses on helping students to examine their own and others' perceptions of women, to reflect on the impact that pregnancy and gynaecological illness can have on a woman and those around her, and to consider some of the influences on health professionals in managing women's health. Poetry, film and images of women from art are all used. The use of images aims to raise student awareness of the potentially adverse consequences of the (human) tendency of doctors to want to put people in boxes or categories. The images are not used in an attempt to promote a politically correct or positive image of women. They are chosen instead in the belief that carefully facilitated discussion of the images will allow students to recognise and challenge, for themselves, some of the set ideas and preconceptions they have inherited as a result of growing up with these, and similar, images. Rather than trying to market a package of 'acceptable' images or representations of women, the images are used in an attempt to show students the subtle way in which exposure to a wide variety of representations of women can influence the way in which they respond and relate to women.

This focus on ideas rather than on facts also implicitly acknowledges the fact that we cannot hope, in two hours, to provide students with meaningful insights

9 Kirklin *et al* (2000) p 52.

into the cultural, religious and ethnic traditions of all the patients whom they will meet. Instead, we are doing something that we consider to be rather more radical: we are reminding these very idealistic students, the vast majority of whom have entered medicine because they want to help people, just how easy it is, despite all one's good intentions, to lose the person behind the disease, the individual behind the stereotype.

During the teaching session, one of these images is handed to each of the 15 students in the group. They are then asked to spend a few minutes writing down some words that describe the woman they see, and then to share these thoughts with the rest of the group. There are, of course, no correct answers, and what we are really trying to do is demonstrate to the students how easy, and potentially useful, it is to start describing the sort of women they are looking at from a 'two dimensional snapshot'.

Some of the images are controversial, even shocking. The fact that these pictorial representations of women have the ability to provoke strong reactions (such as revulsion or sympathy) in themselves is something which it is vital for these students to be made aware of. We hope that by considering different images and representations of women – as mothers, as sexual beings, naked and clothed, emotionally charged or vulnerable, etc – students will develop an insight into the range and variety of values, expectations and reactions that can associate themselves with these images.

This work could easily be criticised for lacking adequate context, both from an art history and anthropological point of view. In other contexts, we do work closely with art historians, including those at the National Gallery in London, and with social, biological and medical anthropologists at UCL. In the setting of our own course, however, the intention is not to teach either art history or anthropology, but rather to allow students to make the link, for themselves, between familiar representations of women in art, their own ideas, and the work of being a doctor.

During this session students are also asked to read Sylvia Plath's 'Morning Song',[10] in which a new mother addresses her newborn child. The tone here is one of awe and wonder. There are many different poems that we could have chosen and from many different cultures. We chose 'Morning Song' because of its evocative and very personal perspective of a new mother and the way in which the poem casts the midwife (representing medical intervention) very much in a cameo role.

Again, each student is asked to read a stanza slowly and clearly, so that the meaning is clear for all those who listen. We ask the students to consider the following questions: What are the mother's emotions with regard to her baby? How does the mother see herself? Does this bring any images to your mind?

What is interesting about this poem is that it helps the students to think beyond the delivery room, where labour plays out one of the set pieces listed in

10 Plath (1961) p 31.

their textbooks, and to envisage the reality of life as a mother, to consider the relationship of mother to child, and to ponder on the altered self-image of a woman who has become a mother. In other words, the students come to see that the medicalised part of this baby's existence is just one line in the story.

A practical approach to improving our national healths should, I would argue, include educational initiatives that enable students to learn to challenge their own preconceptions as well as assimilating professional knowledge, skills and attitudes. Based on an emerging appreciation of the sexual demographics of health, the work described above represents the beginning of attempts by medical educators to draw on the arts and humanities in addressing these important issues and thereby to ensure that healthcare in every country of our globalised world is provided in a truly cross-cultural context.

Bibliography

Anonymous, 'Factoring in gender: women's health research', Conference website, http://info.med.yale.edu/womenshealth (accessed 29 June 2003).

Kirklin, Deborah *et al*, 'Living with and dying from cancer: a humanities special study module' (2000) 26 *Journal of Medical Ethics: Medical Humanities* 51–54.

Kirklin, Deborah, 'The healing environment: without and within', in Kirklin, Deborah and Richardson, Ruth (eds), *The Healing Environment: Without and Within*, 2003, London: Royal College of Physicians, pp 1–9.

Modell, Bernadette *et al*, 'Informed choice in genetic screening for thalassaemia during pregnancy: audit from a national confidential inquiry' (2000) 320 *British Medical Journal* 337–41.

Paluska, Scott A, and D'Amico, Frank J, 'The comfort of family practice residents with health care of patients of the opposite gender' (2000) 32:9 *Family Medicine* 612–17.

Plath, Sylvia, 'Morning song', in Hughes, Ted (ed), *Sylvia Plath: Selected Poems*, 1961, London: Faber and Faber, p 30.

Rohlfs, Izabella *et al*, 'The importance of the gender perspective in health interview surveys' (2000) 14:2 *Gaceta Sanitaria* 146–55.

Sexton, Anne, 'The abortion', in *All My Pretty Ones*, 1961, Boston: Houghton Mifflin, pp 20–21.

Index

For Product Safety Concerns and Information please contact our EU
representative GPSR@taylorandfrancis.com
Taylor & Francis Verlag GmbH, Kaufingerstraße 24, 80331 München, Germany

www.ingramcontent.com/pod-product-compliance
Lightning Source LLC
LaVergne TN
LVHW011125300926
849160LV00008B/515
9781844720170